LUNG CANCER

LUNG CANCER
Clinical Diagnosis and Treatment

Edited by
Marc J. Straus, M.D.

Chief, Section of Medical Oncology
and Associate Professor of Medicine
Boston University Medical Center
University Hospital
Boston, Massachusetts

GRUNE & STRATTON
A Subsidiary of Harcourt Brace Jovanovich, Publishers
New York   San Francisco   London

Library of Congress Cataloging in Publication Data

Main entry under title:

Lung cancer: clinical diagnosis and treatment.

   Includes bibliographical references and index.
   1. Lungs—Cancer.   I. Straus, Marc J.
RC280.L8L77   616.9'94'24   77-3381
ISBN 0-8089-0998-3

Grune & Stratton, Inc.
111 Fifth Avenue
New York, New York 10003

Distributed in the United Kingdom by
Academic Press, Inc. (London) Ltd.
24|48 Oval Road, London NW 1

Library of Congress Catalog Number 77-3381
International Standard Book Number 0-8089-0998-3
Printed in the United States of America

For
Livia, Samuel, and Dora

Contents

Preface

Contributors

1 Respiratory Carcinogenesis   1
Curtis C. Harris, M.D.

2 Growth Characteristics of Lung Cancer   19
Marc J. Straus, M.D.

3 Production of Markers by Bronchogenic Carcinoma: A Review   33
Aron Primack, M.D., Lawrence E. Broder, M.D., and Robert B. Diasio, M.D.

4 Morphology of Pulmonary and Pleural Malignancies   49
Mary J. Mathews, M.D., and Phillip R. Gordon, M.D.

5 Ultrastructure of Lung Neoplasms   71
Bruce Mackay, M.D., Ph.D., Barbara M. Osborne, M.D., and Roma A. Wilson, M.D.

6 Signs and Symptoms of Bronchogenic Carcinoma   85
Martin H. Cohen, M.D.

7 Cytopathologic Diagnosis of Lung Cancer   95
Yener S. Erozan, M.D., and John K. Frost, M.D.

8 Fiberbronchoscopy   107
Bernard R. Marsh, M.D., John K. Frost, M.D., Yener S. Erozan, M.D., and Darryl Carter, M.D.

9 Mediastinoscopy in Assessment of Lung Cancer   113
Edward M. Goldberg, M.D.

10 Roentgenographic Manifestations of Lung Cancer   129
W. Eugene Miller, M.D.

11 Diagnosis in Metastatic Sites   137
Franco M. Muggia, M.D., Heine H. Hansen, M.D., and Lakshman R. Chervu, Ph.D.

12 Staging Lung Cancer   151
David T. Carr, M.D., and Clifton F. Mountain, M.D.

13 Radiotherapy for Lung Cancer   163
Robert E. Lee, M.D.

14 Biologic, Physiologic, and Technical Determinants in Surgical Therapy for Lung Cancer   185
Clifton F. Mountain, M.D.

15 Chemotherapy in Lung Cancer   199
Oleg Selawry, M.D.

16 Immunotherapy and Lung Cancer   223
Evan M. Hersh, M.D., Giora Mavligit, M.D., and Jordan U. Gutterman, M.D.

17 Pleural Effusions   243
Mark G. Janis, M.D., and Marc J. Straus, M.D.

18 Superior Vena Caval Syndrome   249
Robert J. Polackwich, M.D., and Marc J. Straus, M.D.

19 Concept of Lung Cancer Management   261
Marc J. Straus, M.D.

20 Prognostic Factors for Survival Time in Inoperable Lung Cancer   271
Stephen W. Lagakos, Ph.D.

Preface

Five years ago a 63-year-old man named Max was admitted to our medical service at Barnes Hospital with right upper quadrant pain of two-weeks' duration. His liver scan revealed large defects, and his chest x-ray showed a left hilar lesion. Bronchoscopy was performed and revealed small cell carcinoma of the lung. Max was told his diagnosis and that he had only a few months to live.

There was enormous resistance to treating Max. At that time physicians were unwilling to contend with cancer, and furthermore they considered its treatment futile. They spent little time studying the disease, and they were even less inclined to make use of the information that was already available. Clinical oncology then seemed to be developing along very empirical lines, and it was not receiving sufficient input from the basic sciences. And the laboratory scientists were not taking cues from the clinicians to develop a clinically applicable science.

I had spent the previous two years with Dr. Abraham Goldin in Drug Research and Development at the National Cancer Institute, and we had become interested in studying whether or not there were biologic determinants in various tumors that made them vulnerable to specific treatments. In particular we were concerned with the relationship between the dosage and schedule of anticancer drugs and the cytokinetic characteristics of the tumor.

There was reason to believe that because small cell carcinoma proliferated so rapidly it might be responsive to aggressive chemotherapy, as are choriocarcinoma and Burkitt's lymphoma. We accordingly treated Max with a combination of the drugs cyclophosphamide and methotrexate and based the dosage and schedule in part on cytokinetic principles. It was necessary for Max to travel 200 miles every three weeks to receive treatment, so we established relationships with community physicians and local laboratories to facilitate his care. Max was able to continue to run his dairy, the thing he loved most—and he had a complete remission.

Over the ensuing months we worked to refine the lung cancer protocol. The paucity of data on lung cancer was in stark contrast to the commonness of the disease. Little work had been done in lung cancer, and consequently there was little basis from which to select alternative therapies for patients who failed treatment.

Pathologists were beginning to use a new cell typing system for lung cancer. Small cell (oat cell) carcinoma was distinguished by its aggressive behavior and proclivity for early metastasis. Surgeons were no longer operating on most of these cases. In contrast well-differentiated epidermoid carcinoma was the type most strongly associated with surgical cure. New diagnostic techniques, including fiberoptic bronchoscopy and scanning, were becoming widespread. National cooperative cancer trials were becoming more active, and successes in some cancers awakened an interest in lung cancer, too.

In 1974 Dr. Oleg Selawry and I edited an issue on lung cancer for *Seminars in Oncology*. We attempted to provide the clinician with an up-to-date understanding of the approach to diagnosis and treatment of the disease. We included data relevant to understanding the behavior of the disease, such as cytokinetics and marker production.

In the last two years there has been a surge of interest in clinical oncology, and the specialty of medical oncology is maturing. Predictably there are now subspecialty boards in medical oncology given by the American Board of Internal Medicine. Today our housestaff knows far more about lung cancer than simply its four cell types and the names of the common anticancer drugs. There have been several important developments in the understanding and treatment of lung cancer, and there is now greater knowledge of the pathophysiology of the disease and the approaches to optimal diagnosis. There has been a much greater emphasis on systematic trials using combinations of drugs and multimodality therapy which includes radiotherapy and immunotherapy. Important results have been noted in early and late disease.

With great encouragement I have undertaken to update our 1974 work on lung cancer. All of the contributing authors to the *Seminars in Oncology* issue participated in this book, and they have thoroughly revised their subjects and have included much of the relevant data that has been reported to the beginning of 1977. We were given an opportunity to reconsider our previous statements, and we have attempted to avoid unnecessary overlap. I thank these authors for their time and effort and their willingness to modify and replace old dogmas with new concepts.

We have added two chapters on therapeutics, namely the treatment of pleural effusions in lung cancer and a review of the superior vena caval syndrome which is usually caused by lung cancer. Chapters have also been added on roentgenographic manifestations of lung cancer and on ultrastructural studies. We have briefly summarized various approaches to diagnosis and treatment of the disease in a separate chapter. We have attempted to provide a sufficient understanding of the biology of the tumor and of the diagnostic tools and therapeutic modalities so that treatment will not be merely by proscription. Fortunately the specific treatments of choice will be changing anyway.

I would like to thank in particular Dr. Oleg Selawry, my friend and teacher, for his devoted interest in the understanding of this disease and his encouragement of my work. Drs. Clifton Mountain and David Carr provided helpful advice both for this book and the previous monograph. I also would like to thank my secretary, Ms. Donna Beaton, for her special interest and help in putting this book together and our editors at Grune & Stratton for their consistent and professional assistance.

In our study which began with the treatment of Max's lung cancer approximately 90 percent of the patients with small cell carcinoma have responded, some for longer than two years. A high response rate is now commonly seen with vigorous treatment of this disease, and patients who later develop progressive disease often respond again to other regimens. Recently the other cell types have demonstrated better responses, and exciting data have been reported in the treatment of resectable disease with adjuvant therapy.

I perceive an equally important change in the attitude of most physicians. They are becoming patient advocates, and they are pursuing with vigor and humanity the new avenues open to the diagnosis and treatment of lung cancer.

Marc J. Straus, M.D.

Contributors

Lawrence E. Broder, M.D.
Assistant Professor of Oncology
and Associate Chief of Pulmonary Oncology
Comprehensive Cancer Center of the State of
  Florida
University of Miami
School of Medicine
Miami, Florida

David T. Carr, M.D.
Professor of Medicine
Division of Medical Oncology
Mayo Medical School
Rochester, Minnesota

Darryl Carter, M.D.
Associate Professor of Pathology
Department of Pathology
Johns Hopkins University
School of Medicine
Baltimore, Maryland

Lakshman R. Chervu, Ph.D.
Assistant Professor of Radiology
Department of Radiology
Albert Einstein College of Medicine
Bronx, New York

Martin H. Cohen, M.D.
Deputy Chief
National Cancer Institute-
Veterans Administration Medical Oncology
  Service
Veterans Administration Hospital
Washington, D.C.

Robert B. Diasio, M.D.
Assistant Professor of Medicine
Medical College of Virginia
Richmond, Virginia

Yener S. Erozan, M.D.
Associate Professor of Pathology
Division of Cytopathology
Department of Pathology
Johns Hopkins University
School of Medicine
Baltimore, Maryland

John K. Frost, M.D.
Professor of Pathology
Division of Cytopathology
Department of Pathology
Johns Hopkins University
School of Medicine
Baltimore, Maryland

Edward M. Goldberg, M.D.
Professor of Surgery
University of Health Sciences
Chicago Medical School
and Attending Surgeon
Department of Surgery
Michael Reese Hospital and Medical Center
Chicago, Illinois

Phillip R. Gordon, M.D.
Assistant Professor of Pathology
and Associate Pathologist
Mallory Institute of Pathology
Boston University Medical Center
Boston, Massachusetts

Jordan U. Gutterman, M.D.
Associate Professor of Medicine
Department of Developmental Therapeutics
University of Texas System Cancer Center
M. D. Anderson Hospital and Tumor Institute
Houston, Texas

Heine H. Hansen, M.D.
Chief, Chemotherapy Section
Radiotherapy Division
Finsen Institutet
Copenhagen, Denmark

Curtis C. Harris, M.D.
Head, Human Tissue Studies Section
Experimental Pathology Branch
Carcinogenesis Program
National Cancer Institute
National Institutes of Health
Bethesda, Maryland

Evan M. Hersh, M.D.
Professor of Medicine
and Chief, Section of Immunology
and Deputy Head, Department of
    Developmental Therapeutics
University of Texas System Cancer Center
M. D. Anderson Hospital and Tumor Institute
Houston, Texas

Mark G. Janis, M.D.
Instructor of Medicine
Section of Medical Oncology
Department of Medicine
University Hospital
Boston, Massachusetts

Stephen W. Lagakos, Ph.D.
Assistant Professor of Statistical Science
State University of New York at Buffalo
Amherst, New York

Robert E. Lee, M.D.
Consultant in Therapeutic Radiology
Mayo Clinic and Mayo Foundation
Rochester, Minnesota

Bruce Mackay, M.D., Ph.D.
Associate Pathologist
Department of Pathology
University of Texas System Cancer Center
M. D. Anderson Hospital and Tumor Institute
Houston, Texas

Bernard R. Marsh, M.D.
Associate Professor of Laryngology and
    Otology
Department of Laryngology and Otology
Johns Hopkins University
School of Medicine
Baltimore, Maryland

Mary J. Matthews, M.D.
Pathologist
National Cancer Institute
Veterans Administration Medical Oncology
    Service
and Professor of Pathology
George Washington University
School of Medicine
Washington, D.C.

Giora M. Mavligit, M.D.
Associate Professor of Medicine
Department of Developmental Therapeutics
University of Texas System Cancer Center
M. D. Anderson Hospital and Tumor Institute
Houston, Texas

W. Eugene Miller, M.D.
Consultant in Diagnostic Roentgenology
Mayo Clinic
and Assistant Professor of Diagnostic
    Roentgenology
Mayo Medical School
Rochester, Minnesota

Clifton F. Mountain, M.D.
Professor of Surgery
and Chief, Section of Thoracic Surgery
University of Texas System Cancer Center
M. D. Anderson Hospital and Tumor Institute
Houston, Texas

Franco M. Muggia, M.D.
Associate Director for Cancer Therapy
Evaluation Program
Division of Cancer Treatment
National Cancer Institute
National Institutes of Health
Bethesda, Maryland

Barbara M. Osborne, M.D.
Assistant Pathologist
Department of Pathology
University of Texas System Cancer Center
M. D. Anderson Hospital and Tumor Institute
Houston, Texas

Robert J. Polackwich, M.D.
Clinical Associate
Section of Medical Oncology
Department of Medicine
University Hospital
Boston, Massachusetts

Aron Primack, M.D.
Washington Hospital Center
Washington, D.C.

Oleg Selawry, M.D.
Professor of Oncology
Comprehensive Cancer Center of the State of
  Florida
University of Miami
School of Medicine
Jackson Memorial Medical Center
Miami, Florida

Roma A. Wilson, M.D.
Assistant Pathologist
Department of Pathology
University of Texas System Cancer Center
M. D. Anderson Hospital and Tumor Institute
Houston, Texas

LUNG CANCER

Curtis C. Harris

1

Respiratory Carcinogenesis

The environmental determinants for at least 80 percent of lung cancer in man are known. The main etiologic agent is inhaled tobacco smoke. Although a strong association between inhaled tobacco smoke and the risk of developing bronchogenic carcinoma has been established, other carcinogenic substances that cause lung cancer are also being identified, particularly in the workplace. Synergistic interactions among these substances (e.g., asbestos and tobacco smoke) in increasing the risk of cancer illustrate the complexity of this multifactorial disease, lung cancer. The increasing awareness of the danger of occupational lung cancer on the part of the scientific community, workers, labor unions, and industry has stimulated actions that are resulting in gradual improvement in working conditions, with consequent reduction in exposure to known carcinogens.

The magnitude of the lung cancer problem is substantial. The number of deaths in the United States from lung cancer in 1975 has been estimated at 81,000,[1] i.e., approximately 222 per day and 9 per hour. If current trends continue, it is projected that 295,000 new cases of lung cancer will occur in the year 2000.[2] The incidence of lung cancer is increasing in both sexes, and the incidence in the black population is increasing at a greater rate than in the white population.[3] While the human suffering and loss caused by lung cancer cannot be measured, an economic loss of approximately $2 billion per year in the United States has been estimated from reported data.[4] Lung cancer is a worldwide problem, but its incidence is highest in the industrial countries. Although the incidence rates vary from country to country, depending partly on the availability of health care and the adequacy of demographic systems in each country, the death rates are essentially within one order of magnitude (Fig. 1-1). Scotland, England, Wales, and Finland have the highest incidences of lung cancer, while the United States ranks 10th and Mexico ranks 37th among the 40 countries surveyed.

Lung cancer is an insidious disease that develops over a period of 1 to 4 decades and often remains asymptomatic until late in its course. At the time symptoms cause the patient to seek medical care, lung cancer has frequently invaded and metastasized, so that only 25 percent of these patients are surgical candidates. Although some lengthening of useful survival has been obtained with radiotherapy and chemotherapy, the median survival remains appallingly low, less than 1 year. Prevention would thus seem the logical approach to the control of lung cancer.

The comments by Stuart Yuspa, Paul Netteshein, and Umberto Saffiotti were especially helpful. The secretarial assistance by both Maxine Bellman and Pat Hembree is appreciated.

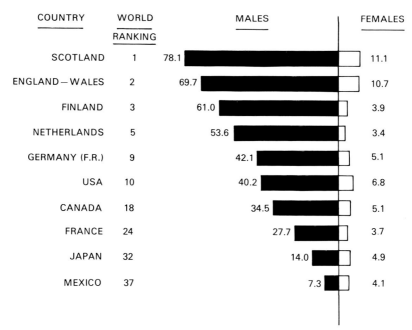

Fig. 1-1.   Death rates (deaths per 100,000 population) from lung cancer in selected countries. (Data from Silverberg E, Holleb AI: Cancer statistics, 1974—Worldwide epidemiology. CA 24:2–21, 1974.)

Respiratory carcinogenesis and epidemiology of lung cancer are active areas of investigation. Several recent reviews, reports, and symposia covering various facets of these investigations are available.[5–11] In this chapter, highlights of recent results and trends will be discussed from the vantage point of an experimental oncologist, with emphasis on methods to both identify high-risk populations and devise means of prophylactic intervention. When compared to the general population, an individual may be at high risk for developing lung cancer because of high levels of exposure to carcinogens and/or because of host factors that increase his susceptibility to the oncogenic effects of environmental carcinogens. Essential components of such a preventive approach must include an understanding of chemical carcinogenesis, the ability to use animal models, the development of model systems using human tissues for studying carcinogenesis, and finally extensive involvement in clinical research.

CHEMICAL CARCINOGENESIS

The majority of human cancers, in particular lung cancer, appear to be caused by exogenous agents, including environmental chemicals. Pub-

lic awareness of this danger, and scientific interest in these findings have resulted in new emphasis on studies of chemical carcinogenesis. In the next two brief sections of this chapter, only salient generalizations are presented. Comprehensive reviews[12,13] and the proceedings of a world symposium[14] are recommended reading for those interested in more detailed information.

Neoplastic Transformation and Tumor Progression

On a simplistic basis, chemical carcinogenesis can be divided into two phases: *neoplastic transformation* and *tumor progression* (Fig. 1-2). The first phase involves the transformation of normal cells to malignant cells. The chemical carcinogens must reach the target cells, usually by passing through a body surface, then interact with cell constituents, and finally transform the cells. The surface area of the lower respiratory tract, which is lined by target epithelial cells, is readily available for direct contact with inhaled carcinogens. However, the journey of the chemical carcinogen to the bronchial target cell can also be indirect (e.g., via ingestion). This type of exposure would be greatly influenced by absorption, distribution, metabolism, and excretion.

CHEMICAL CARCINOGENESIS

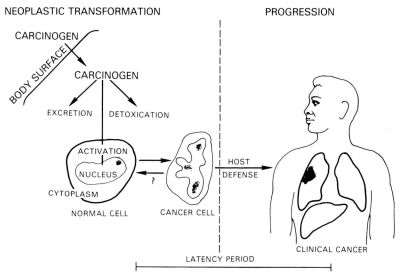

Fig. 1-2. Neoplastic transformation and tumor progression are the two basic phases of carcinogenesis.

Direct and Indirect Chemical Carcinogen

Chemical carcinogens may be classified as either direct- or indirect-acting, depending on their requirements for metabolic activation. *Direct-acting carcinogens* need only to reach the target cell in sufficient concentration to cause the interactions leading to neoplastic transformation. Because of their intense reactivity, direct-acting carcinogens do not generally persist in the general environment. They are mainly synthetic chemicals used (1) in laboratory investigations, (2) in the clinic as alkylating antitumor drugs, and (3) in industrial synthetic processes. Most chemical carcinogens are *procarcinogens* (indirect-acting), and they require metabolic activation, which frequently occurs within the target cell. These carcinogens are more stable chemicals (both naturally occurring compounds and products of an industrialized society) that persist in the environment until they are activated in an exposed individual. As will be discussed in a later section, the metabolic activation of procarcinogens varies among species and among individuals within a single outbred species (e.g., man), which is caused in part by genetic factors.

The binding of the active form of a chemical carcinogen to cellular macromolecules is thought to be an important step in chemical carcinogene-sis. The activated forms of most chemical carcinogens are positively charged (electrophilic) reactants that readily bind to negatively charged cellular macromolecules, including DNA[15] (Fig. 3). The extent to which carcinogens bind to DNA has been correlated with their carcinogenicity in some experimental studies.[12] Deactivation of procarcinogens and direct-acting carcinogens by both enzymatic and nonenzymatic pathways also occurs. Therefore the differential ability of various tissues to activate and deactivate chemical carcinogens may in part account for the organo-tropic specificity of certain carcinogens, including some respiratory carcinogens. Once the critical cellular interactions have induced the transformed state, these malignant cells may progress to clinically evident cancer in the *permissive* host. Tumor progression and the host factors influencing it (e.g., immune surveillance and stimulation) have been the subject of a recent review.[16]

Tumor induction by chemicals is dependent on many factors, including route of exposure, dose, regimen, absorption, distribution, metabolism, and excretion. The portal of entry and the distribution in the body dictate in large part the sites of neoplastic transformation caused by direct-acting carcinogens. After having met the requirement of reaching the target site, chemical carcinogens requiring metabolic activation induce tumors primarily in those tissues containing activating enzymes. In general, tumor incidence is also directly dependent on the dose of the chemical in experimental animals and in man. For example, the risk of bronchogenic carcinoma in man is related to the number of cigarettes smoked,[10,11] and the risk of bladder cancer in industrial workers exposed to aromatic amines correlates with length of exposure.[17] However, in these examples the dose–response relationship is difficult to define both because man is exposed to many chemical carcinogens simultaneously and because the exact dose of each of these carcinogens is difficult to measure.

Modifying factors in chemical carcinogenesis determined by the host include species, strain, sex, hormonal status, age, immunologic competence, and nutritional status.[13] The metabolic and proliferative status of the target cell is also important. Animal models and experimental systems using human tissues are providing new methods to define the role of these host determinants in respiratory carcinogenesis.

ANIMAL MODELS

Animal models have been developed to reproduce human disease in an experimental setting. A hamster model for human bronchogenic carcinoma has been developed by Saffiotti et al.[18] Hamsters were selected as the experimental animals because they have a paucity of both spontaneous tumors and respiratory infections. When given respiratory carcinogens by intratracheal instillation, hamsters develop malignant tumors histologically similar to those found in human lung cancer. Squamous cell carcinoma, adenocarcinoma, and large cell carcinoma are produced, but oat cell carcinoma is not seen. This animal model has been particularly suitable for morphologic and biochemical studies.

Morphogenesis of Squamous Cell Carcinoma

In the hamster model described above, serial-kill studies[19–21] have suggested that the morphogenesis of squamous cell carcinoma is a multistage process similar to that proposed in man by Auerbach.[22] The chemical carcinogens utilized in these experimental studies (benzo[a]pyrene and N-methyl-N-nitrosourea) initially cause mucous

cell hyperplasia and squamous metaplasia in the tracheobronchial epithelium of the hamster. In the areas of squamous metaplasia that persisted after carcinogen administration, significant changes were observed by electron microscopy. These ultrastructural changes were not seen in a reversible form of squamous metaplasia caused by vitamin A deficiency. Persistent alterations in nuclear structure of basal cells and defects in the basal lamina were restricted to areas of squamous metaplasia caused by these chemical carcinogens. In a study similar in design to the one described above, Schreiber et al.[23] followed the carcinogenic process in the hamster by correlating cytologic changes in cells obtained by tracheal washing with histologic changes in the tracheal epithelium. Their study adds further indirect support to the proposed multistage process of morphogenesis.

Binding of Chemical Carcinogens to Cellular Macromolecules

As mentioned in the preceding section (Fig. 1-3), the interaction of chemical carcinogens with cellular macromolecules and structures is believed to be an important step in chemical carcinogenesis. Such interactions in the respiratory tract have been studied in a short-term tracheal culture system developed by Kaufman et al.[24] Using this in vitro system it has been shown that the respiratory epithelium of the hamster has the metabolic capability to activate a procarcinogen (benzo[a]pyrene) to reactive forms that bind to cellular macromolecules. Prior in vivo administration of unlabelled benzo[a]pyrene to donor animals caused a subsequent increase in the in vitro binding of ^{3}H-benzo[a]pyrene to tracheal mucosal cells,[25] as determined by autoradiography, and to their isolated DNA.[26] This binding was reduced by adding an inhibitor of aryl hydrocarbon hydroxylase, 7,8-benzoflavone, to the culture medium;[26] aryl hydrocarbon hydroxylase is a microsomal mixed-function oxygenase that is important in the metabolic activation of benzo[a]pyrene. With an autoradiographic assay to determine intracellular binding sites, binding was observed in both the nucleus and cytoplasm, and the majority of the nuclear binding of ^{3}H-benzo[a]pyrene was in the heterochromatic regions. Further studies have shown that binding of ^{3}H-benzo[a]pyrene to tracheal DNA varies among

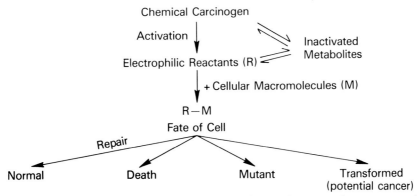

Fig. 1-3. Binding of a carcinogen to cellular macromolecules may have several consequences for the cell. If the cellular damage is faithfully repaired, the cell will return to normal. Severe damage may cause death. Finally, sublethal damage may cause a mutation and/or may transform normal cells into neoplastic cells that may progress into clinically evident cancer.

certain inbred strains of hamsters and and that an inverse relationship exists between the age of the hamster donating the trachea and in vitro binding levels of benzo[a]pyrene to DNA.[27] The usefulness of such data in predicting states of susceptibility to respiratory carcinogenesis in this animal model is currently being studied.

Experimentally induced vitamin A deficiency may be a state in which there is an increased susceptibility to respiratory carcinogenesis.[28] One can speculate that this increased susceptibility may be caused by an enhanced capability of respiratory epithelium in vitamin-A-deficient animals to activate chemical carcinogens into forms that bind to cellular receptors (e.g., DNA), thus leading to neoplastic transformation. With an in vitro tracheal culture system, increased binding of ^{3}H-benzo[a]pyrene to DNA was found in respiratory epithelium taken from vitamin-A-deficient hamsters, as compared to tissue from normal hamsters.[29] Furthermore, this increased binding to DNA in vitamin-A-deficient tracheal epithelium was reduced by adding a vitamin A compound, β-retinyl acetate, to the culture medium.[27] While these studies measure binding to a specific class of macromolecules, they do not identify which cells are responsible for this increased level of binding to macromolecules, and in the tracheal epithelium of the vitamin-A-deficient hamster focal areas of squamous metaplasia are found. Such information can be obtained by autoradiographic techniques. When ^{3}H-benzo[a]pyrene was given by intratracheal instillation to hamsters deficient in vitamin A, more autoradiographic grains were found in the foci of squamous metaplasia than in the nonmetaplastic areas.[30] In addition to increased binding of ^{3}H-benzo[a]pyrene on a cellular basis, increased cell proliferation in the tracheobronchial epithelium was found in vitamin-A-deficient hamsters.[31] Thus vitamin A influences cellular differentiation, rate of cell proliferation, and metabolism of benzo[a]pyrene in the hamster tracheobronchial epithelium, but which of these factors affects the ultimate tumor response is still unclear.

Interaction among Chemical Carcinogens and Physical Carcinogens

Man is exposed to numerous carcinogenic and noncarcinogenic agents. Studies in experimental animals are needed to dissect out the importance of these various exposures. Animal models are being used not only to identify individual carcinogens but also to study the interaction among carcinogens in regard to induction of cancer. Kaufman and Madison[32] have shown that benzo[a]pyrene and N-methyl-N-nitrosourea, each given by intratracheal instillation in a sequential manner, act synergistically to cause lung cancer in the hamster. The mean latency period of the tumors (predominantly squamous cell carcinomas) was approximately 22 weeks in hamsters receiving both chemical carcinogens, compared to approximately 56 weeks in those animals receiving only one carcinogen. Little and associates[33-36] have used the hamster to investigate the pathogenesis of lung cancers induced by alpha radiation emitted from a physical carcinogen, polonium 210. Polonium 210 is found in tobacco smoke. Lung cancers were induced by polonium 210 in hamsters at levels of exposure (15 rads) comparable to those found in the lungs of human cigarette smokers. Furthermore, a synergism between benzo[a]pyrene and polonium 210 was discovered in this animal model. Polonium 210 (total 0.05 μCi) and benzo[a]pyrene (total 4.5 mg) given simultaneously on carrier particles of ferric oxide for 15 weekly instillations caused twice the incidence of lung carcinomas than would be expected from the effect of either carcinogen alone. Asbestos, a fibrous physical carcinogen, may also enhance the tumorigenicity of chemical carcinogens in both man and animal models. Epidemiologic investigations, which will be discussed in more detail in a following section of this chapter, suggest that asbestos workers who smoke cigarettes have a markedly increased risk of lung cancer when compared to either nonsmoking asbestos workers or smokers in the general population. Smith et al[37] have reported results from a preliminary experimental study in hamsters measuring the cocarcinogenicity of asbestos. Chrysotile asbestos, which by itself is a potent carcinogen for mesothelial tissues,[38] increased the incidence of lung carcinomas induced by benzo[a]pyrene (suspended in Tween 60) when both were given by intratracheal instillation. The previously mentioned studies underscore not only the deleterious interaction that can occur by combined administration of chemical carcinogens such as benzo[a]pyrene and N-methyl-N-nitrosourea but also the synergistic effects caused by exposure to both physical carcinogens (oncogenic fibers and radiation) and chemical carcinogens.

Methods for inhalation exposure of respiratory carcinogens have also been developed (see Laskin and Sellakumar[39]). Experimental studies using inhalation methodology are expensive, but they offer theoretical advantages when compared to intratracheal administration of chemical carcinogens by injection. Volatile chemicals are especially suitable for inhalation assays. For example, recently reported studies have described the carcinogenicity of an α-halogen ether, bis(chloromethyl)ether, in rats and hamsters.[40] Both lifetime and limited-period exposures to bis (chloromethyl) ether at levels as low as 0.1 part per million caused squamous cell carcinomas and adenocarcinomas in lungs of rats. α-Halogen

ethers are electrophilic reactants used in industry as intermediates in the synthesis and preparation of water repellants, ion-exchange resins, polymers, and solvents for polymerization reactions. Industrial workers exposed to α-halogen ethers appear to have an increased risk of lung cancer, especially oat cell carcinoma.[41,42]

While tobacco smoke readily induces invasive cancers of the larynx in rodents, it has proved difficult to produce lung cancers experimentally (see Nettesheim and Schreiber[6]). The explanation for this difficulty may be the extensive filtering of the smoke by the well-developed nasal cavities of rodents. Regardless of the explanation, tobacco smoke is a complex mixture of approximately 2000 chemicals, many of which have been shown to be carcinogens (Table 1-1) and tumor promoters in a variety of experimental systems. Unfortunately, a suitable animal model has yet to be found in which lung cancer can be induced by inhalation of this mixture.

In addition to the methods previously described, lung cancer has been produced in animals by other methods and agents.[6,39] For example, beeswax pellets impregnated with carcinogens have been inserted into lungs of rats. Using this method, Stanton et al.[43] have induced lung cancers with very small quantities of tobacco smoke condensates. While there are no data to support a viral etiology of human lung cancer, polyoma virus instilled into the lungs of hamsters will produce tumors,[44] and jaagsietke, a disease of sheep with a high incidence of lung tumors, appears to be caused by a virus.[45]

Table 1-1
Identified Carcinogens in Tobacco Smoke*

Gas phase
  dimethylnitrosamine, diethylnitrosamine, methylethylnitrosamine, N-nitrosopyrrolidine, nitrosopiperidine
Particulate phase
  benzo[a]pyrene, methylbenzo[a]pyrenes, dibenz[a,h]acridine, dibenz[a,j]acridine, dibenz[c]carbazole, β-naphthylamine, benzo[b]fluoranthene, benzo[j]fluoranthene, methylfluoranthene, benz[α]anthracene, chrysene, methchrysenes, nitrosonanabasine, benzo[c]phenanthrene, nitrosonornicotine, polonium 210, arsenic

*Data from Harris[9] and Wynder and Hoffman.[101]

Cocarcinogens in Respiratory Carcinogenesis

Cocarcinogens are agents that have little or no carcinogenic action but augment the carcinogenicity of chemical carcinogens by increasing cancer incidence and/or shortening latency period. Cocarcinogenic agents, as well as states of either increased or decreased susceptibility to respiratory carcinogens, are being identified in animal models. Respiratory infections may be an example of a state of increased susceptibility to respiratory carcinogens. For example, Schreiber et al.[46] have shown in a well-controlled study that a respiratory infection by influenza virus in rats increases the susceptibility to lung cancer caused by systemic administration of N-nitrosoheptamethyleneimine, an organotropic carcinogen. The respiratory infection could have increased the number of susceptible target cells, perhaps by enhancing the rate of cell proliferation and/or altering the metabolic activation of this procarcinogen. In man, chronic bronchitis is frequently found in lung cancer patients, but its role in the pathogenesis of this cancer is uncertain.

The role of air pollution in human lung cancer is controversial. When adjusted for cigarette smoking, a comparison of the rates of lung cancer in urban and rural areas show only small differences ranging from a 1.26-fold to a 2.33-fold increase in urban residents.[47] Data in animal models suggest that air pollutants can augment tumorigenicity of respiratory carcinogens. In inhalation studies, SO_2, a common gaseous air pollutant, enhanced the carcinogenicity of benzo[a]pyrene in a synergistic fashion.[48] Lung cancer was observed only in the group exposed to both SO_2 and benzo[a]pyrene, while no cancers were found in animals exposed to either single agent at the doses tested. In a similar study another common gaseous air pollutant, NO_2, augmented the carcinogenicity of benzo[a]pyrene.[49] Ferric oxide is probably the most common particulate pollutant in the air. When given to hamsters by either inhalation or intratracheal instillation it increased the tumor incidence caused by diethylnitrosamine, a systemically administered respiratory carcinogen.[50,51] Neither SO_2 nor NO_2 nor ferric oxide alone is carcinogenic in experimental animals. The mechanisms by which these cocarcinogenic agents act are unknown. They may act in part by increasing cell proliferation in the respiratory epithelium, by altering metabolism of the carcinogens, and/or by decreasing clearance of the carcinogens by the mucous-ciliary transport mechanism that serves as a host defense factor in the lung. The postulated role of cocarcinogens in the carcinogenesis of human lung cancer has not yet been demonstrated, but assuming that studies in animal models may indicate similar responses in man, cocarcinogens will have to be considered as part of the complex equation defining the risk from exposure to known chemical carcinogens in the workplace and in the general environment.

Vitamin A Prophylaxis in Respiratory Carcinogenesis

Animal models may be useful for devising means of prophylactic intervention in an attempt to interrupt the carcinogenic process. Saffiotti et al.[52] found that high doses of vitamin A (retinyl palmitate) administered by feeding *after* a carcinogenic intratracheal regimen of benzo[a]pyrene and ferric oxide markedly reduced the incidence of squamous metaplasia and lung cancer in the hamster model. In the rat the incidence of pulmonary squamous nodules (precursors to squamous cell carcinoma) was reduced when vitamin A (β-retinyl acetate) was given both *during* and *after* administration of methylcholanthrene.[53] Since the findings in the latter study may in part have been caused by the inhibitory effects of vitamin A compounds on microsomal activation of methylcholanthrene,[54] Nettesheim and associates[55] gave β-retinyl acetate to rats only *after* the carcinogenic regimen of methylcholanthrene. Again, a reduction in both the incidence and the size of the squamous nodules was found. An approach to enhance the anticarcinogenic effects of vitamin A compounds while reducing their toxicity has recently been discussed.[56] This approach has had some success. Bollag[57] recently reported a reduced incidence of skin carcinomas induced by 7,12-dimethylbenz[a]anthracene, followed by promotion with Croton oil when the mice were given an aromatic analogue of vitamin A acid by feeding during the promotion phase of skin carcinogenesis. This analogue had low toxicity for the mouse, as manifested by slight desquamation of the skin. While these studies and others[56] are consistent with an anticarcinogenic effect of vitamin A compounds, there have also been studies suggesting that vitamin A enhances carcinogenesis.[58,59] These conflicting data, as well as the toxicity of vitamin A compounds and the inherent difficulties present in extrapolation among species, require that additional studies be made before clinical trials are undertaken in high-risk patients.

EXPERIMENTAL HUMAN BRONCHIAL STUDIES

Model Systems Using Human Tissues

The extrapolation of carcinogenesis data from studies utilizing experimental animals to man presents a number of complex problems (see Weisburger[13] and Harris[60] for recent reviews). One approach to providing a link between these experimental studies and human cancer is the development of a model system to study carcinogenesis in important human target tissues (e.g., the bronchus). The development of such a system involves three major facets: (1) Obtaining viable human tissues, (2) in vitro maintenance of these tissues, and (3) xenotransplantation of human tissues into immunodeficient animals to assess tumorigenicity of suspected malignant cells transformed in vitro (Fig. 1-4). Assuming that the human tissue can be suitably maintained in such systems, then it can be exposed to carcinogens and to anticarcinogens while in culture and/or as a xenograft. Organ and explant cultures of human tissues have the advantages of retaining normal cellular differentiation and the three-dimensional intercellular relationships. One can also use such cultures to initiate monolayer cell cultures.

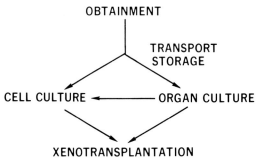

Fig. 1-4. An approach to the use of human tissues in carcinogenesis studies.

Recent studies have indicated that explants of human bronchi can be maintained in a controlled experimental setting.[61,62] Bronchial specimens were taken either at surgery or at "immediate autopsy"[63] from patients with and without lung cancer. The patients had not received previous cancer therapy. Grossly normal-appearing bronchial specimens obtained in this manner were maintained in explant culture for at least 4 months and in athymic nude mice for at least 8 months.

Metabolism of Chemical Carcinogens

The explant cultures of human bronchi have been useful in studying the metabolism of chemical carcinogens. Cultured human bronchial mucosa has the ability to metabolize carcinogenic polynuclear aromatic hydrocarbons into forms that tightly bind to macromolecules, including DNA.[64] Recent investigations have shown that the binding of benzo[a]pyrene to DNA is dependent on the concentration of benzo[a]pyrene, the duration of exposure, and the temperature of incubation.[65] In addition, more benzo[a]pyrene was bound in bronchial epithelial cells than to fibroblasts in the explants. While the intraindividual variation in binding to DNA due to methodology was approximately 10 percent, the interindividual variation was at least 50-fold.[66] This marked interindividual variation may in part reflect the genetic control of benzo[a]pyrene metabolism in the heterogeneous human population; pharmacogenetic studies in fraternal and identical twins have shown that *inter*individual variation in drug metabolism is greater than *intra*individual variation.[67] One can speculate that genetically controlled differences in metabolic activation of procarcinogens may determine, in part, susceptibility.

Several chemicals that have been shown to have an anticarcinogenic effect in experimental animals also inhibit the metabolism of carcinogenic polynuclear aromatic hydrocarbons.[12] The effect of these chemicals on metabolism of benzo[a]pyrene in cultured human bronchial mucosa is currently being studied. For example, 7,8-benzoflavone reduces the level of benzo[a]pyrene bound to DNA of bronchial explants, whereas nicotine causes no change in the level of binding.[65,68] Although a correlation between the binding of a chemical to DNA and its potency as a carcinogen has been suggested in both experimental animals and cell culture systems, this relationship in human cells remains to be proved. Other aspects of metabolism of chemical carcinogens are being studied in human tissues. The activities of aryl hydrocarbon hydroxylase, benzo[a]pyrene 4,5-oxide hydratase, benzo[a]pyrene 4,5-oxide glutathione transferases, all of which are enzymes important in the activation and inactivation of benzo[a]pyrene, can be assayed. The level of metabolites of benzo[a]pyrene can also be measured by high-pressure liquid chromatography. Thus it would appear that methodologies developed for and utilized in studies of carcinogenesis in experimental animals and cell cultures can be successfully extended to similar investigations in human cells and tissues. These investigations should eventually aid in identifying both chemical carcinogens and host factors that determine susceptibility. The current status of this developing area of investigation has recently been reviewed.[69]

HUMAN LUNG CANCER

Respiratory Carcinogens in Man

A variety of agents either have been proved to be or are suspected of being respiratory carcinogens in man (Table 1-2). Tobacco smoke, clearly the dominant etiologic agent, is a complex mixture of both physical and chemical carcinogens (Table 1-1).

The link between cigarette smoking and lung cancer was established initially through retrospective epidemiologic studies in 1950. Confirmation was obtained by both prospective and further retrospective studies in the United States, Canada, Japan, and England.[10,11] The lung cancer mortality rate of male cigarette smokers has been estimated to be 8 to 20 times that of those who have never smoked.[70] The smoker's risk for developing squamous cell carcinoma and oat cell carcinoma (two histologic types of lung cancer rarely found in nonsmokers) is higher than his risk for developing adenocarcinoma and bronchiolar carcinoma.[71] The dose–response relationship between cigarette smoking and lung cancer is illustrated in Fig. 1-5.[72] In addition to the markedly increased risk of lung cancer, cigarette smokers have at least a threefold greater risk of cancer in the larynx, oral cavity, and esophagus than nonsmokers.[72] The risk of lung cancer for cigar and pipe smokers is not as great as that for cigarette smokers, apparently because they inhale less smoke than cigarette smokers. However, smoking more than 5 cigars or 10 pipes per day may be associated with an enhanced risk of lung cancer and (to a more significant extent) an increased risk of cancer of the oral cavity.[73] The carcinogenic hazard of the recently popular small cigars has yet to be determined.

The type of cigarettes smoked may influence risk levels. The risk of lung cancer (squamous cell carcinoma and small cell carcinoma) is less in smokers of filter cigarettes than in those who smoke nonfilter cigarettes (Fig. 1-6).[11,72] While the exact explanation for this diminished risk is uncertain, filter cigarettes do have reduced levels of "tar" and nicotine. Also, the level of tar in nonfilter cigarettes has decreased over the last 15 years because of increased use of reconstituted tobacco. Carcinogenic polynuclear aromatic hydrocarbons (e.g., benzo[a]pyrene) are found in cigarette tar.

Occupationally Related Lung Cancer

In addition to the lung cancer caused by cigarette smoking, lung cancer may be contracted as one of several occupationally related respirato-

Table 1-2
Respiratory Carcinogens in Man

Type of Exposure	Carcinogens
Personal	Tobacco smoke
Occupational and/or environmental	Asbestos, nickel (refining), radon daughters, radiation, bis(chloromethyl)ether, chromates, coke-oven gas, mustard gas, arsenic

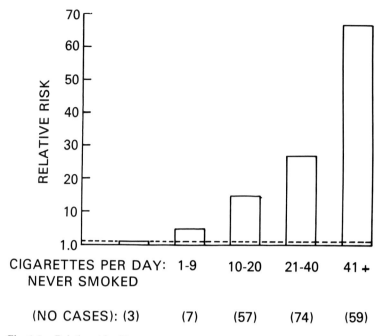

Fig. 1-5. Relative risk of lung cancer correlates with number of cigarettes smoked per day. (Reproduced by permission from Wynder EL, Mabuchi K: Etiological and preventive aspects of human cancer. Prev Med 1:300–334, 1972.)

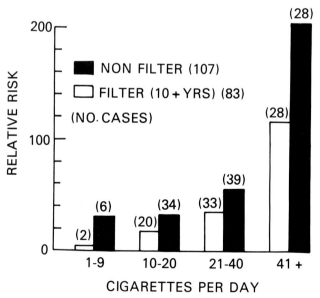

Fig. 1-6. Filter cigarettes appear to be less of a carcinogenic hazard when compared to nonfilter cigarettes. (Reproduced by permission from Wynder EL, Mabuchi K: Etiological and preventive aspects of human cancer. Prev Med 1:300–334, 1972.)

ry diseases of smokers and nonsmokers alike. The list of respiratory carcinogens in both the workplace and the general environment (Table 1-2) is undoubtedly incomplete. One indication of this is a recent epidemiologic study conducted by Hoover and Fraumeni[74] of mortality in United States counties with chemical industries. An increased risk of lung cancer was found to be associated with the manufacturing of industrial gases, pharmaceutical preparations, soaps and detergents, paints, inorganic pigments, and synthetic rubber. Recent preliminary data[75] suggest an increased incidence of lung cancer (particularly adenocarcinoma and large cell carcinoma), as well as liver cancer, in workers exposed to vinyl chloride. The composite risk of cancer in these workers has yet to be determined, since the initial exposure to vinyl chloride in most of the workers was less than 15 years ago, and the latency period for most cancers caused by chemical carcinogens in man is 1 to 4 decades. These preliminary results indicate the urgent need for further investigation into occupational exposure to respiratory carcinogens, and they suggest possible locations to begin such studies.

Exposure to asbestos also increases the risk of lung cancer. A remarkable synergism between asbestos exposure and cigarette smoking has been found.[76] Asbestos workers who smoke cigarettes have an eightfold increased risk of dying of bronchogenic carcinoma as compared with cigarette smokers who do not work with asbestos, and they have 92 times the risk of those who neither smoke cigarettes nor are exposed to asbestos. Asbestos-induced respiratory abnormalities have also been described in members of the families of asbestos workers.[77] Such exposure is believed to occur from asbestos carried on the worker's clothing, as well as from airborne particles when such families reside near asbestos plants. Asbestos has become a common pollutant in our general environment, especially in urban areas, and this asbestos derives from many sources. Recently asbestos has been found in samples of spackling, patching, and jointing compounds purchased in retail stores. Rohl et al.[78] have gone so far as to state that ''measurements suggest that home repair work involving the use of such materials may result in exposure to doses at concentrations sufficient to produce disease.'' Warnock and Churg[79] have recently described an association between the presence of asbestos in the lung and the occurrence of bronchogenic car-

cinoma in an urban population with environmental exposure to asbestos. Only 1 of 30 of these patients with lung cancer had a known occupational exposure to asbestos.

Arsenic is another widespread environmenal contaminant that appears to be a respiratory carcinogen. Urban air and tobacco are contaminated with arsenic. The data suggesting that arsenicals are respiratory carcinogens come primarily from epidemiologic studies of workers exposed to these compounds.[80-84] Lee and Fraumeni[82] reported a threefold increase in the expected incidence of lung cancer among 8000 smelter workers exposed to arsenic trioxide. An eightfold increase was found among workers who were heavily exposed to arsenic and who worked for longer than 15 years in this environment. A positive dose–response relationship between the incidence of lung cancer and exposure to arsenicals during the manufacture of insecticides containing arsenic has also recently been reported;[81] while the influence of other unidentified chemicals and cocarcinogens, especially SO_2, should not be discounted, it would seem likely that arsenic was the principal etiologic agent. This conclusion is supported by other studies showing an increased incidence of lung cancer in other groups of workers exposed to arsenical compounds.[83,84]

Among the most extensively studied occupational groups are the uranium miners of the Colorado plateau. They have an increased risk of lung cancer that is positively related to exposure to radon daughters (e.g., polonium 210) in the mines. Once again, as in the case of asbestos workers, this increased risk was most striking in cigarette smokers. Furthermore, a synergism between tobacco smoke and radon daughters in causing bronchogenic carcinoma (especially oat cell carcinoma) has been demonstrated.[85,86] Radon daughters have also been found in mines other than uranium mines, and it has been suggested that they may in part be responsible for the increased incidence of lung cancer in the miners in Schneeberg and Jachymov, as well as the fluorspar miners of Newfoundland and the hematite miners of England.[87]

Host Determinants in Lung Cancer

Host determinants including genetic factors for human lung cancer are being defined. A familial predisposition to some types of cancer has been found in epidemiologic studies. This predisposition is generally site-specific. First-degree relatives have a greater frequency of cancer of the same site, but not cancers in general.[88] The risk of lung cancer is approximately threefold greater in close relatives of lung cancer patients than in other adults in the general population;[89] in this study the controls were matched by age, sex, residence, and race. The explanation for familial predisposition to lung cancer is complex, and it could be founded in common environment, similar personal habits, and genetic factors. Interaction among environmental and genetic factors responsible for lung cancer is suggested by a study that showed a synergistic increase in risk due to familial predisposition and cigarette smoking.[90]

An association between lung cancer and a number of other diseases (sarcoidosis, scleroderma, and interstitial pulmonary fibrosis) has been noted.[91] A threefold increased risk of lung cancer was found in 2544 patients with sarcoidosis observed over a period of a decade when compared to the general population.[92] The distribution of histologic types of lung cancer was similar to that found in the general population. In contrast, alveolar cell carcinomas were the most common type found in patients with scleroderma (progressive systemic sclerosis),[93] and the risk for developing this malignancy was correlated to the degree of interstitial pulmonary fibrosis. Finally, a rare genetic condition, autosomal-dominant inheritance of interstitial pulmonary fibrosis and abnormal hemoglobin (Malmö), which was described in a Swedish family, may predispose to small cell carcinoma of the lung.[94]

A *homozygous* deficiency of α-antitrypsin (AAT) has been clearly associated with a predisposition for chronic obstructive pulmonary disease (COPD). Individuals with the heterozygous genotype of this condition may also be at greater risk to develop chronic bronchitis and COPD if they smoke cigarettes.[95] A genetic deficiency of AAT could be a predisposing factor to the carcinogenic effects of either tobacco smoke or other respiratory carcinogens. To test this hypothesis, both AAT Pi types and trypsin inhibitory capacity (TIC) were measured in sera from 72 patients with lung cancer and 196 patients with abnormal sputum cytology but no clinical evidence of lung cancer.[96] The distributions of Pi types, which are under genetic control, in these two groups of patients and healthy adults were similar. Thus a genetic deficiency of AAT is probably not a state of increased susceptibility to the carcinogenic effects of respiratory carcinogens such as tobacco smoke.

The susceptibility to bronchogenic carcinoma caused by tobacco smoke could in part be related to an enhanced capability of the host to activate chemical carcinogens. Inducible activity of aryl hydrocarbon hydroxylase, an enzyme that is involved in the activation of polynuclear aromatic hydrocarbons into carcinogenic metabolites, may be increased in the lymphocytes of patients with lung cancer as compared with controls.[97] The inducibility of aryl hydrocarbon hydroxylase in cultured human lymphocytes appears also to be under genetic control,[98] although its exact mode of inheritance is uncertain. Furthermore, it is unknown at present whether levels of aryl hydrocarbon hydroxylase found in the "indicator" cell, the lymphocyte, reflect those found in the target cells, the bronchial epithelium. It is hoped that additional studies in this area will soon clarify the relationship between aryl hydrocarbon hydroxylase levels and cancer susceptibility in man.

PREVENTION

An approach to the prevention of lung cancer is outlined in Table 1-3. Initial efforts are directed at identifying both environmental carcinogens

Table 1-3
An Approach to the Prevention of Lung Cancer

Identification of environmental carcinogens
    Prescreen
        mutagenesis
        in vitro carcinogenesis
    Animal bioassay
    Epidemiology
Identification of individuals at high risk
    Highly susceptible to environmental
        carcinogens
    Exposed to high levels of environmental
        carcinogens
Intervention
    Reduce or eliminate exposure to carcinogens
    Inhibit activation of carcinogens
    Enhance deactivation of carcinogens
    Reverse and/or stabilize preneoplastic lesions

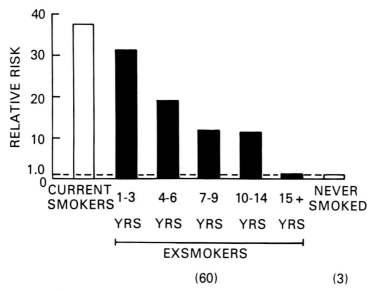

Fig. 1-7. The relative risk of lung cancer in cigarette smokers is compared to the risk in exsmokers. (Reproduced by permission from Wynder EL, Mabuchi K: Etiological and preventive aspects of human cancer. Prev Med 1:300–334, 1972.)

and individuals at high risk, such as (1) those highly susceptible to respiratory carcinogens, (e.g., those individuals in which the balance between metabolic activation and deactivation is tilted toward activation) and/or (2) those exposed to high levels of respiratory carcinogens in their workplaces, in their general environment, and in their personal environments as affected by such habits as tobacco smoking.

Following identification of high-risk individuals, prophylactic intervention could be taken. Reduction or elimination of the respiratory carcinogen is conceptually the simplest form of intervention, but it is often difficult in pragmatic terms. Identification of the subpopulation of individuals highly susceptible to the carcinogenicity of tobacco smoke in the large population of smokers would allow focusing of attention and finite economic resources on this group. Furthermore, within this group of high susceptibility, the knowledge that smoking two packs of cigarettes a day elevates one's lifetime risk of lung cancer nearly 100 percent (instead of current estimates of approximately 10 percent) might be an additional stimulus to heed antismoking efforts. These antismoking efforts need to be based on both an understanding of the hazards of tobacco smoke and a definition of metabolic, physiologic, psychologic, social, and cultural factors that dictate

the response of the smoker. Even if an individual stops smoking completely, it may require 3–4 years before there is an appreciable diminution in risk of lung cancer (Fig. 1-7).[72]

If an individual cannot be persuaded to stop smoking, less harmful ways of smoking can be suggested, and cigarettes with reduced levels of carcinogens could be used. There is already evidence suggesting that filter cigarettes containing lower levels of tar and nicotine are a less carcinogenic hazard than nonfilter cigarettes.[72] Further improvements in cigarette filters are needed. The formulation of a less-hazardous cigarette is an obvious high-priority area for research.

In a select group of highly susceptible individuals, drug therapy could be used to inhibit the activation and/or enhance the deactivation of chemical carcinogens. In experimental systems, prototypes of these drugs may now exist.[56,99] Finally, it may be possible to reverse and/or stabilize preneoplastic lesions before they become malignant.

While lung cancer has a devastating effect on the health of our population, efforts are under way that will eventually reduce its toll. Building on the evidence obtained by epidemiologists and clinicians, experimental oncologists have developed model systems to systems to identify carcinogens as well as to elucidate the mechanisms involved in carcinogenesis. There is promise that high-risk individuals can be identified and that early preneoplastic changes can be recognized and possibly reversed.

Saffiotti[100] has stated that "cancer—in the last quarter of the twentieth century—can be considered as a 'social disease,' a disease whose causation and control are rooted in the technolo-gy and economy of our society. The prevention of cancer is largely an attainable goal, but it requires the coordinated effort of our society in its many components: government, the scientific community, industry, labor and qualified public opinion." Lung cancer appears to be the prime example of this group of societal diseases and one in which prevention is clearly an attainable goal.

REFERENCES

1. Cutler SJ, Scotto J, Devesa SS, et al: Third national cancer survey—an overview of available information. J Natl Cancer Inst. 53:1565–1575, 1974

2. Gori GB, Peters JA: Etiology and prevention of cancer. Prev Med 4:235–246, 1975

3. Burbank F, Fraumeni J: U.S. cancer mortality: Nonwhite predominance. J Natl Cancer Inst 49:649–659, 1972

4. Hodgson T: The economic costs of cancer, in Schottenfeld D (ed): Cancer Epidemiology and Prevention. Springfield, Ill, Charles C Thomas, 1974, p 56

5. Karbe E, Park J (eds): Experimental Lung Cancer, Carcinogenesis and Bioassay, New York, Springer-Verlag, 1974

6. Nettesheim P, Schreiber H: Advances in experimental lung cancer research, in Grundmann E (ed): Handbuch der Allgemeinen Pathologie. Berlin, Springer-Verlag, 1974, pp 603–691

7. Saffiotti U: Experimental respiratory tract carcinogenesis, in Homburger F (ed): Progress in Experimental Tumor Research. Vol. 11. New York, Karger, 1969, pp 302–333

8. Nettesheim P, Hanna M, Deatherage J: Morphology of Experimental Respiratory Carcinogenesis, AEC Series 21. Springfield, Va, US Technical Information Service, 1970

9. Harris C: Cause and prevention of lung cancer. Semin Oncol 1:163–166, 1974

10. Schneiderman MA, Levin DL: Trends in lung cancer mortality, incidence, diagnosis, treatment, smoking, and urbanization. Cancer 30:1320–1325, 1972

11. Wynder EL: Etiology of lung cancer: Reflection on two decades of research. Cancer 30:1332–1339, 1972

12. Heidelberger C: Chemical carcinogenesis. Ann Rev Biochem 44:79–121, 1975

13. Weisburger J: Chemical carcinogenesis, in Holland J, Frei E (eds): Cancer Medicine. Philadelphia, Lea & Febiger, 1973, pp 45–90

14. Ts'o POP, DiPaolo J (eds): Chemical Carcinogenesis. The Biochemistry of Disease, vol. 4. New York, Marcel Dekker, 1974

15. Miller J, Miller E: Some current thresholds of research in chemical carcinogenesis, in Ts'o POP, DiPaolo J (eds): Chemical Carcinogenesis. The Biochemistry of Disease, vol. 4. New York, Marcel Dekker 1974, pp 61–85

16. Farber E: Carcinogenesis—Cellular evolution as a unifying thread: Presidential address. Cancer Res 33:2537–2550, 1973

17. Hoover R, Cole P: Temporal aspects of occupational bladder carcinogenesis. N Engl J Med 288:1040–1043, 1973

18. Saffiotti U, Cefis F, Kolb L: A method for the experimental induction of bronchogenic carcinoma. Cancer Res 28:104–124, 1968

19. Harris CC, Kaufman DG, Sporn MB, et al: Histogenesis of squamous metaplasia and squamous cell carcinomas of the respiratory epithelium in an animal model. Cancer Chemother Rep 4:43–56, 1973

20. Harris CC, Sporn MB, Kaufman DG, et al: Histogenesis of squamous metaplasia in the hamster tracheal epithelium caused by vitamin A deficiency or benzo[a]pyrene–ferric oxide. J Natl Cancer Inst 48:743–761, 1972

21. Harris CC, Kaufman DG, Sporn MB, et al: Ultrastructural effects of N-methyl-N-nitrosourea on the tracheobronchial epithelium of the Syrian golden hamster. Int J Cancer 12:259–269, 1973

22. Auerbach O, Stout A, Hammond E, et al: Changes in bronchial epithelium in relation to lung cancer. N Engl J Med 265:253–259, 1961

23. Schreiber H, Schreiber K, Martin DH: Experimental tumor induction in a circumscribed region of the hamster trachea: Correlation of histology and exfoliative cytology. J Natl Cancer Inst 54:187–197, 1975

24. Kaufman DG, Baker MS, Harris CC, et al: Coordinated biochemical and morphologic examination of hamster tracheal epithelium. J Natl Cancer Inst 49:783–792, 1972

25. Harris CC, Kaufman DG, Sporn MB, et al: Localization of benzo[a]pyrene-3H and alterations in nuclear chromatin caused by benzo[a]pyrene–ferric oxide in the hamster respiratory epithelium. Cancer Res 33:2842–2848, 1973

26. Kaufman DG, Genta VM, Harris CC, et al: Binding of ³H-benzo[a]pyrene to DNA from hamster tracheal epithelial cells. Cancer Res 33:2837–2841, 1973

27. Kaufman D, Genta V, Harris C: Studies on carcinogen binding in vitro in isolated hamster trachea, in Karbe E, Parks J (eds): Experimental Lung Cancer, Carcinogenesis and Bioassay. New York, Springer-Verlag, 1974, pp 564–574

28. Nettesheim P, Williams ML: The influence of vitamin A on the susceptibility of the rat lung to 3-methylcholanthrene. Int J Cancer 17:351–357, 1976

29. Genta VM, Kaufman DG, Harris C, et al: Vitamin A deficiency enhances the binding of benzo[a]pyrene to tracheal epithelial DNA. Nature 247:48–49, 1974

30. Paradise L, Boren H, Wright E, et al: In vivo localization of ³H-benzo[a]pyrene in tracheal epithelium of vitamin A-sufficient and -deficient hamsters: Quantitative autoradiography. Fed Proc 35:567,1976

31. Harris CC, Silverman T, Jackson F, et al: Proliferation of tracheal epithelial cells in normal and vitamin-A-deficient hamsters. J Natl Cancer Inst 51:1059–1062, 1973

32. Kaufman D, Madison R: Synergistic effects of benzo[a]pyrene and N-methyl-N-nitrosourea on respiratory hamsters, in Karbe E, Park J (eds): Experimental Lung Cancer, Carcinogenesis and Bioassay. New York, Springer-Verlag, 1974, pp 207–219

33. Little JB, Kennedy RA, McGandy RB: Lung cancer induced in hamsters by low doses of alpha radiation from polonium 210. Science 188:737–738, 1975

34. McGandy R, Kennedy A, Terzaghi M, et al: Experimental respiratory carcinogenesis: Interaction between alpha radiation and benzo[a]pyrene in the hamster, in Karbe E, Park J (eds): Experimental Lung Cancer, Carcinogenesis and Bioassay. New York, Springer-Verlag, 1974, pp 485–493

35. Kennedy AR, Little JB: Localization of polycyclic hydrocarbon carcinogens in the lung following intratracheal instillation in gelatin solution. Cancer Res 35:1563–1567, 1975

36. Little JB, O'Toole WF: Respiratory tract tumors in hamsters induced by benzo[a]pyrene and ²¹⁰Po radiation. Cancer Res 34:3026–3039, 1974

37. Smith WE, Miller L, Churg J: An experimental model for study of co-carcinogenesis in the respiratory tract, in Nettesheim P, Hanna M, Deatherage J (eds): Morphology of Experimental Respiratory Carcinogenesis. AEC Symposium Series 21, Oak Ridge, Tenn, AEC, 1970, pp 299–316

38. Wagner JC: Mesotheliomas in rats following inoculation of asbestos. Br J Cancer 23:567–581, 1969

39. Laskin S: Sellakumar A: Models in chemical respiratory carcinogenesis, in Karbe E, Park J (eds): Experimental Lung Cancer, Carcinogenesis and Bioassay. New York, Springer-Verlag, 1974, pp 7–19

40. Drew RT, Laskin S, Kuschner M, et al: Inhalation carcinogenicity of alpha halo ether. Arch Environ Health 30:61–72, 1975

41. Figueroa WG, Raszkowski R, Weiss W: Lung cancer in chloromethyl methyl ether workers. N Engl J Med 288:1096–1098, 1973

42. Weiss W, Boucot K: The respiratory effects of chloromethyl methyl ether. JAMA 234:1139–1141, 1975

43. Stanton M, Miller E, Wrench C, et al: Experimental induction of epidermoid carcinoma in the lungs of rats by cigarette smoke condensate. J Natl Cancer Ins 49:867–877, 1972

44. Rabson AS, Branigan WJ, Legallais FY: Lung tumors produced by intratracheal inoculation of polyoma virus in Syrian hamsters. J Natl Cancer Inst 25:937–965, 1960

45. Perk K, Hod I, Presentey B, et al: Lung carcinoma of sheep (jaagsiekte). II. Histogenesis of the tumor. J Natl Cancer Inst 47:197–205, 1971

46. Schreiber H, Nettesheim P, Lijinsky W, et al: Induction of lung cancer in germfree, specific-pathogen-free, and infected rats by N-nitroso-heptamethyleneimine: Enhancement by respiratory infection. J Natl Cancer Inst 49:1107–1114, 1972

47. Lave L, Seskin E: Air pollution and human health. Science 169:723–732, 1970

48. Laskin S, Kuschner M, Drew RT: Studies in pulmonary carcinogenesis, in Hanna MG, Nettesheim P, Gilbert J (eds): Inhalation carcinogenesis. AEC Symposium Series 18, Oak Ridge, Tenn, AEC, 1970, pp 321–352

49. Laskin S, Kuschner M, Sellakumar A, et al: Combined Carcinogen-Irritant Animal Inhalation Studies. OHOLO Biological Conference, Ness Ziona, Israel, 1975

50. Nettesheim P, Creasia D, Mitchell T: Studies on the carcinogenic and cocarcinogenic effects of inhaled synthetic smog and ferric oxide particles. J Natl Cancer Inst 55:159–169, 1975

51. Montesano R, Saffiotti U, Shubik P: The role of topical and systemic factors in experimental respiratory carcinogenesis, in Hanna MG, Nettesheim P, Gilbert J (eds): Inhalation Carcinogenesis. AEC Symposium Series 18, Oak Ridge, Tenn, AEC, 1970, pp 353–375.

52. Saffiotti U, Montesano R, Sellakumar AR, et al: Experimental cancer of the lung. Inhibition by vitamin A of the induction of tracheobronchial squamous metaplasia and squamous cell tumors. Cancer 20:757–864, 1967

53. Cone MV, Nettesheim P: Effects of vitamin A on 3-methylcholanthrene induced squamous meta-

plasia and early tumors in the respiratory tract of rats. J Natl Cancer Inst 50:1599–1606, 1973

54. Hill D, Shen TW: Inhibition of benzo[a]pyrene metabolism catalyzed by mouse and hamster lung microsomes. Cancer Res 35:2717–2723, 1975

55. Nettesheim P, Cone V, Snyder C: The influence of retinyl acetate on the postinitiation phase of lung cancer in rats. Cancer Res 36:996–1002, 1976

56. Sporn MB, Dunlop NM, Newton DL, et al: Prevention of chemical carcinogenesis by vitamin A and its synthetic analogs (retinoids). Fed Proc 35:1332–1338, 1976

57. Bollag W: Prophylaxis of chemically induced epithelial tumors with an aromatic retinoic acid analog (Ro 10-9359). Eur J Cancer 11:721–724, 1975

58. Smith W, Yazdi E, Miller L: Carcinogenesis in pulmonary epithelia in mice on different levels of vitamin A. Environ Res 5:152–163, 1972

59. Smith D, Rogers A, Herndon B, et al: Vitamin A (retinyl acetate) and benzo[a]pyrene induced respiratory tract carcinogenesis in hamsters fed a commercial diet. Cancer Res 35:11–16, 1975

60. Harris C: The carcinogenicity of anticancer drugs: A hazard in man. Cancer 37:1014–1023, 1976

61. Trump B, McDowell E, Barrett L, et al: Studies of ultrastructure, cytochemistry and organ culture of human bronchial epithelium, in Karbe E, Park J (eds): Experimental Lung Cancer, Carcinogenesis and Bioassay. New York, Springer-Verlag, 1974, pp 548–563

62. Barrett L, McDowell E, Frank A, et al: Long-term explant culture of human bronchial epithelium. Cancer Res 36:1003–1010, 1976

63. Trump B, Valigorsky J, Dees J, et al: Cellular change in human disease. A new method of pathological analysis. Hum Pathol 4:89–109, 1974

64. Harris C, Genta V, Frank A, et al: Carcinogenic polynuclear hydrocarbons bind to macromolecules in cultured human bronchi. Nature 252:68–69, 1974

65. Harris C, Frank A, van Haaften C, et al: Binding of ³H-benzo[a]pyrene to DNA in cultured human bronchus. Cancer Res 36:1011–1018, 1976

66. Harris C, Autrup H, van Haaften C: Interindividual variation in benzo[a]pyrene (BP) binding to DNA in cultured human bronchi. Science 193:1067–1069, 1976

67. Vesell E, Passanati G, Greene F, et al: Genetic control of drug levels and of the induction of drug-metabolizing enzymes in man: Individual variability in the extent of allopurinol and nortriptyline inhibition of drug metabolism. Ann NY Acad Sci 179:752–773, 1971

68. Harris C, Autrup H, van Haaften C, et al: Inhibition of benzo[a]pyrene to DNA in cultured human bronchial mucosa, in Nieburgs H (ed):

Proceedings of the 3rd International Symposium on Detection and Prevention of Cancer. New York, Excerpta Medica, 1977

69. Harris C: Chemical carcinogenesis and experimental models using human tissues. Beitr Pathol 158:389–404, 1976

70. U.S. Public Health Service: The health consequences of smoking. A report to the Surgeon General: 1971. Washington, DC, US Department of Health, Education and Welfare, Public Health Service, Publication (HSM) 71-7513, 1972, p 458

71. Harris CC: The epidemiology of different histologic types of bronchogenic carcinoma. Cancer Chemother Rep 4:59–63, 1973

72. Wynder EL, Mabuchi K: Etiological and preventive aspects of human cancer. Prev Med 1:300–334, 1972

73. Wynder EL, Mabuchi K: Lung cancer among cigar and pipe smokers. Prev Med 1:529–542, 1972

74. Hoover R, Fraumeni J: Cancer mortality in the United States counties with chemical industries. Environ Res 9:196–207, 1975

75. Waxweiller R, Stringer W, Falk H, et al: Neoplastic risk among vinyl chloride polymerization. Ann NY Acad Sci 271:40–49, 1976

76. Selikoff I, Hammond E, Churg J: Asbestos exposure, smoking and neoplasia. JAMA 204:106–112, 1968

77. Anderson H, I, Lilis R, Daum S, et al: Household-contact asbestos neoplastic risk. Ann NY Acad Sci 271:311–324, 1976

78. Rohl AN, Langer AM, Selikoff IJ, et al: Exposure to asbestos in the use of consumer spackling, patching, and taping compounds. Science 189:551–553, 1975

79. Warnock M, Churg A: Association of asbestos and bronchogenic carcinoma in a population with low asbestos exposure. Cancer 35:1236–1242, 1975

80. Blot WJ, Fraumeni JF: Arsenical air pollution and lung cancer. Lancet 2:142–143, 1975

81. Ott IG, Holder BB, Gordon HL: Respiratory cancer and occupational exposure to arsenical. Arch Environ Health 29:250–255, 1974

82. Lee AM, Fraumeni JF: Arsenic and respiratory cancer in man: An occupational study. J Natl Cancer Inst 42:1045–1052, 1969

83. Roth F: Bronchial cancer of arsenic-poisoned vintagens. Virchows Arch [Pathol Anat] 331:119–137, 1958

84. Hill A, Faning E: Studies in the incidence of cancer in a factory handling inorganic compounds of arsenic. I. Mortality experience in the factory. Br J Ind Med 5:1–6, 1948

85. Lundin FE, Wagoner JK, Archer G: Radon Daughter Exposure and Respiratory Cancer: Quantitative and Temporal Aspects. Springfield,

Va, US Technical Information Service, US Department of Commerce, 1971

86. Saccomanno G, Archer VE, Auerbach O, et al: Histological types of lung cancer among uranium miners. Cancer 27:515–523, 1971

87. Fraumeni J: Chemicals in the induction of respiratory tract cancer, in: Excerpta Medica International Congress Series 351, vol. 3, Proceedings XI International Cancer Congress, Florence. New York, Excerpta Medica, 1974, pp 327–335

88. Fraumeni J: Genetic factors, in Holland J, Frei E (eds): Cancer Medicine. Philadelphia, Lea & Febiger, 1973, pp 7–15

89. Lynch H: Recent Results in Cancer Research. vol 12. New York, Springer-Verlag, 1967, p 186

90. Tokuhata G, Lilienfeld A: Familial aggregation of lung cancer in humans. J Natl Cancer Inst 30:289–298, 1963

91. Mulvihill JJ: Genetic factors in pulmonary neoplasms, in Schimke RN (ed): Birth Defects, Cancer and Genetics. New York, National Foundation–March of Dimes, 1976, pp 99–111

92. Brincker H, Wilbek E: The incidence of malignant tumours in patients with respiratory sarcoidosis. Br J Cancer 29:247–251,1974

93. Godean P, de Saint-Maur P, Herreman G, et al: Carcinoma bronchiolo-alveolaire et scleroderma. Sem Hop Paris 50:1161–1168, 1974

94. Berglund S: Erythrocytosis associated with haemoglobin Malmö, accompanied by pulmonary changes, occurring in the same family. Scand J Haematol 9:355–369, 1972

95. Lieberman J: Alpha$_1$-antitrypsin deficiency. Med Clin North Am 57:691–714, 1974

96. Harris C, Cohen M, Connor R, et al: Serum alpha$_1$-antitrypsin in patients with lung cancer or abnormal sputum cytology. Cancer 38:1655–1657, 1976

97. Kellermann G, Shaw C, Luyten-Kellermann M: Aryl hydrocarbon hydroxylase inducibility and bronchogenic carcinoma. N Engl J Med 289:934–937, 1973

98. Kellermann G, Luyten-Kellermann M, Shaw C: Genetic variations in human lymphocytes. J Human Genet 25:327–331, 1973

99. Wattenberg LW: Inhibition of carcinogenic and toxic effects of polycyclic hydrocarbons by phenolic antioxidants and ethoryquin. J Natl Cancer Inst 48:1425–1431, 1972

100. Saffiotti U: Prevention of occupational cancer—Toward an integrated program of governmental action: Role of the National Cancer Institute. Ann NY Acad Sci 271:393–395, 1976

101. Silverberg E, Holleb AI: Cancer statistics, 1974—Worldwide epidemiology. CA 24:2–21, 1974

102. Wynder E, Hoffman D: Experimental tobacco carcinogenesis. Science 162:862–871, 1968

Marc J. Straus

2

Growth Characteristics of Lung Cancer

The trend in treatment of lung cancer has been toward the use of more complicated protocols, including adjuvant therapy for early disease, multimodality therapy, and combination chemotherapy. The designs of these new strategems are in part based on some general conceptions of the growth behavior of tumors. For instance, a basis for the use of surgery and adjuvant chemotherapy is that clinically nondetectable foci of tumor remaining after surgery are thought to be more susceptible to chemotherapeutic cell kill, as compared with larger populations of tumor cells. There are some experimental data to support this concept,[1] but clinically there have been conflicting results.[2,3] A clear understanding of the relationship between the cytokinetic growth parameters of the microscopic tumor and the selective effects of various types of drugs in inhibiting or killing tumor cells is needed. There is presently no adequate way to study these relationships in the common solid tumors. It is therefore necessary to develop cytokinetic principles for macroscopic disease and attempt to apply them first to the therapeutic design of treatment for advanced disease, where drug–tumor cell interactions can be tested more easily.

There are a number of features of lung cancer that lend themselves to cytokinetic study. First, it is a common disease usually diagnosed initially by the presence of a lesion on a standard chest x-ray. These lesions can often be measured, and tumor volume growth determinations can be made. Second, the tumor is often directly available for histologic and cytokinetic analysis by fiberoptic bronchoscopy of primary lesions or biopsy of exophytic lesions. Third, with close to 25,000 patients undergoing thoracotomy annually in this country, the potential exists for acquiring sufficient tumor tissue for cytokinetic analysis. In this chapter we will review the cytokinetic parameters that have thus far been studied in human lung cancer and their application to therapeutic designs.

DEFINITIONS OF TUMOR GROWTH

Tumor growth is a dynamic process in which the growth rate of the entire tumor or subpopulations of cells may change as a function of tumor age, size, or other variables. Nevertheless, it may be possible to describe some basic principles of growth that underlie the kinetic behavior of all tumors. The time required for the total population of tumor cells to double in volume is called the doubling time (DT). The cycle that cells undergo from mitosis to mitosis (generation time T_c) is divided into discrete phases: G_1, S (DNA synthetic period), G_2, and M (mitosis), as originally described.[4] The times during which cells traverse the phases of the cycle are designated T_{G1}, T_S, etc., and are classically determined by pulsing the

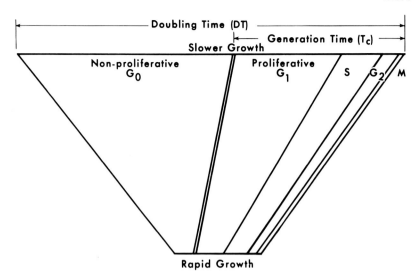

Fig. 2-1. Schematic representation of the relationships of cytokinetic parameters in rapid tumor growth and slower growth.

cells with tritiated thymidine (^{3}H-TdR) and analyzing the cells autoradiographically (ARG).[5]

The relationships of the cytokinetic parameters in rapid tumor growth and slower growth are shown schematically in Fig. 2-1. A certain population of cells is nonproliferative, and some of these cells have the potential to reenter the proliferative cycle. As the tumor grows there is usually slowing of growth. The major increment of cells is in the nonproliferative fraction. The T_c also tends to increase, and of the proliferative cells the proportion of cells in phase G_1 increases the most.

The labeling index (LI) measures the fraction of cells of a population that take up detectable amounts of radioactive label; in Fig. 1 the LI is best described simplistically as T_S/DT.

MEASUREMENTS OF TUMOR GROWTH AND THEIR APPLICATION

In this section we have comprehensively analyzed the English literature on cell kinetic determinations of human lung cancer and their application to therapy. This represents an update of a previous review,[6] with particular emphasis on new in vivo cytokinetic studies.

Doubling Time

In 1956 the classic article[7] by Collins et al. described the use of serial x-ray measurements to determine the DT of metastatic lung lesions in 24 patients (Fig. 2-2). Growth rates in this group of patients ranged from a DT of 11 days to a DT of 164 days (Table 2-1). Collins showed that differences in mean DT for various cell types may exist. He also illustrated clearly that by the time the diagnosis of a lesion is made by x-ray, the majority of the doublings in the life of the tumor have already occurred. Assuming a single cancer cell is 10 μ in diameter, it will take 20 doublings to grow to a nodule 1 mm in diameter. After 10 more doublings a 1-cm nodule containing 10^9 cells and weighing approximately 1 g will be present. These simplified determinations disregard the presence of stroma and other noncancer tissue. Following the report of Collins et al. there have been a number of articles over the years that have been concerned with DT in lung cancer primary and metastatic lesions.[8–29]

The selection process for identifying "measurable lesions" probably varies greatly. Nevertheless, Breur's contention[24] that measurements on a given film are usually reproducible within 1 mm has been true for most studies. Brenner et al.[27] noted an error of 7–10 percent in diameter measurements. Schwartz[11] showed that accurate DT measurements were facilitated by the finding that 50 percent of patients had lesions visible on chest x-rays 2 years earlier. Riegler[20] was able to show that with careful x-ray follow-up a number of patients had peripheral lesions that developed in a central direction. Thus far, accurate DT measurements have depended on establishment of strict criteria by one or more investigators in individual institutions. New standards of DT measurements suitable for application in interinstitutional studies must be developed and tested.

The mathematical formula of Meyer[15] for calculating DT is simple to use: $DT = t \log (\frac{2}{3}\log) (D_t/D_0)$, where t is the time between measurements, D_0 is the diameter at first measurement, and D_t is the diameter at last measurement.

DT distributions were found to be log-normal[9,19,22] for primary or metastatic growths. This distribution was found when metastatic lesions in the lung were evaluated separately on the basis of the organ in which the primary cancer originated (e.g., breast, colorectal). Analyses of our composite data of primary lung cancer (Table 2-2) show that the distribution also occurs when cell types are separated.

Collins et al.[7] and others[8,10,11] demonstrated that during the time interval that measurements were made, growth of lesions was exponential. A few exceptions were reported. Garland et al.[14] noted a decrease in lesion size in 2 of 22 patients and a variation in growth rate in others. Schwartz[11] noted that 4 patients had tumors with slowing growth rates when the tumors were very large. The curve of Welin et al.[30] shows an early lag phase for tumor growth. Of great importance is the demonstration by Breur[25] and Brenner et al.[27] that after reduction in tumor volume with a course of radiation therapy or chemotherapy the growth rate resumed at the initial exponential rate.

The corollary of assuming exponential growth from one cell to death is that the total duration of tumor growth in an individual can be estimated. The duration from one cell to a 2-cm nodule is estimated at 25 years for adenocarcinoma and 8 years for undifferentiated and squamous cell carcinoma.[10,14,15] The similarities in growth times reported by various authors for individual cell types are due to the similarities in mean DTs (Table 2-2).

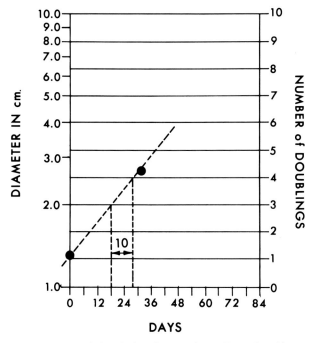

Fig. 2-2. DT of metastatic lung lesions in 24 patients. (Reproduced by permission from Collins VP, Loeffler RK, Tivey H: Observations on growth rates of human tumors. Am J Roentgenol Radium Ther Nucl Med 76:988–1000, 1956.)

Table 2-1
Doubling Times (Days) of Cancer Metastatic to Lung: Primary Tumor*

Author	No. of Patients	Testis No.	Testis Mean	Testis Range	Breast No.	Breast Mean	Breast Range	Colorectal No.	Colorectal Mean	Colorectal Range	Soft Tissue and Osseous No.	Soft Tissue and Osseous Mean	Soft Tissue and Osseous Range	Comments
Collins[7]	24	9	36	11–153	2	56	28–84	4	84	43–123	23	42		Most rapidly growing metastasis is measured
Spratt[9]	118	10	48		29	82		10	109					
Joseph[17]	113	7		13–58	9		11–100	15		11–150	64		5–340	25 cases of osteogenic sarcomas had DTs of 11–360 days
Chahinian[19]	20	2	24	22–26	1	100	100	4	63	42–90	1	40	40	Average DT of 20 cases; was 40 days
Breur[24]	86	9	40	4–205	6	196	23–745	2	94	63–135	16	104	20–212	Fibrosarcoma
											13	50	17–253	Osteosarcoma Mean DT of 7 cases of embryonal carcinoma was 17 days
Brenner[27]	30				4	170	31–335	1	59					9 cases of metastatic hypernephroma had a mean DT of 123 days
Band[28]	15				4	67	38–102				15	42	11–120	8 cases of osteosarcoma, 2 fibrosarcoma, 2 Ewing's sarcoma
Israel[29]	5				4	67	38–102				1	22	22	Osteosarcoma
Total	411	37	39	10–205	59	102	11–745	36	92	11–150	133	58	5–340	Joseph's data[17] are not included in computation of means

*Detailed information is given only for patients with the four primary tumor types indicated. Composite data for various other primaries would be too small for meaningful comparisons.

22

Table 2-2
Doubling Times (Days) of Primary Lung Cancer

Author	No. of Patients	Undifferentiated			Small Cell			Large Cell			Epidermoid			Adenocarcinoma			Comments
		No.	Mean	Range	No.	Mean	Range	No.	Mean	Range	No.	Mean	Range	No.	Mean	Range	
Meyer[8]	22				2	23.5	23–24	2	80	48–112	11	136	42–381	7	184	58–590	Fair correlation of poor survival and rapid DT, or initial lesion > 4.0 cm in diameter
Schwartz[11]	12										10	82	27–200	2	72	17–126	DT ≥ 58 days; no response to treatment
Spratt[9]	34	13	93								13	70		8	118		Unclassified tumors were "undifferentiated"
Spratt[10]	22	9	90								6	93		7	269		
Garland[14]	41	9	124	34–480							22	126	39–333	7	224	28–480	Two tumors were mixed
Weiss[16]	19	2	89	55–123				1	115		8	113	61–204	7	236	146–307	Two tumors were mixed; good correlation between rapid DT and poor survival
Chahinian[19]	30				3	39	17–71				21	95	7–275	3	61	46–74	3 tumors were of unknown histology
Israel[29]	10										8	59	27–110	2	95	55–135	
Total	190	33	100	34–480	5	33	17–71	3	92	48–112	99	100	7–381	43	183	17–590	Mean DT of adenocarcinoma significantly longer (p <0.01) than the mean of each of the other cell types

By the time a tumor is 1 cm in diameter, most doublings in the overall growth of the tumor have already occurred. We have no evidence that growth to 1 cm is exponential or even that growth starts with one cell. Growth characteristics of dysplastic cells and in situ tumors are unknown. We have suggested that in the spontaneous AKR mouse tumor the early growth may include a lag phase.[30] We have also demonstrated in a solid tumor animal model[31] that early tumor growth includes a lag phase, and the total growth curve therefore is not best fit by a Gompertz function.

In human tumors it is clear that in a number of patients the average rate of tumor growth prior to diagnosis is more rapid than the exponential rate measured after diagnosis. In these patients it is seen that if tumor growth from one cell had occurred at the measured exponential rate, the tumor would have had to have started prior to conception of the individual.

There is consistent agreement that the DTs of primary lesions, such as pulmonary,[16-18] colorectal,[9,32] and breast,[33] are substantially lower than the DTs of their respective lung metastases. The reasons for this are speculative, but it is generally noted that in animal tumors (such as AKR) the transplanted tumors grow more rapidly than the spontaneous counterparts. It is unclear whether a relationship exists between the rate of the DT of the primary tumor and the rate of the DT of its metastasis.

DT OF PRIMARY AND METASTATIC LUNG LESIONS

We have compiled DT measurements for 601 patients from the English literature (Tables 2-1 and 2-2). For the 411 patients with metastatic lesions the detailed information for testicular, breast, colorectal, soft tissue, and osseous metastases is further abstracted (Table 2-1). The mean DT of metastases in 37 patients with testicular cancer was 39 days. This is considerably less than the mean value of approximately 100 days for breast and colorectal tumors. There is overlap of DT measurements when the four metastatic tumors are compared (Table 2-1) because the range of DTs is fairly broad for each group.

We have separated primary lung cancer data by cell type (Table 2-2). Although pathologic classifications have changed since 1956 and there has only recently been moderate concurrence by pathologists,[34,35] there is still a trend in the data.

The mean DT of adenocarcinoma (183 days) is significantly longer than those of epidermoid carcinoma (100 days) and undifferentiated carcinoma (100 days). The latter two DTs are longer than the DT of small cell carcinoma (33 days). These data are in close agreement with those reported by Charbit et al.[22] The numbers for small cell carcinoma are scant, but they confirm our clinical impression and support other kinetic data.[36-38]

SYMPTOMS AND PROGNOSIS

An early diagnosis after the onset of clinical illness[11] and/or a brief duration of symptoms prior to diagnosis[33] are associated with more rapidly growing tumors. Chahinian[19] reported that in general the worst symptoms occurred in patients with tumors with more rapid DTs. He noted that tumors with more rapid DTs were smaller than tumors with slower DTs when initially found. It may be that rapid DT tumors present smaller because they are symptomatic sooner. A rationale for earlier symptoms may be the difficulty the body has in instituting adaptive measures to cope with very rapid growth. More rapidly proliferating tumors may metastasize sooner.[11] The implication is clear that patients with more rapidly growing tumors do worse. In cases where the DTs are similar the patients with the larger lesions do worse. It should be possible to develop a prognosis chart that assigns appropriate weightings to the DT and the size of the tumor at diagnosis.

Breur showed that with increasing DT the times from first treatment to death, from first symptom to death, and from first symptom to first treatment increased.[24] Joseph et al.[17] divided patients into three DT categories (Table 2-3). The interval from the primary lesion resection to diagnosis of metastases was 4.8 months for the group with DT ≤ 20 days, and it increased to 29.5 months for the group with DT > 40 days. The 1-year survival in untreated patients in these two groups was 11 and 86 percent, respectively. In treated patients the 1-year survival similarly increased from 28 to 100 percent. In the studies of Weiss et al.[16,18] the growth rate was the best prognostic factor. In Schwartz's study[11] patients with DT > 58 days had no response to therapy. We will discuss the implication of this finding later.

There is good correlation between tumor size at time of diagnosis or resection of a primary lung

Table 2-3

Comparison of Tumor Doubling, Onset of Pulmonary Metastases, and Survival*

DT (days)	No. of Patients	Primary Lesion Resection to Metastases Mean Interval (months)	Solitary Focus to Multiple Foci Mean Interval (months)	Percentage Survival in Untreated Patients			Percentage Survival in Treated Patients		
				Patients	*6 months*	*1 year*	*Patients*	*6 months*	*1 year*
20	71	4.8	3.0	64	63	11	7	86	28
21–40	17	11.1	4.9	11	90	45	6	100	82
40	25	29.5	5.2	14	100	86	11	100	100

*Adapted by permission from Joseph WL, Morton DL, Adkins PC, et al: Prognostic significance of tumor doubling time in evaluating operability in pulmonary metastatic disease. J Thorac Cardiovasc Surg 61:23–32, 1971.

25

lesion and patient survival. In the report of Jackman et al.[12] the 5-year survival rates in patients with resected peripheral bronchogenic carcinoma 2.0 cm in diameter or less, 2.1–3.0 cm, and 3.1–4.0 cm were 68, 46, 41 percent, respectively. In the study of Steele et al.[13] the 4-year survival rates in patients with tumors 2 cm or less, 2.5–4.0 cm, and 4.5–6.0 cm were 53, 41, and 29 percent, respectively. In Meyer's combined study of patients with resected and nonresected tumors there was a similar relationship.[8] These data[8,12,13] are skewed because they are mostly based on resected tumors. Small cell carcinoma, which is rarely resected, has the most rapid DT; it is diagnosed at a smaller size initially and has the poorest prognosis if untreated.

There is a further correlation in primary lung cancer and metastatic tumors to the lung between more rapid DTs and younger age.[9,19,24,33] In these studies the dividing line between younger and older patients varies from 29 years[9] to 59 years.[19] For some studies,[19] however, one factor is the inclusion of metastatic testicular tumors that are rapidly growing in general and tend to occur in younger men.

Summarizing this section, we may say that the DT varies considerably, even within a given cell type, and it may be of more prognostic importance than cell type per se. Something intrinsic to the cell type determines its particular distribution of DTs, but when DTs are matched from different cell types, prognosis does not seem to differ. This point needs further study. The DT independent of tumor size at diagnosis has a marked effect on prognosis. Increased tumor size at diagnosis may independently imply a poor prognosis for selected patients with particular cell types. Age as a prognostic determinant independent of DT is of little value. Whether age for a given cell type influences DT is uncertain. Again, the appropriate correlative studies need to be done.

DT AND RESPONSE TO THERAPY

If diameter measurements are carefully made over a sufficiently long interval, the effects of radiotherapy[25] or chemotherapy[27] on tumor growth may be determined. The effects of radiation therapy simultaneously on two or more lesions have been studied.[25] It may be possible to correlate a reduction in tumor mass with increases in survival rates and response rates to therapy.

Israel et al. have demonstrated a very practical use of DT.[29,39] In patients with measurable lesions who undergo therapy it is often possible to demonstrate a response within a week by examination of careful sequential measurements. Moreover, those patients who respond and then demonstrate a regrowth slope similar to the initial slope are considered to be treatment failures.

Currently on most cancer protocols a progression of disease is defined as a 50 percent diameter square increase in the tumor. Patients may not have therapy altered until this mass increase is reached. Israel's thesis merits further consideration, particularly since it permits alteration of the treatment at a much earlier juncture. Its limitation is that only a small porportion of patients have easily measurable lesions.

BENIGN VERSUS MALIGNANT LESIONS

Another interesting association reported by Nathan et al.[26] related DT to prediction of the presence of benign versus malignant lung lesions. Every lesion (10 of 10) with DTs less than or equal to 7 days and 17 of 18 lesions with DTs greater than 500 days were benign. In patients age 40 years and above with solitary cancer nodules, none had a DT less than 37 days. In all 27 patients with malignant lung lesions under age 40 years the DTs were less than 200 days. Rapid DTs were usually due to pneumonia, pulmonary infarcts, and abscesses. Very slow DTs (> 7 months) were usually seen with granulomas or benign tumors.

DT AND OTHER KINETIC FACTORS

Autoradiographic studies have been performed on tumors of patients that were previously evaluated for DT. There is disagreement whether mitotic indices have any correlation with DTs.[18,24] Malaise et al., in a recent study, pooled data from the literature on labeling indices (LI) in human tumors.[23] The highest LIs were observed in embryonal tumors: 30 percent. The LIs in squamous cell tumors and adenocarcinomas were 8.3 and 2.1 percent, respectively. There was a fair relationship between increasing DT and decreasing LI. There was a high correlation between an increasing rate of cell loss and an increasing LI.

In another study, Breur related the radiosensitivity of human tumors to DT.[25] From DT measurements of 16 patients being treated for pulmonary metastases, he calculated that the D_{37} (the dose of radiation that reduces the population of cells 37 percent of the initial number) extended from 299 rads to 2558 rads. The D_{37} was based on fractionated daily doses of 100–150 rads. Patients, in general, who had embryonal carcinoma had the lowest D_{37}. There was a strong correlation between a low D_{37} and a short DT. High values of D_{37} contradict the small differences found in experiments with cell cultures that generally have a D_{37} between 100 and 200 rads for mammalian cells. Breur calculated that $D_{37} = 220$ rads + 10 DTs. It must be understood that Breur's D_{37} calculations are based on volume changes and may not accurately reflect actual percentages of cells killed, particularly since resorption of dead cells is so variable. Nevertheless, this approach is interesting and may be applicable to the calculation of cell kill. The data[25] also suggest that accurate dose–response calculations in human cancer are possible if kinetic determinations become more sophisticated than DT measurements.

Kinetic Studies

The value of measuring DTs is clear, and yet it is a crude parameter at best. It tells us nothing about rates of proliferation and death of subpopulations of cells and response to treatment of subpopulations. Human studies to ascertain cell cycle times using classic autoradiographic means have been few.[36–38,40–47]

Labeling studies may involve in vivo injection of ^{3}H-TdR, in vitro incubation of cells in ^{3}H-TdR, or intralesional injection of the isotope. The intralesional dose is generally 2–100 μCi ^{3}H-TdR.[45] While this dose is "low," there may be problems with variable diffusion of the isotope. In vitro studies involve no radiation hazard and are easier to do. However, an important consideration is that the cells may be perturbed in an in vitro environment. Some of our results[38] suggest that in vitro data yield lower values in general as compared with in vivo data. More accurate studies make intravenous injection of isotope necessary, and these are cumbersome to perform. These studies require doses of 5–60 mCi for adequate labeling. We have performed extensive radiation dosimetry studies with ^{3}H-TdR in man that support its safety in this experimental setting.[50,51]

LABELING INDEX

The labeling index (LI) has been the most frequently studied kinetic parameter using labeling techniques. Most of the LIs have been taken in skin cancers, particularly melanoma,[48,49] and most of the studies have been performed by in vitro labeling of tumor biopsies.

We have pooled the data on LI in lung cancer (both in vitro and in vivo) by cell type (Table 2-4). The LI of small cell carcinoma is relatively high compared to the LIs of other tumors such as melanoma[48,49] and breast cancer,[52] where many more patients have been studied. No doubt the average LI of all patients with small cell carcinoma would be lower than 10–20 percent; otherwise the DT would probably be less than 10 days. There is perhaps a selection bias in that patients with accessible tumors may have the more rapidly proliferating neoplasms.

Although there are not yet enough lung cancer LI data, in general the LI may be a more

Table 2-4
Kinetic Data in Lung Cancer

Cell Type	Doubling Time		Labeling Index		Cell Cycle Parameters (Hours)			
	(days)	(No. patients)	(%)	(No. patients)	T_c	T_S	G_1	G_2+M
Small cell	33	(5)	12	(1)	64	19	38	7*
			22	(3)				
			15	(17)				
Epidermoid	100	(99)	31	(1)	14	5	5	4†
Adenocarcinoma	183	(43)	33	(1)				
Large cell	92	(3)	10	(1)				
			20	(1)	124	20	98	6‡

*Data from Muggia et al.[37]
†Data from Terz el al.[46]
‡Data from Straus and Moran.[38]

sensitive and prognostically important tool than DT. High LIs more accurately signify a worse prognosis if untreated. Of greater importance may be the use of sequential LIs. In one study where the LI fell after treatment, the patient responded, and a rise in LI was predictive for rapid progression.[49] However, the change in LI that is seen after treatment depends on when the specimen is taken. A drug that is S-phase-specific would be expected to lower LI initially. However, if the tumor is sufficiently reduced in size, recruitment of cells in the S phase may follow, and a subsequent LI may be increased. This phenomenon has been noted in an in vivo study of ovarian tumor treated with ARA-C[42] and in ENT tumors following radiotherapy.[53] Therefore LI studies may necessitate serial samples in a given patient if they are to have optimal prognostic importance.

GROWTH FRACTION

The growth fraction (GF) can be measured by continuous infusion of ^{3}H-TdR in vivo, usually for 2 to 4 days. All proliferative cells then may be labeled. There are some investigators who think that GF is the most important single kinetic parameter, since it is "most highly correlated with growth rate."[23] Nevertheless, GF is usually calculated indirectly based on assumptions for T_S, etc. Some direct measurements have been surprisingly high.[53]

CELL CYCLE DISTRIBUTIONS

Determination of cell cycle distributions requires in vivo ^{3}H-TdR, with serial sampling of the tumor. The current data in solid tumors are very sparse. It is impossible to describe cell cycle distributions accurately based on most of the reported percentage labeled mitosis (PLM) curves.[44,46] There are, however, some data with reasonable PLM curves.[40,43] Since some PLM curves have been derived by sampling several separate tumor sites, a clear curve implies that in these cases there is relative homogeneity of tumor growth from site to site. We have analyzed the variation of tumor growth within single exophytic lesions and from lesion to lesion.[38] Accurate PLM curves require frequent sampling[38,43] and at times several simultaneous samples per time point.

There are only three PLM curves in lung cancer,[37,38,46] two performed by injection of systemic ^{3}H-TdR[38,46] and one performed by intrale-

sional injection[37] (Table 2-4). The curve by Terz has few points, and it has been suggested that a second wave of the curve was missed (Table 2-4). Thus rapid generation time (T_c) of 14 hr is calculated in the patient with epidermoid carcinoma. This is much more rapid than one would expect, and it is likely that the second wave was not missed and the T_c is closer to 40 hr. Muggia's patient with small cell carcinoma was only sampled for 44 hr, so that any estimate of T_c is conjectural (Table 2-4). Nevertheless, it is reasonable to assume from the data that T_c is greater than 48 hr.

We have described the PLM curve of a patient with large cell anaplastic carcinoma of the lung[38] (Fig. 2-3). The separate sites were sampled for 200 hr. Not only was a clear PLM curve obtained, but the cell cycle characteristics of the three sites were similar. The T_c was 124 hr and T_S was 20 hr (Table 2-4). These curves are very similar to previously published well-described curves. The T_S of the 2 melanoma patients described by Shirakawa et al.[43] were 20 and 24 hr. Their T_c were approximately 3 days. In Bresciani's study of 5 patients the T_S ranged from 18 to 34 hr.[40]

It may be that tumors of similar histopathologic types manifest similar PLM curves.[54] In general, leukemias tend to have narrow first waves in the PLM curve, indicating a short T_S ($\approx$ 5–10 hr). Solid tumors have had broader first waves, and T_S has usually been longer ($\approx$ 20 hr). It is conceptually possible that PLM curves will be similar from patient to patient and that LI and DT will differ markedly. In the latter two situations nonproliferative cells are taken into account (Fig. 2-1). In PLM curves only the proliferative cells are analyzed.

The implication is that the greater the homogenicity in cell cycle distribution from patient to patient the greater the likelihood that therapy can be designed effectively for a disease without having to tailor it to the individual patient. Our current studies include analysis of PLM curves in a series of patients with each of the four histopathologic types of lung cancer and the perturbation effects on the cell cycle of various chemotherapeutic agents.

Another important kinetic tool is cytofluorometry, which measures the DNA content distribution of single cell suspensions. This has not yet been applied to human solid tumors. It has great potential in analyzing drug effects.

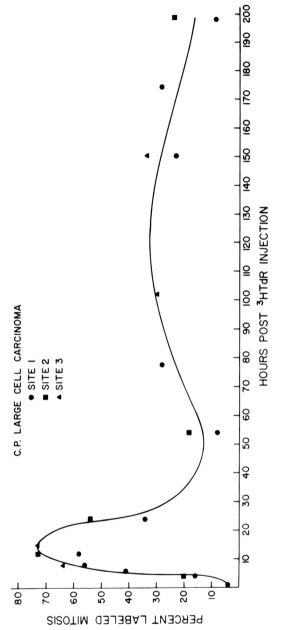

Fig. 2-3. PLM curve of patient with large cell anaplastic carcinoma of the lung.

PROTOCOLS BASED ON CELL KINETICS

There have been few protocols clinically that have attempted to design treatment schedules based on cell kinetic considerations. One is constrained first to do phase I and II clinical studies in order to determine which drugs have clinical effects in a particular tumor. Generally one then combines two or more of the most effective drugs, usually with different mechanisms of actions.

In lung cancer the most responsive tumor is the most rapidly proliferating: small cell carcinoma. Many agents can induce a response. The challenge is to provide optimal therapy with known modalities. We designed a protocol in which patients with extensive disease were treated with Cytoxan and methotrexate (see Chapter 15). The Cytoxan was given every 3 weeks. Eight days after beginning Cytoxan, methotrexate was begun. This was based on data that indicated a rise in LI 8 days following Cytoxan.[56,57] Doses were modified further so as to achieve high levels of drug with acceptable toxicity. Thus far, of 11 patients with small cell carcinoma, 10 have responded (7 completely); 5 of 7 patients with large cell carcinoma, 5 of 8 with adenocarcinoma,

and 0 of 2 with epidermoid carcinoma responded, with a median survival time of about 1 year. This represents a substantial increase in survival, but the role that cell kinetics rationale has played is hypothetical.

The applications of cell kinetics are in their infancy. In the meantime, with our present information, it is sometimes possible to plan more sensible therapeutic approaches. We know, for instance, that in certain cell types individual drugs have demonstrated therapeutic effectiveness. There are also experiments that have demonstrated the importance of dose size and interval between doses for a given drug.[58] Further, the sequence in which combinations of therapy are given is crucial.[59,60] In some patients with very long DT it might be reasonable to withhold treatment if the cell type is generally refractory to treatment. Of it may be possible to switch therapy before progression has occurred by the usual criteria. In patients with high LI, aggressive therapy with "shorter courses" seems warranted. No change in LI over 2 weeks suggests that one should rapidly change to alternative therapy.

The better the cell kinetics data we collect the more likely it is that we can learn how to use them. There seems little likelihood that an empirical approach to lung cancer treatment will provide substantial successes.

REFERENCES

1. Straus MJ, Sege V, Choi SC: The effect of surgery and pretreatment or posttreatment adjuvant chemotherapy on primary tumor growth in an animal model. J Surg Oncol 7:497–512, 1975
2. Brunner KW, Marthaler TH, Muller W: Unfavorable effects of long term adjuvant chemotherapy with endoxan in radically operated bronchogenic carcinoma. Eur J Cancer 7:285–294, 1971
3. Fisher B, Carbone P, Economou SG, et al: L-phenylalanine mustard (L-PAM) in the management of primary breast cancer. N Engl J Med 292:117–122, 1975
4. Howard A, Pelc SR: Synthesis of deoxyribonucleic acid in normal and irradiated cells and its relation to chromosome breakage. Heredity (Lond) [Suppl] 6:261–273, 1953
5. Quastler H, Sherman FG: Cell population kinetics in the intestinal epithelium of the mouse. Exp Cell Res 17:420–438, 1959

6. Straus MJ: The growth characteristics of lung cancer and its application to treatment design. Semin Oncol 1:167–174, 1974
7. Collins VP, Loeffler RK, Tivey H: Observations on growth rates of human tumors. Am J Roentgenol Radium Ther Nucl Med 76:988–1000, 1956
8. Meyer JA: Growth rate versus prognosis in resected primary bronchogenic carcinomas. Cancer 31:1468–1472, 1973
9. Spratt JS Jr, Spratt TL: Rates of growth of pulmonary metastases and host survival. Ann Surg 159:161–171, 1964
10. Spratt JS Jr, Spjut HJ, Roper CL: The frequency distribution of the rates of growth and the estimated duration of primary pulmonary carcinomas. Cancer 16:687–693, 1963
11. Schwartz M: A biomathematical approach to clinical tumor growth. Cancer 14:1272–1294, 1961
12. Jackman FJ, Good CA, Clagett OT, et al: Survival

rates in peripheral bronchogenic carcinomas up to four centimeters in diameter presenting as solitary pulmonary nodules. J Thorac Cardiovasc Surg 57:1–8, 1969

13. Steele JD, Kleitsch WP, Dunn JE Jr, et al: Survival in males with bronchogenic carcinomas resected as asymptomatic solitary pulmonary nodules. Ann Thorac Surg 2:368–376, 1966

14. Garland LH, Coulson W, Wollin E: The rate of growth and apparent duration of untreated primary bronchial carcinoma. Cancer 16:694–707, 1963

15. Meyer JA: The concept and significance of growth rates in human pulmonary tumors. Ann Thorac Surg 14:309–322, 1972

16. Weiss W, Boucot KR, Cooper DA: Growth rate in the detection and prognosis of bronchogenic carcinoma. JAMA 198:1246–1252, 1966

17. Joseph WL, Morton DL, Adkins PC, et al: Prognostic significance of tumor doubling time in evaluating operability in pulmonary metastatic disease. J Thorac Cardiovasc Surg 61:23–32, 1971

18. Weiss W, Boucot KR, Cooper DA: Survival of men with peripheral lung cancer in relation to histologic characteristics and growth rate. Am Rev Respir Dis 98:75–86, 1968

19. Chahinian P: Relationship between tumor doubling time and anatomoclinical features in 50 measurable pulmonary cancers. Chest 61:340–345, 1972

20. Riegler LG: A roentgen study of the evolution of carcinoma of the lung. J Thorac Cardiovasc Surg 34:283–297, 1957

21. Dawson JM, Hall TC, Schneiderman MA, et al: Objective evaluation of change in tumor size in lung cancer patients with nonmeasurable disease. Cancer 19:415–420, 1966

22. Charbit A, Malaise EP, Tubiana M: Relation between the pathological nature and the growth rate of human tumors. Eur J Cancer 7:307–315, 1971

23. Malaise EP, Chavaudra N, Tubiana M: The relationship between growth rate, labelling index and histological type of human solid tumors. Eur J Cancer 9:305–312, 1973

24. Breur K: Growth rate and radiosensitivity of human tumors. I. Growth rate of human tumors. Eur J Cancer 2:157–171, 1966

25. Breur K: Growth rate and radiosensitivity of human tumors. II. Radiosensitivity of human tumors. Eur J Cancer 2:173–188, 1966

26. Nathan MH, Collins VP, Adams RA: Differentiation of benign and malignant pulmonary nodules by growth rate. Radiology 79:221–231, 1962

27. Brenner MW, Holsti LR, Perttala Y: The study by graphical analysis of the growth of human tumors and metastases of the lung. Br J Cancer 22:1–13, 1967

28. Band PR, Kocandrle C: Growth rate of pulmonary metastases in human sarcomas. Cancer 36:471–474, 1975

29. Israel L, Chahinian P, Accard JL, et al: Growth curve modification of measurable tumors by 75 mg/m² of CCNU every 3 weeks. Eur J Cancer 9:789–797, 1973

30. Straus MJ, Choi SC, Goldin A: Increased lifespan in AKR leukemia mice treated with prophylactic chemotherapy. Cancer Res 33:1724–1728, 1973

31. Straus MJ, Shackney S: Comparative analysis of methods of measuring tumor growth using the Ca755 mouse carcinoma. (in preparation)

32. Welin S, Youker J, Spratt JS, et al: The rates and patterns of growth of 375 tumors of the large intestine and rectum observed serially by double contrast enema study (Malmö technique). Am J Roentgenol Radium Ther Nucl Med 90:673–687, 1963

33. Kusama S, Spratt JS Jr, Donegan WL, et al: The gross rates of growth of human mammary carcinoma. Cancer 30:594–599, 1972

34. Yesner R: Observer variability and reliability in lung cancer diagnosis. Cancer Chemother Rep [Part 3] 4:55–58, 1973

35. Matthews MJ: Morphology of lung cancer. Semin Oncol 1:175–182, 1974

36. Muggia FM, DeVita VT: In vivo tumor cell kinetic studies: Use of local thymidine injection followed by fine-needle aspiration. J Lab Clin Med 80:297–301. 1972

37. Muggia FM, Krezoski SK, Hansen HH: Cell kinetics studies in patients with small cell carcinoma of the lung. Cancer 34:1683–1690, 1974

38. Straus MJ, Moran RE: Cell cycle parameters in human solid tumors. Cancer (in press)

39. Israel L, Chahinian P: Evaluation of the survival gain in 22 measurable lung tumors treated with chemotherapy. An approach towards quantitative evaluation of cancer treatments in man. Eur J Cancer 5:631, 1969

40. Bresciani F, Paoluzi R, Benassi M, et al: Cell kinetics and growth of squamous cell carcinomas in man. Cancer 33:28–37, 1974

41. Bennington JL: Cellular kinetics of invasive squamous carcinoma of the human cervix. Cancer Res 29:1082–1088, 1969

42. Clarkson B, Ota K, Ohkita T, et al: Kinetics of proliferation of cancer cells in neoplastic effusions in man. Cancer 18:1189–1213, 1965

43. Shirakawa S, Luce JK, Tannock I, et al: Cell proliferation in human melanoma. J Clin Invest 49:1188–1199, 1970

44. Friedman M, Nervi C, Casale C, et al: Significance of growth rates, cell kinetics, and histology in the irradiation and chemotherapy of squamous cell carcinoma of the mouth. Cancer 31:10–16, 1973

45. Young RC, DeVita VT: Cell cycle characteristics of human solid tumors in vivo. Cell Tissue Kinet 3:285–290, 1970

46. Terz JJ, Curutchet HP, Lawrence W Jr: Analysis of the cell kinetics of human solid tumors. Cancer 28:1100–1110, 1971

47. Frindel E, Malaise E, Tubiana M: Cell proliferation kinetics in five human solid tumors. Cancer 22:611–620, 1968

48. Livingston RB, Ambus U, George SL, et al: In vitro determination of thymidine-^{3}H labeling index in human solid tumors. Cancer Res 34:1376–1380, 1974

49. Murphy WK, Livingston RB, Ruiz VG, et al: Serial labeling index determination as a predictor of response in human solid tumors. Cancer Res 35:1438–1444, 1975

50. Straus MJ, Tehada F, Krezoski S: Systemic tritiated thymidine for cell cycle analysis in human solid tumors, in Proceedings XI International Cancer Congress, Florence. New York, Excerpta Medica, 1974 (abstract)

51. Straus MJ, Straus SE, Battiste L, et al: The uptake excretion and radiation hazards of tritiated thymidine in humans. Cancer Res 37:610–618, 1977

52. Silvestrini R, Sanfilippo O, Tedesco G: Kinetics of human mammary carcinomas and their correlation with the cancer and the host characteristics. Cancer 34:1252–1258, 1974

53. Tubiana M, Richard JM, Malaise E: Kinetics of tumor growth and of cell proliferation in U.R.D.T. cancers: Therapeutic implications. Larynogoscope 85:1039–1052, 1975

54. Shackney SE: A cytokinetic model for heterogeneous mammalian cell population. II. Tritiated thymidine studies: The percent labeled mitosis (PLM) curve. J Theor Biol 44:49–90, 1974

55. Straus MJ: Combination chemotherapy in advanced lung cancer with increased survival. Cancer 38:2232–2242, 1976

56. Nordenskjold B, Zetterberg A, Lowhagen T: Measurement of DNA synthesis by ^{3}H-thymidine incorporation into needle aspiration from human tumors. Acta Cytol 18:215–221, 1974

57. Straus MJ: unpublished observations

58. Straus MJ, Mantel N, Goldin A: Effects of priming dose schedules in methotrexate treatment of mouse leukemia L1210. Cancer Res 31:1429–1433, 1971

59. Straus MJ, Mantel N, Goldin A: The effect of the sequence of administration of Cytoxan and methotrexate on the life-span of L1210 leukemic mice. Cancer Res 32:200–297, 1972

60. Vietti T, Eggerding F, Valeriote F: Combined effect of X radiation and 5-fluorouracil on survival of transplanted leukemic cells. J Natl Cancer Inst 47:865–870, 1971

Aron Primack
Lawrence E. Broder
Robert B. Diasio

3

Production of Markers by Bronchogenic Carcinoma: A Review

Many biologic products have been found to be produced by malignancies or in association with malignant disease. These products fall into several main categories: hormones, antigens, enzymes, fetal proteins, and others. These compounds have been termed marker substances, and they mark the existence, progression, or regression of certain types of cancer. Such compounds may be of significance to the researcher in developing theories about the biology of cancer and to the clinician in the diagnosis and localization of the carcinoma, as well as in evaluation of the effects of various therapeutic modalities.

The following is not only a compilation of personal data but also a review of the literature concerning those marker substances that have been found present in patients with bronchogenic carcinoma. Wherever possible, the microscopic type of lung cancer responsible for production of the individual markers will be noted, using the classification of the World Health Organization.[1] This review is divided into three sections: ectopic hormone production, fetal proteins, and other

compounds. Some of the syndromes of neuro-muscular origin[2] associated with lung cancer are discussed elsewhere in this book.

HORMONE PRODUCTION

The phenomenon of hormone production by nonendocrine tumors has been recognized for nearly 50 years. The general aspects of ectopic hormone production have previously been reviewed.[3-16]

As a specific class of marker substances, ectopic hormones occupy a unique position both clinically and theoretically. The physician caring for the cancer patient is often alerted to the presence of an endocrine marker by abnormal physical findings (e.g., Cushingoid features, increased skin pigmentation) or abnormalities in routine laboratory studies (e.g., hypokalemic alkalosis, hypercalcemia, hyponatremia), in contrast to the situation with the other classes of tumor markers (such as enzymatic markers), which are much more frequently clinically silent. Furthermore, the physican may be faced with metabolic derangements secondary to the ectopically secreted hormones that demand immediate attention (a situation not typical of the other classes of markers).[3] From a theoretical point of view, the

The authors acknowledge the assistance of Mr. Jeffrey Lee and Ms. Elaine Bild, both of whom were helpful in assisting with the research. The authors also wish to thank Ms. Susan Jones for her help in editing and typing the manuscript.

study of ectopic hormones is of immense interest in regard to an understanding of tissue dedifferentiation, as well as the basic biology of tumors.

In order for hormone production to qualify as being ectopic in its origin from an otherwise nonendocrine tumor, at least one of the following criteria must be met: (1) demonstration of hormone production by tumor cells in vitro; (2) demonstration of an arteriovenous gradient across the tumor, with the hormone concentration being higher in the venous than in the arterial blood; (3) demonstration of reduction of hormone level with surgical removal of the tumor, with increased levels reappearing when there is documented recurrence of tumor.

Of the many tumors that have been shown to produce hormones ectopically, bronchogenic carcinoma holds a special place. It has been estimated that perhaps as many as 10 percent of all such tumors produce ectopic hormones,[3] and with the development of newer, more sensitive assays the figure may be found to be even higher. Furthermore, many lung carcinomas have been shown to produce multiple hormones. As will be shown subsequently, almost all the major hormones (particularly peptide hormones) have been identified as being produced by lung carcinoma. The only major hormones not yet demonstrated to be ectopically produced by lung tumors are thyrotropin, secretin, and cholecystokinin. Table 3-1 lists the hormones that have been found to be ectopically produced by bronchogenic carcinoma, with a summary of production by cell type.

Adrenocorticotropic Hormone

One of the ectopic hormones most frequently observed in association with bronchogenic carcinoma is that associated with adrenocorticotropin production. With the development of a radioimmunoassay for corticotropic hormone (ACTH),[17] increasing numbers of patients with this syndrome have been described. This hormone is most frequently noted in patients with the small cell variant of bronchogenic carcinoma.

Elevated rates of cortisol production have been reported in patients with carcinoma of the lung;[18] but response to dexamethasone suppression has led to the conclusion that there is increased ACTH production by the normal mechanism and that there is no ectopic production in these patients. Therefore increased ACTH levels alone are not indicative of ectopic production.

Belsky and Marks[19] noted an exaggerated plasma corticoid response to ACTH in 33 percent of lung cancer patients and in 29 percent of ill noncancerous control patients. These investigators also found stored ACTH in the pituitaries in higher amounts in patients with adrenal hyperplasia. They concluded that these findings may indicate general illness, not necessarily carcinoma. Kawai and Tamura[20] reported 23 patients with lung cancer in whom 14 exhibited one or more abnormalities of adrenocortical function. Elevated levels of ACTH associated with bronchogenic carcinoma have been demonstrated to decrease with removal of the tumor. ACTH has been identified within lung tumor specimens, and its presence has been explained by either increased binding (trapping) or ectopic production.[21]

In 14 cases of documented small cell carcinoma elevated levels of serotonin, as well as ACTH, were found in the tumor tissue.[22,23] Studies conducted at the NCI-VA Oncology Branch also indicate that serotonin may occasionally be elevated in patients with bronchogenic carcinoma.* In other cases small cell carcinomas producing ACTH have been reported in studies using electron microscopy.[22,24] Neurosecretory-type granules are seen in these tumors. There is the possibility that the cell of origin of small cell carcinoma and carcinoid is the same, i.e., the argentaffine Kulchitsky cell,[25]

Specific study of the 17-ketosteroids in 3 patients with ACTH-producing small cell carcinomas[26] showed a specific pattern of production. Further enzyme studies will be needed to determine if there is one pattern that is more often seen that could add to the usefulness of steroid production as a marker.

The clinical differences between ectopic ACTH and Cushing's syndrome have been adequately described, and a summary will suffice here. In the ectopic syndrome, males are affected more commonly than females, and on the average the patients are older than those with Cushing's syndrome. In patients with ectopic ACTH production the clinical course of the endocrine syndrome is often rapid. The electrolytic disturbance of hypokalemic alkalosis is much more common than in Cushing's disease. In our experience the

---

*Broder, L. E., personal communication, 1976.

Table 3-1
Number of Reported Patients with Ectopic Hormone Production in Bronchogenic Carcinoma by Cell Type

Hormone	Histologic Cell Type						Reference Numbers
	Epidermoid	Small Cell	Adeno-carcinoma	Large Cell Anaplastic	"Undifferentiated"	Not Specified	
ACTH	8	75	3		3	56	19,21–24,26,32,33,94,149–172
hCG	3	1	2	5		4	37,52,173–176
hGH		2	5	4			59–64
MSH		13					32–35,168
PTH	9	1				29	65,68,71,72,76–81
ADH	1	9		1	2	10	69,92,93,96,98,111,113,176–184
Prolactin					1		113
Insulin					1		119
Glucagon					1		119
Serotonin		14					23,33,58,114
hPL	1	1		2	1		56,67
Calcitonin	1	24	3				84,86–89
Estradiol	1		3				115
Renin		1					118
Erythropoietin				1		4	120–122

presence of the syndrome portends a poor prognosis.

Laboratory evidence for ectopic production of ACTH includes elevated serum and urinary hydroxysteroid and ketosteroid levels. The serum levels of ACTH are higher than in Cushing's syndrome, and ectopic production is not suppressed even with high-dose dexamethasone. As with Cushing's syndrome, there may be a hyperresponsiveness of the adrenal glands to an ACTH stimulation test. Multiple endocrine syndromes, including excess ACTH, MSH, and PTH or ADH in bronchogenic carcinoma patients, have been reported.[3]

The recent discovery of the existence of a precursor form of ACTH, called "big ACTH," promises to have a major impact on the study of ectopic hormones. This compound appears to be a larger molecule than ACTH, and it lacks significant bioactivity.[27] There is evidence that trypsin degradation of "big ACTH" releases a hormone with ACTH-like activity on starch gel electrophoresis that is further trypsin-degraded at the same rate as ACTH.[28] "Big ACTH" has been identified in all four major cell types of lung cancer.[28-31] Studies performed thus far suggest that the incidence of elevated levels of "big ACTH" in lung cancer may approach 90 percent.[29,31] Unfortunately this compound is present in many nonneoplastic conditions involving the lung, although the values tend not to be as high.[29] Additional studies are needed.

Other recent developments include the finding of corticotropin-releasing-factor-like activity in a patient with small cell carcinoma of the lung.[30]

Melanocyte-Stimulating Hormone

Thirteen patients with ectopic melanocyte-stimulating hormone (MSH) production have been reported.[32-35] All were patients with small cell carcinoma, and many showed measurable levels of ACTH. MSH itself is identical with a portion of ACTH, and thus the activity measured may indicate ACTH. However, a separation of MSH and ACTH has been accomplished, and the MSH/ACTH ratio was > 1 in the 7 patients in one report.[34] Shapiro and Nicholson[35] showed differences between MSH from a patient with oat cell carcinoma of the lung and MSH of normal pituitary origin.

Human Chorionic Gonadotropin

The association between pulmonary neoplasms and gynecomastia was reported as early as 1915.[36] Recently a number of reports have appeared describing production of hCG by all cell types, predominantly the anaplastic large cell type. Faiman and Colwell[37] reported finding an arteriovenous gradient across the tumor, thus proving true ectopic production. hCG has been found in the serum of approximately 7–10 percent of patients with bronchogenic carcinoma.[38-40]

Glycoprotein-tropic hormones have been shown to be composed of two subunits. The nonspecific α subunit is common to all, but the β subunit is specific for each separate hormone.[41-44] Tashjian and Weintraub[45] have recently shown unbalanced synthesis of these subunits. Weintraub and Rosen[46] and Vaitukaitis[47] have reported isolated subunit production in patients with bronchogenic carcinoma. Specific immunoassay may lead to an increase in the number of biologic markers that can be found.[48]

Multiple hormone production has been described in 1 patient, a 45-year-old man with large cell anaplastic bronchogenic carcinoma: hCG, human placental lactogen (hPL), estrogens, and placental alkaline phosphatase (PAP).[49] This tumor is now being grown in cell culture,[50] and it continues to produce these markers in vitro. Studies are now being performed to determine its specific growth and hormone characteristics and their relationships to its environment and to drugs.[51]

The interest in hCG as a tumor marker is heightened by the fact that no hCG is normally seen in males or nonpregnant females. Therefore any hCG found in this patient population is significant. Furthermore, it may be a very early sign, as exemplified by Rosen's finding of hCG production in a patient with gynecomastia who 13 months later developed clinically overt epidermoid carcinoma of the lung.[52]

Gynecomastia may not necessarily be only related to hCG, as evidenced by the work of Posternak,[53] who reported 100 patients with biopsy-proven bronchogenic carcinoma encompassing all cell types. Of these, 6 patients were found to have true gynecomastia, but none showed abnormal excretion of gonadotropins. It is speculative but interesting to wonder if any of these patients represented unbalanced synthesis.

Gynecomastia has been found in malnutrition per se.[54] Further clinical correlations are needed to determine if there are, indeed, any clinical signs of the low levels of ectopic hCG found in these patients.

To determine whether the hCG found in patients with bronchogenic carcinoma is ectopically produced or is in fact an indication of trophoblastic transformation of aberrancy, Beck and Porteous[55] studied three large cell anaplastic tumors that were associated with hCG production. The absence of the immunologically reactive growth hormone that is normally expected in placental tissue indicated that the hCG was ectopically produced.

Human Placental Lactogen

Human placental lactogen (hPL) (chorionic somatomammotropin) has been described in the serum of 5 patients with bronchogenic carcinoma.[56-58] In a series of 200 lung cancer patients studied by Weintraub et al.* hPL was present in 1.5 percent. This indicates a specific marker of nontrophoblastic origin in patients with lung cancer, since this hormone is not normally present at any level in men or nonpregnant women. Recently a discordance of the three markers hPL, hCG, and placental alkaline phosphatase (PAP) has been reported.[56] The use of multiple assays will undoubtedly increase the number of cancer patients showng at least one significant tumor marker.

Human Growth Hormone

Elevated serum human growth hormone (hGH) levels have been seen in patients with small cell carcinoma, adenocarcinoma, and large cell anaplastic carcinoma of the lung.[59-64] Production of hGH by a large cell anaplastic carcinoma in tissue culture has been reported,[62] thus proving true ectopic production. Several patients with hypertrophic osteoarthropathy accompanying bronchogenic carcinoma have been studied, but elevated serum hGH levels have not been found.[61-64]

*Weintraub, B., Rosen, S. W., Broder, L. E., Muggia, F. M., and Primack, A., manuscript in preparation.

Parathyroid Hormone

There have been numerous reports of hypercalcemia in patients with bronchogenic carcinoma without apparent bone involvement.[65-68] The serum of these patients often shows a biochemical pattern typical of hyperparathyroidism, with elevated calcium and low phosphorus indicative of possible ectopic production of parathyroid hormone (PTH).[69,70] These changes have reverted to normal in patients after treatment.[71] Incidence studies suggest that 6–16 percent of patients with bronchogenic carcinoma (cell types not specified) have hypercalcemia without evidence of bone involvement.[71,72]

With the recent development of radioimmunoassay techniques it has become possible to measure small quantities of immunologically similar compounds.[73-75] A specific difficulty at the present time is the lack of human PTH for study; therefore serum PTH values are now determined by using an antibody directed against animal PTH. Using this technique, PTH-like material has been found most often in patients with epidermoid carcinoma.[65,76-81] This is in agreement with our own clinical observations, where hypercalcemia without autopsy evidence of osseous metastases is a hallmark of epidermoid carcinoma. Conversely, hypercalcemia is uncommon in patients with small cell carcinoma, despite the high incidence of bone metastases associated with this cell type.

Recently some immunologic differences have been noted between ectopic PTH and naturally occurring PTH.[82] This may reflect a true difference; it may indicate a pro-PTH, as has been seen with other hormones; or it may reflect technical problems with the radioimmunoassay.

More studies will be needed to define the cause of hypercalcemia in patients with cancer. For example, a recent paper has indicated that there may be a role for prostaglandins as mediators of hypercalcemia in patients with bronchogenic carcinoma.[83] Further refinements in the diagnosis of bone involvement as well as the determination of PTH will aid our understanding of the hypercalcemia in bronchogenic carcinoma.

Calcitonin

Since the first report demonstrating ectopically produced calcitonin from a small cell carcinoma a few years ago,[84] there have followed several additional reports, with currently 28 cases in the literature.[85-90] Most of these have been in patients with small cell carcinoma. That these tumors are indeed producing calcitonin is supported by the demonstration of elevated levels in the venous effluent from the tumor, while peripheral venous levels and thyroid venous samples are lower. Furthermore, calcitonin levels have been shown to fall with objective tumor response to chemotherapy.[85,91]

Antidiuretic Hormone

Winkler and Crankshaw[92] observed hypochloremia in a patient with carcinoma of the lung in 1938. Schwartz and Bennett[93] reported two cases of bronchogenic carcinoma presenting with hyponatremia and inappropriate urinary sodium loss and hypertonic urine. It was postulated that there was sustained, inappropriate secretion of antidiuretic hormone (ADH) (SIADH) in these subjects. Since that report several patients who apparently have this syndrome have been studied.[69,94-98] Ivy[99] reviewed this syndrome and reported a 59-year-old man with SIADH who presented with neurologic signs 3 months prior to discovery of an undifferentiated small cell bronchogenic carcinoma. Other reviews have also appeared.[100-102]

The syndrome of SIADH consists of hyponatremia, a urine hypertonic to serum, and normal renal and adrenal function. ADH has been shown in man to be synonymous with arginine vasopressin.[103] The serum levels of arginine vasopressin have usually been shown to be normal, but they do not react normally in response to hydration.[104] There are several possible explanations for this syndrome. The identification of ADH in the tumor tissue lends credence to the view that this hormone is produced ectopically by the tumor. In vitro production of the hormone vasopressin has been reported, further substantiating ectopic production.[105] Care must be taken in labeling ADH as ectopic in origin, since thoracic–CNS connection or metastases to the CNS may also cause inappropriate secretion of ADH. Olson et al.[106] reported a patient with adenocarcinoma of the bronchus that had metastasized to the hypothalamus and invaded the neurohypophyseal tract. They postulated that "the strategic location of the tumor was responsible for the SIADH."

Several cases have shown ADH in significant quantities in tumor tissues.[96,107,108] This may represent production or trapping. Dutaw and Delson[96] reported three new cases of SIADH and summarized the results of others. The histologic cell type in 87 percent of the cases of patients was undifferentiated small cell carcinoma; the cell type was adenocarcinoma in 8 percent and epidermoid carcinoma in only 5 percent.

In addition, Rees et al.[109] and Daly et al.[110] each described a patient with oat cell bronchogenic carcinoma who developed a renal tubular defect to explain the hyponatremia associated with aminoaciduria and increased phosphate excretion. The SIADH syndrome has been described with infection (including tuberculosis and cerebrovascular disease) and with drugs (notably chlorpropamide, cyclophosphamide, and vincristine). Therefore many other conditions must be ruled out before ascribing the etiology of this condition to the neoplasm itself.

In addition to ADH, the neurophysins (the group of polypeptides that act as binding proteins for the hormones vasopressin and oxytocin) have been isolated from bronchogenic carcinoma tissue.[111,112]

Prolactin

Turkington[113] reported serum levels of prolactin in a patient with undifferentiated bronchogenic carcinoma. Prolactin levels in the tissue were not studied. The sera of 20 other patients with bronchogenic carcinoma were screened for prolactin activity, but none was detected.

5-Hydroxytryptophan

The carcinoid syndrome has been described in patients with small cell bronchogenic carcinoma.[58,114] Bronchial adenomas are deliberately omitted from this review. Serotonin has been found in 14 cases of small cell carcinoma, and electron microscopic study has been done.[114] We have studied serotonin levels in 49 lung cancer patients and have found slight elevations of serotonin in about 25 percent in all cell types.* There has been much speculation as to the similarities and differences of small cell bronchogenic carcinoma and carcinoid tumors.[25]

*Broder, L. E., personal communication, 1976.

Estradiol

Kirschner and Cohen[115] reported a case of bronchogenic carcinoma with ectopic gonadotropin secretion that was also associated with elevated urinary estradiol production. Further studies are needed for proof that this hormone is indeed potentially ectopically produced by lung carcinoma. Of concern is the fact that unlike the previously described ectopic hormones, all of which are peptide hormones, estradiol is a steroid. Synthesis of such a compound would require all the enzymes needed in the biosynthesis of steroids.[3]

Hypoglycemic Factor

One case of hypoglycemia with bronchogenic carcinoma (cell type epidermoid) has been reported.[116] Hypoglycemia has been associated with other types of pulmonary neoplasms, e.g., fibrosarcoma and fibroma.[117]

Renin

Another hormone whose status remains unclear regarding ectopic production by lung carcinoma is renin, or more properly a substance with reninlike activity. One case has recently been noted in the literature in which a patient with small cell carcinoma of the lung presented with increased plasma renin levels unresponsive to changes in salt intake.[118]

Insulin and Glucagon

A liver metastasis in a patient with an undifferentiated lung cancer showed elevated levels of insulin and glucagon as compared to the surrounding normal liver tissue.[119] Biologic activity of these hormones indicated no difference from the normal pancreatic hormones.

Erythropoietin and Erythrocythemia

Erythrocythemia has been observed in patients with several types of malignant and nonmalignant tumors. The results in hematologic remissions following removal of the tumor have suggested a causal relationship apparently due to the elaboration of an erythropoietic factor by the tumor. Because of inadequacies in the assay for erythropoietin, many of the erythropoietic factors have not been determined in patients reported with erythrocythemia. Literature data indicate that 5 patients have been reported with bronchogenic carcinoma, making it a marker not commonly associated with lung cancer.[120-122]

Gastrin

Gastrin has not heretofore been mentioned in the literature as being associated with bronchogenic carcinoma. However, in a study conducted at the NCI-VA Oncology Branch approximately 10 percent of patients with bronchogenic carcinoma had minimally elevated levels of serum gastrin.*

FETOPROTEINS

Recently two fetal antigens have been described and extensively studied: α-fetoprotein (AFP)[123] and carcinoembryonic antigen (CEA).[124]

AFP

AFP is an alpha globulin found in serum in fetal life. Production normally stops within weeks after birth, but AFP has been found in adults with cancer, notably hepatocellular carcinoma, in up to 75 percent of cases.[125] However, AFP is much less common in bronchogenic carcinoma. Corlin and Tompkins[126] reported one case, and this was a patient with known liver metastases. Waldmann et al. studied 150 patients with bronchogenic carcinoma and found that 7 percent of these had minimal levels of AFP present in their serum.[127] There was no preference for any specific cell type.

CEA

CEA was first studied as a marker for gastrointestinal neoplasms.[124] More recently, elevated serum levels (> 2.5 ng/ml) have been found in 60–86 percent of patients with bronchogenic carcinoma.[40,128,129]

Of considerable interest is the possibility that plasma CEA levels may be of value in prognosis and in evaluating response to therapy. Concan-

*Broder, L. E., personal communication, 1976.

non et al. studied 142 patients with bronchogenic carcinoma.[130] They concluded that the CEA test did not correlate well with patient survival or with the stage of disease at the time of diagnosis. Thus the pretherapy CEA may not be of value as a diagnostic or prognostic test in the management of a significant number of patients with bronchogenic carcinoma. Broder et al.[40] studied 69 previously untreated patients with bronchogenic carcinoma. They found a subsequent decrease in CEA levels in 8 of 9 patients associated with objective tumor response.

Currently the search continues for additional markers more specific for lung carcinoma. Yachi et al.[131] isolated two antigens (X and Y) from extracts of human lung cancers. These were not found in nonmaligant tissues, and they did not have the properties of CEA, in that the antigens described by Yachi were not soluble in perchloric acid.

OTHER COMPOUNDS

Placental Alkaline Phosphatase

Placental alkaline phosphatase (PAP) is not normally found in adult men or nonpregnant women, but it has been found in a patient with bronchogenic carcinoma.[132] This enzyme has been useful in monitoring the progression or regression of tumor growth. In a series of bronchogenic carcinoma patients, PAP was found in about 3 percent.*

Polyamines

Polyamines are small organic cations that may possibly be regulators of growth processes.[133] There is a parallelism of polyamine synthesis in many systems. There are several polyamines, including spermine, spermidine, and putrescine. In mammalian cells there is no apparent degradation of these compounds, and accumulation occurs shortly after tissue growth stimulation in both normal and neoplastic cells.

*Weintraub, B., Rosen, S. W., Broder, L. E., Muggia, F. M., and Primack, A., manuscript in preparation.

When amino acid analyzer and gas–liquid chromatology techniques are employed, the three polyamines are found in small quantities in normal human urine. In general, putrescine, spermidine, and possibly spermine urinary levels are elevated in cancer patients.[134-137] Preliminary work suggests a correlation between response to chemotherapy and polyamine levels.[138] These polyamines are therefore nonspecific, but they may aid in diagnosis and follow-up of patients with cancer and may help investigators define growth regulation.[139]

Histaminase

Histaminase (diamine oxidase) has been found to be elevated in medullary thyroid carcinoma tissue,[140,141] a neoplasm thought to be of neural crest origin.[142,143] Small cell carcinoma of the lung displays properties similar to those of medullary thyroid carcinoma, as indicated previously; it is also thought to be a tumor of neural crest origin. Recently 32 percent of 25 patients with bronchogenic small cell carcinoma were found to have elevated levels of histaminase in their plasma.[144] These data support the proposed embryologic relationship between small cell carcinoma of the lung and medullary thyroid carcinoma.

DISCUSSION

The preceding review has listed numerous markers that are found in patients with bronchogenic carcinoma and that are useful in many ways, both practical and theoretical. There are several classes of markers, and their significances differ. Hormones fall into two general classes: those that are normally found in these patients and those that are not normally found. The major interest, of course, is in those that are not normally found, since in these cases there is no background because they are specific for malignancy and they will not normally be attributed to overproduction by the normal gland. These specific hormones include hCG and hPL.

Fetal antigens, to date, have not been specific for a given tumor type, but the search for such specific antigens in lung cancer should be continued. Other avenues of research include specific separation of CEA into its subunits.

Polyamines and other markers are also non-specific, but they have the advantage of being elevated in a high percentage of patients. Thus, this may be a biochemical parameter to follow in the future in some patients with lung cancer. It is thought that the patients most likely to benefit from polyamine marker evaluation are those who have high tumor loads or in whom the tumor is turning over quite rapidly, as in small cell carcinoma.

A carcinoma must be of fairly large bulk to be detected by the current techniques. It is estimated that most tumors measure 1 cm in diameter (corresponding to approximately 10^9 cells) at the time of detection. Each diagnostic method has its limitations. In order for a lesion to appear on a radionuclide scan, the lesion must be greater than 2 cm in diameter. Fortunately, newer techniques in computerized axial tomography may decrease this minimal lesion size below 1 cm in diameter. X-ray ordinarily does not detect chest lesions of less than 1 cm. With accurate biochemical measurement it is conceivable that detection of fewer cells and smaller tumors could be accurately and specifically noted. Although at this time markers are often accurate diagnostic tools for malignancy, their sensitivity must be improved, and more markers must be found in order to use this technique in a greater number of patients.

The use of markers for estimation of tumor response to treatment is currently under intense investigation. Patients are screened for markers prior to treatment. Serial measurements are obtained in marker-positive patients and are correlated with other parameters of tumor response and with survival. Preliminary results are promising in several types of markers in bronchogenic carcinoma. This aspect of markers is best known in patients with choriocarcinoma, where hCG acts as a specific marker as the disease activity changes.[16] More recently, Salmon et al.[145] have shown the correlation of immunoglobulins with cell number in multiple myeloma. However, it must be pointed out that the problem in lung cancer may be quite different from that in the other tumor types. For example, the hCG levels found in patients with bronchogenic carcinoma are lower than those found for choriocarcinoma,

and they often show significant discordances in relation to response or progression of disease. We still have not approached the sophistication of Salmon et al.[145] in the correlation of a marker level with cell number.

Marker substances may aid in the detection of metastatic or primary disease by their measurement in other body fluids, e.g., cerebrospinal fluid.[146] The other area in which markers may be of benefit is the evaluation of bronchial secretions. Techniques are now being developed to measure marker substances in bronchial secretions, and this may be a step toward localization of early disease in bronchogenic carcinoma.

Marker substance study may aid in the delineation of genetic and biochemical changes that occur as cells undergo malignant degeneration. One possible explanation of the mechanism of marker production is de-repression of a genome responsible for production of that given substance. This is supported by the finding of markers that are identical by all possible tests, including radioimmunoassay, to the substances that are produced in their normal settings. There have been ectopic hormones studied that were not immunologically identical to the active hormones produced normally. This may indicate production of a "parent" compound that undergoes metabolism to its normal active compound, as with "big insulin"[147] and more recently "big ACTH,"[30] or it may indeed represent production of a new but similar compound that would imply a different genetic makeup in the malignant cell. In addition, marker substances may help describe growth characteristics of tumors and aid in the rational timing of chemotherapy.

The mechanism of production of these markers is as yet unknown, but the most widely held view favors the mechanism of gene derepression, as reviewed recently.[148] This could explain the production of all markers, since all cells are derived from a single cell, which at one time contained the genetic material needed for all cellular metabolism. With continuation of the present impetus in this area, new markers will be found, and some will have increased specificity. These will aid all oncologists, both scientifically and therapeutically.

REFERENCES

1. Kreyberg L: Histological Typing of Lung Tumors. International Histological Classification of Tumors. Geneva, Rotosadag, 1967, p 19

2. Brain DM, Norris FH Jr (eds): The Remote Effects of Cancer on the Nervous System, vol. 1. New York, Grune & Stratton, 1965

3. Rees LH, Ratcliffe JG: Ectopic hormone production by non-endocrine tumours. Clin Endocrinol (Oxf) 3:263–299, 1974

4. Nathanson L, Hall TC: A spectrum of tumors that produce paraneoplastic syndromes. Lung tumors: How they produce their syndromes. Ann NY Acad Sci 230:367–377, 1974

5. Lipsett MB: Humoral syndromes associated with nonendocrine tumors. Ann Intern Med 61:733–756, 1964

6. Lipsett MB: Hormonal syndromes associated with neoplasia. Adv Metab Disord 3:111–152, 1968

7. Liddle GW, Nicholson WE: Clinical and laboratory studies of ectopic humoral syndromes. Recent Prog Horm Res 25:383–414, 1969

8. Amatruda TT: Nonendocrine secreting tumors, in Bondy PK, Rosenberg LE (eds): Duncan's Diseases of Metabolism (ed 6). Philadelphia, WB Saunders, 1969, pp 1227–1244

9. Sachs BA: Endocrine disorders produced by nonendocrine malignant tumors. Bull NY Acad Med 41:1069–1086, 1965

10. Myers WPL, Tashima CK: Endocrine syndromes associated with nonendocrine neoplasm. Med Clin North Am 50:763–778, 1966

11. Bower BF, Gordon GS: Hormonal effects of nonendocrine tumors. Ann Rev Med 16:83–118, 1965

12. Williams MJ, Sommers SC: Endocrine and certain other changes in men with carcinoma of the lung. Cancer 15:109–117, 1962

13. Wichert PV: Paraneoplasticsche Syndrome. Med Klin 66:1461–1465, 1971

14. Greenberg E, Woolner L: A review of unusual systematic manifestations associated with carcinoma. Am J Med 36:106–120, 1964

15. Knowles JH, Smith LH: Extrapulmonary manifestations of bronchogenic carcinoma. N Engl J Med 262:505–510, 1960

16. Ross GT: Chemotherapy of metastatic and nonmetastatic gestational trophoblastic neoplasms. Tex Rep Biol Med 24[Suppl 2]:326–328, 1966

17. Yalow RS, Glich SM: Radioimmunoassay of human plasma ACTH. J Clin Endocrinol Metab 24:1219–1255, 1964

18. Saez S: Adrenal function in cancer: Relation to the evolution. Eur J Cancer 7:381–387, 1971

19. Belsky JL, Marks LJ: Plasma 17-hydroxycorticosteroid responsiveness to ACTH in patients with bronchogenic carcinoma. Metabolism 11:435–442, 1962

20. Kawai A, Tamura M: Studies on adrenal cortical functions in patients with lung cancer. Metabolism 18:609–619, 1969

21. Sachs B, Becker N, Bloomberg AE, et al: "Cure" of ectopic ACTH syndrome secondary to adenocarcinoma of the lung. J Clin Endocrinol Metab 30:590–597, 1970

22. Hattori S, Matsuda M, Tateishi R, et al: Oat-cell carcinoma of the lung. Cancer 30:1014–1024, 1972.

23. Horai T, Nishihara H, Tateishi R: Oat-cell carcinoma of the lung simultaneously producing ACTH + seratonin. J Clin Endocrinol Metab 37:212–219, 1973

24. Corrin B, McMillan M: Fine structure of an oat-cell carcinoma of the lung associated with ectopic ACTH syndrome. Br J Cancer 24:755–758, 1970

25. Bensch KG, Corrin B: Oat-cell carcinoma of the lung. Its origin and relationship to bronchial carcinoid. Cancer 22:1163–1172, 1968

26. Cawley JP, Tretbar HA, Musser BO: Gas-liquid chromatographic studies of urinary 17-ketosteroids in three patients with adrenocorticotropin-producing bronchogenic carcinoma. Am J Clin Pathol 51:86–94, 1969

27. Gewirtz G, Yalow RS: Ectopic ACTH production: Big and little forms. Endocrinology 92[Suppl]:A-52, 1973

28. Schneider B, Gewirtz G: Big ACTH: Conversion to biologically active ACTH by trypsin. Endocrinology 92[Suppl]:A-52, 1973

29. Ayvazian LF, Schneider B, Gewirtz G, et al: Ectopic production of big ACTH in carcinoma of the lung. Am Rev Respir Dis 111:279–287, 1975

30. Yalow RS, Berson SA: Characteristics of "big ACTH" in human plasma and pituitary extracts. J Clin Endocrinol Metab 36:415–423, 1973

31. Gewirtz G, Yalow RS: Ectopic ACTH production in carcinoma of the lung. J Clin Invest 53:1022–1032, 1974

32. Liddle GW, Givens JR, Nicholson WE, et al: The Ectopic ACTH syndrome, in: Proceedings of Second International Congress of Endocrinology. 83:1063–1067, 1961

33. Imura H, Matsukura S, Yamamoto H, et al: Studies on ectopic ACTH-producing tumors. II. Cancer 35:1430–1437, 1975

34. Shimizu N, Ogata E: Studies on the melanotropic activity of human plasma and tissue. J Clin Endocrinol Metab 25:948–990, 1965

35. Shapiro M, Nicholson WE: Differences between ectopic MSH and pituitary MSH. J Clin Endocrinol Metab 33:377, 1971

36. Locke EA: Secondary hypertrophic osteoarthro-

pathy and its relationship to club-fingers. Arch Intern Med 15:659–713, 1915

37. Faiman C, Colwell JA: Gonadotropin secretion from a bronchogenic carcinoma. N Engl J Med 277:1395–1399, 1967

38. Vaitukaitis JL, Ross GT: Recent advances in evaluation of gonadotropic hormones. Ann Rev Med 24:295–302, 1973

39. Braunstein GD, Vaitukaitis JL, Carbone PP, et al: Ectopic production of human chorionic gonadotropin by neoplasms. Ann Intern Med 78:39–45, 1973

40. Broder LE, Waalkes TP, Primack A, et al: Biologic markers in the evaluation of disease status of patients with advanced bronchogenic carcinoma. Proc Am Assoc Cancer Res 16:223, 1975

41. Swaminathan N, Bahl OP: Dissociation and recombination of the subunits of human chorionic gonadotropin. Biochem Biophys Res Commun 40:422–427, 1970

42. Morgan FJ, Canfield RE: Nature of the subunits of human chorionic gonadotropin. Endocrinology 88:1045–1053, 1971

43. Pierce JG: The subunits of pituitary thyrotropin—their relationship to other glycoprotein hormones. Endocrinology 89:1331–1344, 1971

44. Saxena BB, Rathnam P: Dissociating phenomenon and subunit nature of follicle-stimulating hormone from human pituitary glands. J Biol Chem 246:3549–3554, 1971

45. Tashjian AH, Weintraub BD: Subunits of human chorionic gonadotropin unbalanced synthesis and secretion by clonal cell strains derived from a bronchogenic carcinoma. Proc Natl Acad Sci USA 70:1419–1422, 1973

46. Weintraub BD, Rosen SW: Ectopic production of the isolated beta subunit of human chorionic gonadotropin. J Clin Invest 52:3135–3142, 1973

47. Vaitukaitis JL: Immunologic and physical characterization of HCG secreted by tumors. J Clin Endocrinol Metab 37:505–514, 1973

48. Weintraub BD, Rosen SW: Competitive radioassays and "specific" tumor markers. Metabolism 22:1119–1127, 1973

49. Muggia FM, Rosen SW, Weintraub BD, et al: Ectopic placental proteins in nontrophoblastic tumors—serial measurements following chemotherapy. Cancer 36:1327–1337, 1975

50. Rabson AS, Rosen SW: Production of human chorionic gonadotropin "in vitro" by a cell line derived from a carcinoma of the lung. J Natl Cancer Inst 50:669–674, 1973

51. Broder LE, et al: The effect of antineoplastic agents on cell growth (CG) and alpha subunit production (AP) in a human bronchogenic carcinoma cell line in vitro. Proc Am Assoc Cancer Res 17:741, 1976 (abstract)

52. Rosen SW, Becker CE: Ectopic gonadotropin production before clinical recognition of bronchogenic carcinoma. N Engl J Med 279:640–641, 1968

53. Posternak F: Gynecomastie et cancer bronchique: syndrôme paraneplasique ou non? Schweiz Med Wochenschr 100:501–506, 1970

54. Klatskin G, Salter WT, Humm FD: Gynecomastia due to malnutrition. I. Clinical studies. Am J Med Sci 213:19–30, 1947

55. Beck SJ, Porteous IB: Gonadotropin-secreting bronchial carcinoma: Aberrant endocrine activity or trophoblastic differentiation. J Pathol 101:59–62, 1970

56. Sussman HH, Weintraub BD: Relationship of ectopic placental alkaline phosphatase to ectopic chorionic gonadotropin and placental lactogen: Discordance of three "markers" for cancer. Cancer 33:820–823, 1974

57. Weintraub BD, Rosen SW: Ectopic production of human chorionic somatomammotropin by nontrophoblastic cancers. J Clin Endocrinol Metab 32:94–101, 1971

58. Gowenlock MB, Platt DS: Oat cell carcinoma of the bronchus secreting 5-hydroxytryptophan. Lancet 1:304–306, 1964

59. Beck C, Burger HG: Evidence for the presence of immunoreactive growth hormone in cancers of the lung and stomach. Cancer 30:75–79, 1972

60. Cameron DP, Burger HG: On the presence of immunoreactive growth hormone in a bronchogenic carcinoma. Ann Med 18:143–146, 1969

61. Dupont B, Hoyer I: Plasma growth hormone and hypertrophic osteoarthropathy in carcinoma of the bronchus. Acta Med Scand 188:25–30, 1970

62. Greenberg PB, Beck C: Synthesis and release of human growth hormone from lung carcinoma in cell cultures. Lancet 1:350–352, 1972

63. Sparagana M, Phillips G: Ectopic growth hormone syndrome associated with lung cancer. Metabolism 20:730–736, 1971

64. Steiner H, Dahlback O: Ectopic growth-hormone production and osteoarthropathy in carcinoma of the bronchus. Lancet 1:783–785, 1968

65. Sherwood LM, O'Riordan JLH: Production of parathyroid hormone by nonparathyroid tumors. J Clin Endocrinol Metab 27:140–146, 1967

66. Myers WPL: Hypercalcemia in neoplastic disease. Arch Surg 80:308–318, 1960

67. Myers WPL: Hypercalcemia in neoplastic disease. Cancer 9:1135–1140, 1956

68. Plimpton CH: Hypercalcemia in malignant disease without evidence of bone destruction. Am J Med 21:750–759, 1956

69. Lafferty FW: Pseudohyperparathyroidism. Medicine 45:247–260, 1966

70. Zilva JF, Nicholson JP: Plasma phosphate and potassium levels in the hypercalcemia of malignant disease. J Clin Endocrinol Metab 36:1019–1026, 1973

71. Carey VCI: The incidence of hypercalcemia in

association with bronchogenic carcinoma. Am Rev Respir Dis 93:584–586, 1966

72. Azzopardi TC, Whittacker RS: Bronchial carcinoma and hypercalcemia. J Clin Pathol 22:718–724, 1969

73. Reiss E, Canterbury JM: Blood levels of parathyroid hormone in disorders of calcium metabolism. Am Rev Med 24:217–232, 1973

74. Tashjian AH, Levine L: Immunochemical identification of parathyroid hormone in nonparathyroid neoplasms associated with hypercalcemia. J Exp Med 119:467–484, 1964

75. Tashjian AH, Munson PL: Assay of human parathyroid hormone. Ann Intern Med 60:523–526, 1964

76. Turkington RW, Goldman JK: Bronchogenic carcinoma stimulating hyperparathyroidism. Cancer 19:406–414, 1966

77. Connor TB, Thomas WCM, Howard JE: The etiology of hypercalcemia associated with lung carcinoma. J Clin Invest 35:697–698, 1956

78. Berson SA, Yalow RS: Parathyroid hormone in plasma in adenomatous hyperparathyroidism, uremia, and bronchogenic carcinoma. Science 154:907–909, 1966

79. Riggs BJ, Arnaud CD: Immunologic differentiation of primary hyperparathyroidism from hyperparathyroidism due to nonparathyroid cancer. J Clin Invest 50:2079–2083, 1971

80. Snedecor PA, Baker HW: Pseudohyperparathyroidism due to malignant tumors. Cancer 17:1492–1496, 1964

81. Massaro DJ, Owen JA: Persistent hypercalcemia associated with bronchogenic carcinoma and primary chief cell hyperplasia of the parathyroids. Am Rev Respir Dis 85:727–734, 1962

82. Strott CA, Nugent CA: Cushing's syndrome caused by bronchial adenomas. Am J Med 44:97–104, 1968

83. Seyberth HW, Segre GV, Morgan JL, et al: Prostaglandins as mediators of hypercalcemia associated with certain types of cancer. N Engl J Med 293:1278–1282, 1975

84. Silva O, Becker K, Primack A, et al: Ectopic production of calcitonin. Lancet 1:317, 1973

85. Silva OL, Becker KL, Primack A, et al: Ectopic secretion of calcitonin by oat-cell carcinoma. N Engl J Med 290:1122–1124, 1974

86. Coombes RC, Hillyard C, Greenberg PB, et al: Plasma-immunoreactive-calcitronin in patients with nonthyroid tumours. Lancet 1:1080–1083, 1974

87. Cattan D, Vesin P, Rougier PH, et al: Letter: Hyperthyrocalcitoninaemia, Schwartz-Bartter syndrome, and oat-cell carcinoma. Lancet 1:938, 1974

88. Milhaud G, Calmette C, Taboulet J, et al: Letter: Hypersecretion of calcitonin in neoplastic conditions. Lancet 1:462–463, 1974

89. Whitelaw AGL, Cohen SL: Ectopic production of calcitonin. Lancet 2:443, 1973

90. Silva OL, Becker KL, Primack A, et al: Increased serum calcitonin levels in bronchogenic cancer. Chest 69:495–499, 1976

91. Silva OL, Broder LE, Becker KL: Calcitonin as a marker for lung cancer. Proc Am Soc Clin Oncol 17:C-160, 1976 (abstract)

92. Winkler AW, Crankshaw OF: Chloride depletion in conditions other than Addison's disease. J Clin Invest 17:1–6, 1938

93. Schwartz, WB, Bennett W: A syndrome of renal sodium loss and hyponatremia probably resulting from inappropriate secretion of antidiuretic hormone. Am J Med 23:529–542, 1957

94. White G: Diabetes insipidus associated with edema. N Engl J Med 250:633–636, 1954

95. Schwartz WB, Tassel D, Bartter FC: Further observations on hyponatremia and renal sodium loss probably resulting from inappropriate secretion of antidiuretic hormone. N Engl J Med 262:743–749, 1960

96. Dutaw G, Delson G: Le syndrôme de Schwartz-Bartter. Etude pharmacologique et histologique de trois observations. Poumon Coeur 27:237–245, 1971

97. Roberts, HJ: The syndrome of hyponatremia and renal loss probably resulting from inappropriate secretion of antidiuretic hormone. Ann Intern Med 51:1420–1426, 1959

98. Ross EJ: Hyponatraemic syndromes associated with carcinoma of the bronchus. Q J Med 32:297–320, 1963

99. Ivy HK: Renal sodium loss and bronchogenic carcinoma. Arch Intern Med 108:115–123, 1961

100. Barjon P, Mion H: Le syndrôme de Schwartz-Bartter. PoumonCoeur 17:213–236, 1971

101. Bartter FC, Schwartz WB: The syndrome of inappropriate secretion of antidiuretic hormone. Am J Med 42:790–806, 1967

102. Hayduk K, Kaufmann W: Das Schwartz-Bartter syndron. Dtsch Med Wochenschr 97:1357–1360, 1972

103. Catt KJ: An ABC of Endocrinology (ed 1). Boston, Little, Brown, 1971, pp 17–18

104. Baumann G, Dingman JF: Plasma arginine vasopressin (AVP) in the inappropriate ADH syndrome (SIADH). Clin Res 18:354, 1970

105. George JM, Capen CC: Biosynthesis of vasopressin (AVP) "in vitro" bronchogenic carcinoma. J Clin Invest 51:141, 1972

106. Olson R, Buchan GC, Porter GA: The syndrome of inappropriate antidiuretic hormone secretion. Arch Intern Med 124:741–747, 1969

107. Barraclough MA, Jones TT, Lee T: Production of vasopressin by anaplastic oat cell carcinoma of the bronchus. Clin Sci 31:135–144, 1966

108. Utiger RD: Inappropriate antidiuresis and carcinoma of the lung: Detection of arginine vasopres-

sin in tumor extracts by immunoassay. J Clin Endocrinol Metab 26:970–974, 1966

109. Rees T, Rosalki SB, MacLean ADW: Hyponatraemia and impaired renal tubular function with carcinoma of bronchus. Lancet 2:1005–1009, 1960

110. Daly JJ, Nelson MA, Rose DP: Hyponatraemia with carcinoma of the bronchus. Postgrad Med 39:158–159, 1963

111. Legros JJ, Louis F: Identification of a vasopressin-neurophysin and of an oxytocin-neurophysin in man. Neuroendocrinology 13:371–375, 1974

112. Hamilton BPM, Upton GV, Amatruda TT: Evidence for the presence of neurophysin in tumors producing the syndrome of inappropriate antidiuresis. J Clin Endocrinol Metab 35:764, 1972

113. Turkington RW: Ectopic production of prolactin. N Engl J Med 285:1455–1458, 1971

114. Williams ED, Azzopardi JG: Tumors of the lung and the carcinoid syndrome. Thorax 15:30–36, 1960

115. Kirschner MA, Cohen FB: Estrogen production and its origin in men with gonadotropin-producing neoplasms. Endocrinology 92[Suppl]:A-55, 1973

116. Thorne G: C.P.C. N Engl J Med 268:1129–1139, 1963

117. Lowbeer L: Hypoglycemia producing extrapancreatic neoplasms. Am J Clin Pathol 35:233–244, 1961

118. Hauger-Klevene JH: High plasma renin activity in a oat cell carcinoma: A renin-secreting carcinoma. Cancer 26:1112, 1970

119. Unger RH, Bochner J: Identification of insulin and glucagon in a bronchogenic metastasis. J Clin Endocrinol Metab 24:823–831, 1964

120. Donati RM, McCarthy JM, Lange RD, et al: Erythrocythemia and neoplastic tumors. Ann Intern Med 58:47–55, 1963

121. Videbaek A: Polycythemia vera; coexisting with malignant tumors (particularly hypernephroma). Acta Med Scand 138:239–245, 1950

122. Hammond D, Winnick S: Paraneoplastic erythrocytosis and ectopic erythropoietins, in: Paraneoplastic Syndromes. Ann NY Acad Sci 230:219–227, 1974

123. Abeler GI, Perova SD, Karamkova NI, et al: Embryonal serum alpha-globulin and its synthesis by the transplantable mouse hepatoma. Biokhimiia 28:625–634, 1963

124. Gold P, Freedman SO: Demonstration of tumor specific antigens in human colonic carcinomata by immunological tolerance and absorption techniques. J Exp Med 121:439–462, 1965

125. Vogel CL, Primack A, McIntire KR, et al: Serum alpha fetoprotein in 184 Ugandan patients with hepatocellular carcinoma. Clinical laboratory and histopathological conditions. Cancer 33:959–964, 1974

126. Corlin RF, Tompkins RK: Serum alpha-fetoglobulin in a patient with hepatic metastases from bronchogenic carcinoma. Dig Dis 17:553–555, 1972

127. Waldmann TA, McIntire KR, Suer ME, et al: Radioimmunoassay of fetaprotein in the diagnosis of malignancy. Miles International Symposium (in press)

128. Concannon JP, Dalbow MH, Frich JC: Carcinoembryonic antigen (CEA) plasma levels in untreated cancer patients and patients with metastatic disease. Radiology 108:191–193, 1973

129. MacSween JM, Warner NL, Mackay IR: The detection of carcinoembryonic antigen in whole serum for patients with malignant and nonmalignant disease. Clin Immunol Immupathol 1:330–345, 1973

130. Concannon JP, Dalbow MH, Liebler GA, et al: The carcinoembryonic antigen assay in bronchogenic carcinoma. Cancer 34:184–192, 1974

131. Yachi A, Matsuura Y, Carpenter CM, et al: Immunochemical studies on human lung cancer antigens soluble in 50-percent saturated ammonium sulfate. J Natl Cancer Inst 40:663–682, 1968

132. Sussman H, Rosen SW: Discordant secretion of placental alkaline phosphatase (PAP), chorionic gonadotropin (HCG) and somatomammotropin (HCS) in patients with cancer. Clin Res 19:497, 1971

133. Russell DH: Polyamines in growth—normal and neoplastic, in Russell DH (ed): Polyamines—Normal and Neoplastic. New York, Raven, 1973, p 1

134. Russell DH: Increased polyamine concentrations in the urine of human cancer patients. Nature 233:144–145, 1971

135. Russell DH, Levy CC, Schimpf SC, et al: Urinary polyamines in cancer patients. Cancer Res 31:1555–1559, 1971

136. Bremer JH, Kohne E, Endres W: The excretion of diamines in human urine. II. Cadaverine, putrescine, 1,3-diamminopropane, 2,2'-dithiobis(ethylamine) and spermidine in urine of patients with cystinuria and cystinlysinuria. Clin Chim Acta 32:407–418, 1971

137. Chayen R, Dreyfuss G, Dreyfuss R, et al: Urinary polyamines in cancer. Isr J Med Sci 9:564, 1973

138. Denton MD, Glazer H, Smith F, et al: Polyamine levels in patients with neoplastic disease. Clin Res 21:644, 1973

139. Russell DH, Durie BGM, Salmon SE: Polyamines As Predictors of Success and Failure in Cancer Chemotherapy. Lancet, II:797–799, 1975

140. Baylin SB, Beaven MA, Engelman K, et al: Elevated histaminase activity in medullary carcinoma of the thyroid gland. N Engl J Med 283:1239–1244, 1970

141. Baylin SB, Beaven MA, Buja LM, et al: Histami-

nase activity: A biochemical marker for medullary carcinoma of the thyroid. Am J Med 53:723–733, 1972

142. Pearse AGE: The cytochemistry and ultrastructure of polypeptide hormone-producing cells of the APUD series and the embryologic, physiologic, and pathologic implications of the concept. J Histochem Cytochem 17:303–313, 1969

143. Welbourn RB, Pearse AGE, Polak JM, et al: The APUD cells of the alimentary tract in health and disease. Med Clin North Am 58:1359–1374, 1974

144. Baylin SB, Abeloff MD, Wieman KC, et al: Elevated histaminase (diamine oxidase) activity in small-cell carcinoma of the lung. N Engl J Med 293:1286–1290, 1975

145. Salmon SE, McIntyre OR, Ogawa M: IgE myeloma: Total body tumor cell number and synthesis of IgE and DNA. Blood 37:696–705, 1971

146. Snitzer LS, McKinney EC: Carcinoembryonic antigen in cerebrospinal fluid. Proc Am Soc Clin Oncol 17:C-51, 1976 (abstract)

147. Steiner DF, Clark JL, Nolan C, et al: Proinsulin and the biosynthesis of insulin. Recent Prog Horm Res 25:207–282, 1969

148. Frenster JH, Herstein PR: Gene De-repression. N Engl J Med 288:1224–1229, 1973

149. Clinicopathological conference. A case of endocrine dysfunction with lung carcinoma. Br Med J 1:281–286, 1970

150. Knight RA, Ratcliffe JG: Tumor ACTH concentrations in ectopic ACTH syndrome and in control tissues. Proc R Soc Med 64:1266–1267, 1971

151. Andersen AE, McHugh PR: Oat cell carcinoma with hypercortisolemia presenting to a psychiatric hospital as a suicide attempt. J Nerv Ment Dis 152:427–431, 1971

152. Izumi AK, Richman SP: Ectopic adrenocorticotropic hormone syndrome. Arch Dermatol 102:556–559, 1970

153. Sasano N, Fukuda T: Pathology of ectopic ACTH syndrome with emphasis on pituitary Crooke cells and adrenocortical hyperplasia related to ACTH activities in tumor tissues. Tohoku J Exp Med 99:361–380, 1969

154. McMillan M, Maisey MN: Effects of aminoglutethimide in a case of ectopic ACTH syndrome. Acta Endocrinol 64:676–686, 1970

155. Hauer-Klevene JH: Asymptomatic production of ACTH radioimmunoassay in squamous cell, oat-cell, and adenocarcinoma of the lung. Cancer 22:1262–1267, 1968

156. Luton JP, Chaumerliac P: Les hypercorticismes paraneoplastiques. Sem Hop Paris 8:111–120, 1972

157. Davidson C: Diabetes insipidus with an ACTH-secreting carcinoma of the bronchus. Br Med J 1:287–288, 1972

158. Thorne MG: Cushing's syndrome associated with bronchial carcinoma. Guys Hosp Rep 101:251–272, 1952

159. Spaulding WB, Oille WA, Gornall AG: Mineralo-cortoid-like disturbance associated with adrenal metastases from a bronchogenic carcinoma. Ann Intern Med 42:444–451, 1955

160. Meador CK, Liddle GW: Cause of Cushing's syndrome in patients with tumors arising from "nonendocrine" tissue. J Clin Endocrinol Metab 22:693–703, 1962

161. Kovach RD, Kyle LH: Cushing's syndrome and bronchogenic carcinoma. Am J Med 24:981–988, 1958

162. Christy NP: Adrenocorticotropic activity in the plasma of patients with Cushing's syndrome associated with pulmonary neoplasms. Lancet 1:85–86, 1961

163. Brown BM: A case of pluriglandular syndrome. Lancet 2:1022–1023, 1928

164. Thompson GS, Horwick L: Carcinoma of bronchus and Cushing's syndrome. Lancet 2:534–536, 1962

165. Sederberg-Olson P, Binder C, Kehlet H, et al: Episodic variation in plasma corticosteroids in subjects with Cushing's syndrome of differing etiology. J Clin Endocrinol Metab 36:906–910, 1973

166. O'Riordan JLH, Blanshard GP: Corticotropin-secreting carcinomas. Q J Med 35:137–147, 1966

167. Nichols J, Gourley W: Adrenal-weight-maintaining corticotropin in carcinoma of lung. JAMA 185:696–698, 1963

168. Liddle GW, Island DP: Nonpituitary neoplasm and Cushing's syndrome. Arch Intern Med 111:471–475, 1963

169. Liddle GW, Givens JR: The ectopic ACTH syndrome. Cancer Res 25:1057–1061, 1965

170. Island DP, Shimizu N: A method for separating small quantities of MSH and ACTH with good recovery of each. J Clin Endocrinol Metab 25:475–483, 1965

171. Gault MH, Kinsella TD: Carcinoma of lung with adrenal hyperfunction and hypercalcemia treated by parathyroidectomy. Can Med Assoc J 92:317–324, 1965

172. Friedman M, Mikhail JR: Cushing's syndrome associated with carcinoma of the bronchus in a patient with normal plasma electrolytes. Br Med J 1:27–29, 1965

173. Cottrell JC, Becker K: The histology of gonadotropin-secreting bronchogenic carcinoma. Am J Clin Pathol 52:720–725, 1969

174. Fusco FD, Rosen SW: Gonadotropin-producing anaplastic large cell carcinomas of the lung. N Engl J Med 275:507–515, 1966

175. Grillo IA: Endocrine manifestation of pulmonary carcinoma in a Nigerian. Br J Cancer 25:266–269, 1971

176. Bower BF, Mason DM: Measurement of antidiuretic activity (ADA) in plasma and tumor in carcinoma of the lung with inappropriate antidiuresis. Clin Res 12:121, 1964

177. Epstein S, Ranchod M, Goldswain P: Pituitary insufficiency, inappropriate antidiuretic hormone and carcinoma of the bronchus. S Afr Med J 47:664, 1973

178. Amatruda TT, Mulrow PJ: Carcinoma of the lung with inappropriate antidiuresis. N Engl J Med 269:554–549, 1963

179. Ivy HK: The syndrome of inappropriate secretion of antidiuretic hormone. Med Clin North Am 52:817–827, 1968

180. Fontenaille C, Mollet E, Marchetti J: Etude du systeme renine-angiotensine-aldosterone dans 2 cas de syndrôme de Schwartz-Bartter. Presse Med 78:965–968, 1970

181. Akown G, Faye CL: Deux syndrôme de Schwartz-Bartter (S.B.). Presse Med 78:2382, 1970

182. Dongradi G, Poisson M, Bueve-Meryl JP, et al: Association d'un cancer du poumon et de pluiseurs syndromes paraneoplasiques. Ann Med Interne (Paris) 122:959–964, 1971

183. Turner P, Williams R: Unexplained steatorrhoea in the syndrome of hyponatraemia and carcinoma of bronchus. Br Med J 1:287–290, 1962

184. Vorheer H, Massry SG, Utiger RD, et al: Antidiuretic principle in malignant tumor extracts from patients with inappropriate ADH syndrome. J Clin Endocrinol Metab 28:162, 1968

Mary J. Matthews
Phillip R. Gordon

4

Morphology of Pulmonary and Pleural Malignancies

Lung cancers include a wide spectrum of neoplasms that may be of entodermal, mesodermal, or possibly neuroectodermal derivation. Carcinomas arising from the bronchial or bronchioloalveolar surface epithelium and from bronchial mucous glands constitute 90–95 percent of these tumors.[1] The four major cell types include epidermoid (squamous cell) carcinoma, small cell (oat cell) carcinoma, adenocarcinoma, and large cell (anaplastic) carcinoma. If strict criteria are applied for diagnosis, approximately 2–4 percent of these tumors will be found to be composed of a combination of glandular and squamous epithelium (adenosquamous cell carcinoma).[2] Carcinoids constitute up to 5 percent of surgically excised lung tumors. The majority are centrally located and are of bronchial gland origin. Their occasional peripheral locations, multicentric patterns, eccentric clinical and biologic behaviors, and complex relationships with small cell carcinomas underscore the need for better definition and understanding of these neoplasms. Mesotheliomas, although uncommon, appear to be increasing in incidence.[3] These tumors present difficult clinical and light-microscopic diagnostic problems that potentially may be resolved at ultrastructural levels.

This chapter will discuss the pathology, behavior, and diagnostic problems encountered in the neoplasms cited above. The embryology and histology of the lung and pleura will be described briefly. Pathogenetic mechanisms, classification, and incidence of the major types of lung cancer will be reviewed.

EMBRYOLOGY

The laryngotracheobronchial tree is entodermal in origin; it originates as a ventral diverticulum of the foregut.[4] The diverticulum elongates caudally and proliferates laterally to form lung buds. The lung buds dichotomously branch to form bronchopulmonary buds. Splanchnic mesenchyme surrounding these structures gives rise to the future fibroelastic, vascular, muscular, and cartilaginous components of the lung. At approximately the 5th week of fetal life the mesenchyme invests the proliferating buds to form the future visceral pleura. The parietal pleura is derived from the corresponding somatic mesenchyme.

By the 13th week of fetal life the basic structure of the pulmonary conducting system has formed. The lung resembles a tubular or ductal structure lined by cuboidal or columnar epithelial cells and surrounded by a dense, poorly vascularized mesenchyme. Glycogen, ciliary processes, and neurosecretory granules may be identified in the epithelial cells by electron microscopy.[5,6] By the 16th to 17th weeks approximately 24 bronchial branchings have occurred.

Between the 24th and 28th weeks the respira-

49

tory portion of the lung is identifiable. Terminal bronchioles that previously terminated in alveolar buds have proliferated and dilated, giving rise to the respiratory bronchioles with their attending alveolar ducts, sacs, and alveoli. Bronchioles are lined by ciliated and glycogen-containing cuboidal ("Clara") cells that proliferate over the distal airways, forming two distinct types of epithelial cells.[5] The type I pneumocyte is a thinned epithelial cell with attenuated cytoplasm, designed to protect the underlying vascular bed. The type II pneumocyte is a cuboidal epithelial cell containing numerous cytoplasmic organelles and osmiophilic lamellar bodies, the apparent source of surfactant. The two cell types form a continuous membrane. The mesenchyme becomes loose and vascularized, and capillaries come into intimate contact with the lining alveolar cells. There is sufficient surfactant production and adequate vascular bed to permit survival of a premature infant. The processes of air space dilatation and epithelial and vascular proliferation continue until approximately the 8th postnatal year.

HISTOLOGY

The bronchial mucosa is lined by pseudostratified columnar epithelium that rests on a thin basement membrane. Electron micrographs permit identification of at least three distinct types of columnar cells (goblet, ciliated, and brush border types).[7] Two types of basal cells have also been identified: short basal or reserve cells and granular basal cells. These cells rest on a basement membrane and give the mucosa its pseudostratified appearance. Tonofilamentous structures, the precursors of keratin, are occasionally found in the short basal cells. It is presumed that these cells serve as reserve cells that mature to or give rise to the columnar epithelial cells. Also, in response to chronic injury the cells have the potential to form squamous cells. The granular basal cells have elongated nuclei and pseudopodal cytoplasmic processes that interdigitate between columnar cells. Membrane-limited electron-dense granules measuring up to 170 μ are present in the cytoplasmic processes. A thin halo surrounds the electron-dense core. These granules are similar to the neurosecretory granules identified in the argentaffine or Kulchitsky cells of the intestines, the C cells of the thyroid, pancreatic islet cells, adrenal medullary cells, autonomic

neurons, and other related cells. Terzakis et al. have identified similar granules in mature goblet cells of the bronchial mucosa.[8] The granular basal cells are referred to as Kulchitsky or K-type cells.[9] Tateishi has identified tadpole-shaped argyrophilic cells, the light-microscopic counterpart of K-type cells, in bronchial and bronchiolar mucosa, particularly in relationship to zones of goblet cell hyperplasia.[10] It has been speculated that cells with this variety of granules are neuroectodermal in origin and have endocrine and/or chemoreceptor functions. The cells are capable of synthesizing a variety of polypeptide compounds and hormones or their precursors. Serotonin, acetylcholine, kinin activators, ACTH, and ADH are a few of the products presumably produced and secreted by these cells.[11,12]

The bronchial mucous glands, embedded in the submucosa of the bronchi, are composed of lobules of serous and mucous glands that communicate with the bronchial lumen via mucous gland ducts. Bensch initially identified K-type cells overlying the basement membranes of these glands.[13]

Bronchioles are lined by pale vacuolated Clara cells, low columnar ciliated epithelial cells, and basal cells, some of which (as shown by electron microscopy) contain neurosecretory granules.[14] Goblet cells are not present in these structures, except as a metaplastic response to inflammation or injury. Alveolar lining cells are flat and difficult to identify in normal lungs by light microscopy. By electron microscopy these cells are seen to be identical to the pneumocytes described in the preceding section.

The pleura is lined by a single layer of flattened mesothelial cells that rests on a thin connective tissue lamina. Immediately beneath this there are two layers of elastic fibers separated by a loose fibrous tissue. The subpleural tissues are rich in lymphatics and blood vessels. By electron microscopy mesothelial cells are seen to have an abundance of variable-size microvilli projecting from their surfaces.[7,15]

PATHOGENESIS

Carcinomas involving the conducting system of the lung most commonly arise in segmental and subsegmental bronchi in response to repetitive injury and chronic inflammation. Macholda has stressed that at sites of segmental bronchial bifurcations the air flow is altered and the flow of mucus is reduced.[16] Bronchial epithelium at these sites is particularly susceptible to injury. Columnar cells lose their ciliary processes or desquamate. Carcinogenic agents are likely to be deposited and absorbed in these zones. Basal cells initially respond by proliferating an abundance of mucin-secreting goblet cells. With progressive insult, the columnar cells are replaced by an orderly arranged metaplastic stratified squamous epithelium. Eventually the epithelium becomes disorganized, and nuclear atypia and mitoses may be recognized in the basal half of the mucosa (atypical metaplasia or dysplasia). Carcinoma in situ (intraepithelial carcinoma) is characterized by cellular disorganization, nuclear atypia, and atypical mitoses through the full thickness of the mucosa. Later the integrity of the basement membrane may be lost and frank infiltration of neoplastic cells into the underlying stroma may occur. This entire process may take from 10 to 20 years. Such changes have been observed in humans as well as in experimental animal models,[17-20] and they particularly apply in the induction of epidermoid bronchogenic malignancies. Carcinogenic agents implicated in such a process include occupational and atmospheric pollutants such as metabolites of polycyclic hydrocarbons, arsenic, asbestos, chromates, nickel, coal tar, copper, radioactive chemicals, and products of tobacco smoke[21,22] (see Chapter 1).

Spencer has estimated that one-third of epidermoid carcinomas are peripheral in origin and are unrelated to the bronchial tree.[23] It is likely that additional mechanisms pertain in this group. Pulmonary bullae, emphysema, bronchiectasis, and tuberculosis have been associated with peripheral epidermoid malignancies.[24-27]

The pathogenesis of small cell carcinoma is not understood. It is presumed that the tumors arise from the basal reserve cells, and particularly from the granular basal cells (K-type cells) identified in bronchial and bronchiolar mucosa and bronchial mucous glands. The high incidence of this type of malignancy in smokers, particularly in miners who smoke and are simultaneously exposed to radiation particles, suggests a mechanism similar to the epidermoid malignancy described above.[28] Although basal cell hyperplasia, squamous metaplasia, and/or dysplasia may be identified in the bronchial mucosa of patients with small cell tumors, it is difficult if not impossi-

ble to identify the site of origin of these tumors in the bronchial mucosa. Usually a discrete lamina separates the mucosa from the underlying infiltrating malignancy. It is equally difficult to prove their origin from bronchial mucous glands by usual light-microscopic techniques. Spencer has stated that at least one-fifth of these tumors arise in peripheral locations.[23]

The mechanisms of development of adenocarcinomas and large cell carcinomas of the lung are equally obscure. In the United States a small portion of these tumors can definitely be identified as arising from the bronchial surface epithelium or underlying mucous glands. The majority of these tumors are peripheral in location and are unrelated to bronchial structures, except by contiguous growth. Spencer and Woolner have estimated that over three-fourths of these tumors arise in peripheral locations.[23,29] Factors associated with their induction are variable and are probably additive. Exogenous agents implicated include pneumonconiotic dusts, asbestos, cadmium, beryllium, chemical gases, mineral oils, viruses, and mycobacteria.[23] Chronic interstitial pulmonary diseases, such as scleroderma, rheumatoid lung disease, interstitial pneumonitis, and sarcoidosis, which may terminate in focal or diffuse rigidity and honeycombing of the lungs, have been associated predominantly with adenocarcinoma and less commonly with other cell types.[30-33] Pulmonary scars and fibrosis resulting from pulmonary infarcts, tuberculosis, chronic lung abscesses, and other necrotizing pulmonary diseases have been cited as predisposing factors.[30-34] In each of these conditions there is implied destruction, fibrosis, and reconstruction of the pulmonary airways into essentially nonfunctional spaces.

The progressive pulmonary fibrosis, avascularity, and local tissue anoxia stimulate proliferation of the bronchioloalveolar epithelium. Hyperplastic cells extend by contiguity over the adjoining walls or into the newly formed pulmonary spaces, resulting in adenomatous foci that are difficult on occasion to distinguish from bronchioloalveolar carcinomas.[35,36] Frequently these cells become metaplastic and mucous-producing. In some instances basal-type cells proliferate or form peribronchiolar cell nests measuring up to 3 mm in diameter that are similar in appearance and pattern to carcinoids. Such focal zones of hyperplasia have been termed tumorlets by Whitwell.[37] In other instances bronchiolar and reconstructed alveolar walls may be lined by metaplastic stratified squamous epithelium. It is possible that these hyperplastic or metaplastic processes may be the precursor states of the variable tumor types arising in the periphery of the lung.

CLASSIFICATION OF MAJOR TYPES OF LUNG CANCER

There has been a steady increase in the number of pathologists who have accepted the concept and attempted to utilize the WHO histologic classification of lung tumors published in 1967.[38] This classification was initially devised in 1958. A modified form was used by Yesner, Gerstl, and Auerbach, beginning in 1958, to evaluate surgical material submitted by the VA Lung Cancer Chemotherapy Study Group (VALG).[39] This panel found that substantial agreement could be obtained in the differentiated malignancies and in the so-called oat cell subtype of small cell carcinomas. No significant consistency was achieved in the poorly differentiated or anaplastic large cell tumors or in the various subtypes of small cell carcinoma. Yesner suggested that this lack of consistency may have occurred because the modified classification lacked distinctive criteria for poorly differentiated epidermoid tumors and/or required the use of mucin stains to detect poorly differentiated adenocarcinomas. These latter neoplasms are placed in the large cell category in the WHO classification if no glands are identified in the tissue specimen.

In 1972 the pathology panel of the Working Party for Therapy of Lung Cancer (WP-L), in conjunction with the pathology panel assembled at the International Workshop for Therapy of Lung Cancer, agreed on a classification of lung tumors that adhered closely to the WHO classification.[40] The major modifications included combining the fusiform, polygonal, and tubular forms of small cell carcinoma into an intermediate group and subtyping adenocarcinomas according to differentiation and papillary pattern. As in the WHO classification, stratification and intercellular bridge and/or keratin formation were required for poorly differentiated epidermoid carcinomas.

Table 4-1

Comparison of the World Health Organization (WHO), Veterans Administration Lung Cancer Chemotherapy Study Group (VALG) and Working Party for Therapy of Lung Cancer (WP-L) Lung Cancer Classifications

WHO	VALG	WP-L
I. Epidermoid carcinoma	1. Squamous cell carcinoma (a) with abundant keratin (b) with intercellular bridges (c) without keratin or bridges	10. Epidermoid carcinoma 11. Well differentiated 12. Moderately differentiated 13. Poorly differentiated
II. Small cell carcinoma 1. Fusiform 2. Polygonal 3. Lymphocytelike 4. Others	2. Small cell carcinoma (a) with oat cell structure (b) with polygonal cell structure	20. Small cell carcinoma 21. Lymphocytelike 22. Intermediate cell
III. Adenocarcinoma 1. Bronchogenic a. Acinar b. Papillary 2. Broncioloalveolar	3. Adenocarcinoma (a) acinar (b) papillary (c) poorly differentiated	30. Adenocarcinoma 31. Well differentiated 32. Moderately differentiated 33. Poorly differentiated 34. Bronchiolopapillary
IV. Large cell carcinoma 1. Solid tumor with mucin 2. Solid tumor without mucin 3. Giant cell 4. Clear cell	4. Large cell undifferentiated	40. Large cell carcinoma 41. With stratification 42. Giant cell 43. With mucin formation 44. Clear cell

Acinar formation was a prerequisite for diagnosing poorly differentiated adenocarcinomas. Table 4-1 contrasts the 1967 WHO classification with the VALG and WP-L modifications. Morphology in this chapter is based on these classifications, particularly the WP-L modification.

INCIDENCE OF LUNG CANCER BY CELL TYPE

The relative frequency of incidence of the four major cell types of lung cancer varies according to the source and type of material. Biopsy and cytology specimens may be subject to misinterpretation if insufficient material is submitted for evaluation, if bronchial brushings are poorly fixed, or if sputa or other cytologic fluids contain only a few diagnostic neoplastic cells. Surgical or technical crushing of tissues, extensive tumor necrosis, and staining artifacts may also make interpretation of biopsy specimens difficult if not impossible. Differentiated malignancies and small cell tumors tend to be diagnosed as readily and as accurately in cytologic specimens as in minute biopsies, particularly if representative portions of the tumor have not been sampled in the biopsies.

Table 4-2 compares the incidences of lung cancer, based on biopsy and cytology material, reported by Mountain et al. in their TNM system for staging of lung cancer,[41] by Yesner et al. in the VALG studies reported in 1965,[39] and by Feinstein et al. in the Yale–West Haven VAH data published in 1974.[42] Preliminary data are also presented for similar material being studied by the pathology panel of the WP-L.[43] Percentages have been rounded to the nearest whole number for simplicity. There appears to have been a significant reduction in the percentage of epidermoid carcinomas from 1965 to 1974 as reported by Yesner. The increase in the percentage of adeno-

carcinoma is striking. The increased incidence of small cell tumors in the WP-L series is partially due to early activation of chemotherapy and radiotherapy protocols for this responsive group of neoplasms.

It is clear that surgical lung specimens do not give a true perspective on the incidence of lung cancer. Patients with small cell carcinoma are rarely considered surgical candidates if the tumor can be diagnosed by other techniques. A small percentage of these are resected when located in peripheral zones. Table 4-3 contrasts the incidence of lung cancer by cell type in surgical specimens reported by Hinson et al.[44] in London and in a similar group of specimens removed by the VA Surgical Adjuvant Group (VASAG) monitored by Higgins and Shields. Sections from this latter group were reviewed by the WP-L reference pathologist.[45] The predominance of epidermoid malignancies in the Hinson study is striking. The proportions of well-differentiated, moderately differentiated, and poorly differentiated epidermoid carcinomas appear consistent in the two groups. Although there are relatively few small cell tumors in either series, it is interesting that the so-called lymphocytelike tumor or oat cell tumor is present in a relatively small percentage in both groups. Whether this relates to the peripheral nature of these surgically resected tumors or whether it is due to a fairly precise definition of the lymphocytelike subtype is difficult to determine. The paucity of adenocarcinomas in the London study is also striking. Since only 3 of 64 patients had positive bronchial biopsies, it is presumed that these tumors were peripheral in location. The variation in the subtyping is not understood. A reluctance to interpret adenocarcinomas as bronchiolar in origin may play some role in this discrepancy. If the tumors are, in fact, distinct bronchogenic adenocarcinomas, they represent a different form than is seen in the United States.

Table 4-2

Incidence of Lung Cancer by Cell Type in Biopsy and Cytology Specimens

Cell Type	TNM (2155 Cases)	VALG (1965) (1120 Cases)	Yale–VA (1974) (449 Cases)	WP-L (383 Cases)
Epidermoid carcinoma	46%	49%	36%	38%
Small cell carcinoma	17%	19%	22%	29%
Adenocarcinoma	24%	16%	29%	23%
Large cell carcinoma	9%	16%	13%	9%

Table 4-3

Incidence of Lung Cancer by Cell Type in Surgical Lung
Specimens

Cell Type	London (740 Cases)	VASAG (244 Cases)
Epidermoid carcinoma	71%	56%
Well differentiated	19%	14%
Moderately differentiated	45%	53%
Poorly differentiated	35%	33%
Small cell carcinoma	12%	3%
Lymphocyte type	37%	13%
Intermediate	63%	87%
Adenocarcinoma	9%	28%
Well to poorly differentiated	92%	46%
Papillary	8%	54%
Large cell carcinoma	7%	10%
Adenosquamous carcinoma	1%	2%
Others	1%	1%

It is possible that autopsies most closely
reflect the incidence of lung cancer by cell type.
Table 4-4 compares Auerbach's most recent
autopsy study of 662 patients with lung cancer
treated at the VAH, East Orange, New Jersey,
over a period of 17 years[46] with a similar study of
418 patients treated over a 10-year period at the
VAH, Washington, D.C.[47] Because of the VAH
population, the studies were basically limited to
males. Twelve of 80 patients in the Washington,
D.C. study with large cell carcinoma showed rare
glandular maturation in one or rarely two distant
metastatic foci. Because of the predominant anaplastic nature of the tumors, it was elected to
retain these tumors in the large cell category. If
the percentages are corrected for these 12 cases,
adenocarcinomas will represent 29 percent of the

tumors and large cell carcinomas 16 percent. The
overall similarity of percentages in the two groups
is impressive.

EPIDERMOID CARCINOMA

The majority of central epidermoid carcinomas are susceptible to early diagnosis through
monitoring of sputum cytology in high-risk
patients. The earliest form of carcinoma (intraepithelial, noninfiltrating) may present grossly as
localized, slightly red granular plaques or as gray
white leukoplakic foci that may spread from subsegmental or segmental bronchial junctures proximally or distally for distances up to several centimeters.[14] Infiltrating malignancies present as

Table 4-4

Incidence of Lung Cancer by Cell Type in Autopsy
Material.

Cell Type	VAH (N.J.) (662 Cases)	VAH (D.C.) (418 Cases)
Epidermoid carcinoma	35%	30%
Small cell carcinoma	25%	24%
Adenocarcinoma	25%	26% (29%)*
Large cell carcinoma	14%	19% (16%)*
Mixed	1%	

*See text.

bulky fungating gray white or yellow intraluminal bronchial masses. The tumors tend to grow centrally toward the main stem bronchus, obstruct bronchial lumina, and locally invade underlying bronchial cartilages, lymph nodes, and adjoining lung parenchyma. Macholda has attributed this central growth of tumors to the more adequate blood supply present in the proximal segments of the bronchial tree.[16] A small percentage of epidermoid malignancies are papillary in type, and they present as a cauliflowerlike intraluminal growth. Approximately 10 percent of the more distal epidermoid tumors may show central necrosis, caseation, and cavitation. Paulson reports that almost one-half of operable superior sulcus or Pancoast tumors are of this cell type.[48] Organizing pneumonia and abscesses may be identified in the distal obstructed lungs. Coexistent diseases such as emphysema, bronchiectasis, and granulomata may be present. Anthracosilicotic nodules are frequently seen.

In almost all epidermoid malignancies the bronchial mucosa adjacent to the mass shows evidence of squamous metaplasia, dysplasia, or frank intraepithelial neoplasia. These changes assist in confirming the primary nature of the tumor, and they exclude the possibility of a metastatic lesion or bronchial invasion by a primary esophageal malignancy. In well-differentiated infiltrating malignancies there is an abundance of keratin formation. Cells grow in stratified or pseudoductal patterns and may form small whorls or nests. Squamous cells are connected by intercellular bridges that give the cells a prickle appearance, resembling the malpighian layer of the skin. Individual cells may show evidence of intracellular keratinization or may coalesce to form epithelial pearls, which are small foci composed of degenerated and necrotic malignant cells and keratotic debris. Atypical mitotic figures are present and may be abundant. Nuclei are enlarged and have irregular membranes and dense chromatin patterns. Giant nuclei and multinucleated giant cells may be observed. In the cavitary lesions there is extensive central keratinization and necrosis that give this type of tumor its characteristic caseous gross appearance. Calcification of the necrotic debris occurs, but in insufficient quantity to be radiologically apparent. Epidermoid tumors involving the superior sulcus also tend to be well differentiated. Papillary tumors that form exophytic intraluminal bronchial masses are composed of fibrous fronds lined by

multiple layers of neoplastic squamous epithelial cells resting on a basement membrane. There may be only limited superficial infiltration of the stroma in this type of tumor. Moderately differentiated neoplasms show less evidence of keratin formation, less cellular organization, and more marked nuclear atypia (Fig. 4-1). Few tumors, except for the Pancoast and cavitary types, are well differentiated. The majority of tumors overlap in subtype, not only in primary but also in metastatic foci. This pleomorphic lack of uniformity is a distinguishing feature of lung cancers, regardless of type.

In poorly differentiated tumors, stratification, intercellular bridge formation, and/or occasional foci of individual cell keratinization are demonstrable. The tumors are composed predominantly of anaplastic cells that show no attempt at maturation. Nuclei may be bizarre and enlarged, with prominent nucleoli and/or acidophilic inclusions. Giant cells may be present. The cytoplasm is variable in appearance. Some sheets of cells may have clear empty cytoplasm, reminiscent of hypernephroid neoplasms. Special stains may identify glycogen in some of these cells. Fat droplets, usually identified in renal tumors, are not present.

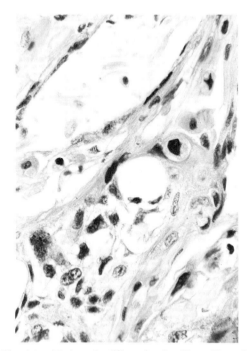

Fig. 4-1. Moderately differentiated epidermoid carcinoma, lung (H&E, × 400).

Bronchial biopsies and cytologic examination of sputa and bronchial washings or brushings constitute the most frequent and effective methods of identifying epidermoid malignancies. Discrepancies in diagnosis almost inevitably occur in the interpretation of poorly differentiated tumors. In some instances cytologic diagnoses may more accurately reflect the proper typing of the tumor than diagnoses rendered on the basis of minute or inadequate bronchial biopsies. It is important to stress that biopsies from metastatic sites, such as the liver, lymph nodes, or bone, may be inadequate for typing, particularly if only anaplastic portions of the tumor have been sampled. In such instances pulmonary cytology may be more reliable in indicating cell type.

Epidermoid carcinomas, when moderately differentiated or well differentiated in type, tend to be locally invasive. Mediastinal invasion may result in superior vena cava obstruction, particularly if the tumor is located in the right upper lobe.[49] In a retrospective study of 131 patients who died within 1 month of a curative surgical resection,[50] 44 patients (33 percent) had evidence of residual disease. In 22 patients the tumor was limited to mediastinal lymph nodes or the region of the bronchial stump. The remaining 22 patients had evidence of extrathoracic extension to abdominal lymph nodes, adrenals, liver, and kidneys. The alternate lung was involved in 3 cases. The development of discriminate staging procedures to identify these early sites of metastases seems important to the appropriate surgical, radiotherapeutic, and chemotherapeutic management of these patients.

In the autopsy study[47] at the Washington, D.C., VAH, 126 patients had epidermoid carcinoma. The tumor was restricted to the thorax in 58 cases (46 percent). The tumors variously invaded mediastinal lymph nodes and soft tissues, the pericardium, pleura, chest wall, and/or ribs. Extrathoracic metastases to the liver, adrenals, kidneys, and bones occurred in 20–25 percent of the cases. The alternate lung was involved in 21 percent. Auerbach reported a similar distribution of metastases in his recent autopsy series,[46] except that 37 percent had metastases to the liver and 35 percent to the central nervous system. Of 35 NCI-VA lung cancer protocol patients treated for epidermoid carcinoma,[47] 6 patients had poorly differentiated tumors. In none of these cases was the tumor limited to the thor-ax. In 5 of the 6 patients there was evidence of metastases to the mucosa and/or submucosa of the small bowel.

SMALL CELL CARCINOMA

Small cell carcinoma may provoke minimal bronchial changes, or the mucosa may be slightly lifted to form a soft white velvety plaque that obliterates normal bronchial markings. Kato et al. reported that in 41 cases in which the bronchial mucosa appeared normal, bronchial biopsies were positive in 22 cases.[51] The tumors tend to spread early and rapidly in a centrifugal pattern and extensively invade the adjoining bronchial, hilar, and mediastinal lymph nodes and soft tissues. Superior vena cava compression, with or without bland or tumor thrombi, may be present. Metastases frequently occur before pulmonary symptoms are recognized. Grossly the tumors tend to be bulky, soft, and gray white. In zones of necrosis the tumor may have a glossy mucoid cut surface. Frequently the tumor forms red hemorrhagic masses and nodules. Bronchial lumina may be stenosed circumferentially late in the course of the disease, but bulky intraluminal masses are rarely produced.

The classic oat cell or lymphocyte type of small cell tumor is composed of cells with small round to oval to spindled nuclei and scant indistinct cytoplasm (Fig. 4-2). The cells are almost twice the size of a lymphocyte. Nuclei are vesicular; they have indistinct nucleoli and a fine salt-and-pepper chromatin distribution. In areas of necrosis or in small biopsies, cells tend to have dense smudged hyperchromatic nuclei. Cells are arranged in clusters, ribbons, trabeculae, or small nests and are supported by a thin vascular fibrous matrix. Mitotic figures may be difficult to identify, particularly in biopsy specimens. In zones of necrosis a basophilic smudgy or granular material is frequently deposited in necrotic tissues and blood vessel walls; it is similar to the encrustation of calcium on elastic fibrils in pulmonary calcinosis. Azzopardi has demonstrated that this material is Feulgen-positive and DNA in character.[52] The staining is presumably caused by excess amounts of DNA liberated by the degenerating and necrotic cells. Cells tend to crush readily, pariticularly in small biopsy specimens, making identification of much of the tumor difficult.

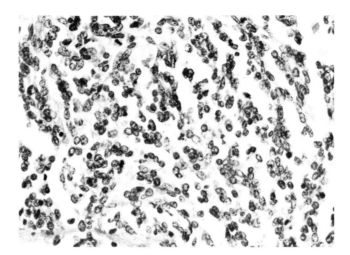

Fig. 4-2. Small cell carcinoma, lymphocytelike type (H&E, × 400).

This crush phenomenon is almost pathognomonic of small cell carcinomas, although lymphoid tissue may also present such artifacts. Isolated neoplastic cells unrelated to the crush zones must be identified before a diagnosis can be established. Silver stains used to identify neurosecretory granules are uniformly negative, although these granules are routinely found in electron micrographs of these tumors.

In the WP-L classification the intermediate form of small cell carcinoma includes tumors composed of cells with larger, more fusiform, and/or polygonal nuclei (Fig. 4-3). Nucleoli are small and indistinct. Nuclear chromatin is stippled. The majority of cells appear devoid of cytoplasm. Some cells, however, do have distinct cytoplasmic structures, and on occasion the cells may fuse to form multinucleated giant cells. The cells may form stratifying nests, cords, rosettes, or tubules. Mitotic figures may be identified. In autopsy and biopsy material there is frequently an admixture of the two subtypes. In some tumors there may be small foci of large cell carcinoma, or cells may show an abrupt transition to squamous epithelium. The rosette or tubular pattern may mimic adenocarcinoma, particularly in metastatic sites. When this pattern is prominent, the tumor is frequently diagnosed as an adenocarcinoma. These varying attempts at maturation to form glands or squamous or anaplastic large cell patterns suggest to some researchers an entodermal derivation of the tumor.[53] It is probable that small cell tumors are derived from both granular and small basal reserve cells, thus explaining the multipotential of a few of these neoplasms.

It is worth reemphasizing that regardless of subtype it is essentially impossible to recognize the primary site of origin of these tumors. Bronchial mucosal changes overlying the tumor imply chronic injury to the respiratory tract and give

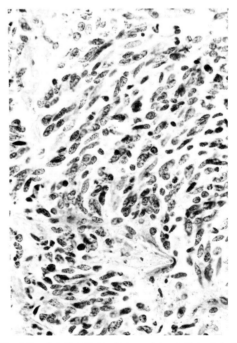

Fig. 4-3. Small cell carcinoma, intermediate spindle cell type (H&E, × 400).

indirect evidence of the primary nature of the tumor.

An attempt has been made to identify differences in behavior at autopsy between the two subtypes of small cell tumors.[47] None has been found. It is apparent, however, that there is a small subset of this type of tumor that responds poorly, if at all, to therapy. There is another small subset in which patients survive beyond all reasonable expectations. It is possible that malignant carcinoids represent some percentage of these subset populations.

Bronchial biopsies, cervical or mediastinal lymph node biopsies, bronchial washings, and sputa provide the most effective means of diagnosing small cell tumors. Cytologic diagnosis, in experienced hands, is as accurate as tissue diagnosis. Discrepancies in diagnosis may occur if cells with distinct cytoplasm are interpreted as large cell tumors, if the dysplastic squamous cells frequently associated with this neoplasm are interpreted as malignant, or if clusters of naked cells (similar in size to lymphocytes or smaller than lymphocytes) are overinterpreted.

Small cell tumors, in addition to their extensive mediastinal invasive tendencies, metastasize widely and early. Of 19 patients with this cell type who underwent curative pneumonectomy or lobectomy and died within 1 month of surgery, there was evidence of residual disease in 13.[50] In 12 of the 13, abdominal lymph nodes, liver, adrenals, brain, and kidney were involved in metastases. The same pattern was manifest in the Washington, D.C., VAH autopsy study of 102 patients with small cell carcinoma.[47] The liver (74 percent), adrenals (55 percent), abdominal lymph nodes (52 percent), pancreas (41 percent), bone (37 percent), and central nervous system (29 percent) were the predominant sites of metastases.

One-fourth of the patients with bony metastases demonstrated marked osteoblastic activity and new bone formation, similar to that seen in bony metastases from the prostate or breast. Pancreatic involvement was associated with peripancreatic lymph node disease. In the earliest forms of pancreatic metastases, parenchymal lymphatics were dilated and plugged with neoplastic cells, thus suggesting a retrograde extension into the pancreas. In almost all cases there was an associated focal acute pancreatitis with fat necrosis. In 3 cases the pancreatitis was massive and hemorrhagic. In 11 cases the tumors in the pancreas were massive. It is possible that these latter cases

represented primary pancreatic neoplasms. The difficulty in establishing the primary nature of this tumor in the lung has been mentioned. The same difficulty pertains to the pancreas. Endocrine organs were also the sites of metastases in a significant number of cases: thyroid (18 percent), pituitary (15 percent), testes (7 percent), parathyroid (1 percent). The ovary of 1 female was also involved. Of greater interest, the tumor metastasized to pituitary adenomata in two instances and to thyroid and parathyroid adenomata in two other instances. The association of these adenomata with small cell carcinoma would tend to reinforce the concept of neurocrestopathies and the interrelationship of multiple endocrine organs and neural-crest-derived cells.[11]

ADENOCARCINOMA

A small percentage of adenocarcinomas of the lung arise from the bronchial surface epithelium or underlying mucous glands. Bronchi present as thick, firm, gray white pipe-stemmed structures with narrowed or stenosed lumina. It is difficult in many instances to distinguish this neoplasm from pancreatic, renal, breast, and colonic tumors that metastasize to bronchi.[54] The majority of adenocarcinomas arise in peripheral locations that are unrelated to bronchi except by contiguous growth or lymphatic dissemination.[23,55–59] The tumors tend to provoke a desmoplastic response, and grossly they present as firm circumscribed subpleural masses with gray white mucoid cut surfaces. The overlying pleura tends to be thickened and puckered. The lesions are frequently smaller in size than tumors of other cell types, although occasionally giant forms may be seen. DeLarue has estimated that 5 percent of such large tumors may cavitate.[55] In some instances the tumors may be overlooked at autopsy or may be mistaken for subpleural scars. Tumors associated with preexisting scars tend to have a central pigmented core. The tumors tend to invade the overlying pleura. In about 5 percent of the cases the tumor may disseminate over the pleural surface forming a thick 1–2-cm gray white pannus.[60] It is difficult at times to distinguish this form from malignant mesotheliomas or carcinomas metastatic to the pleura from extrathoracic sites. With careful search a subpleural parenchymal lesion can usually be identified.

In classic bronchioloalveolar malignancies

the tumors may resemble the subpleural nodules described above. Less often the tumors present as multicentric unilateral or bilateral nodules, or at autopsy they may be mistaken for a confluent or lobar type of pneumonia with mucoid gray cut surfaces suggesting *Klebsiella* infection. Coexistent chronic pulmonary disease, fibrosis, and/or honeycombing may be identified in the uninvolved portions of the lung.

In adenocarcinomas arising from bronchial surface epithelium a transition may be observed from a hyperplastic columnar epithelial lining to a frankly neoplastic epithelium that proliferates to form acinar structures. Rarely the cells may be thrown into papillary folds that project into the lumina. Adenocarcinomas arising from bronchial mucous glands tend to form lobules of neoplastic glands, which may be mucin-producing or may be arranged in a complicated cribriform pattern. In a number of cases no distinct bronchogenic or bronchiogenic origin can be determined. The pulmonary parenchyma adjacent to peripheral tumors usually show foci of fibrosis with hyperplasia and atypia of cells lining bronchioles, alveoli, or pulmonary spaces. In scar-related tumors the central core is composed of fibrocollagenous connective tissue within which elastic fibers and an abundance of pigment granules may be identified. Spencer relates this accumulation of pigment in the scar to lymphatic blockage produced by the fibrosing process.[23] About the periphery of the lesion cells propagate along preexisting alveolar walls and spaces in single or multiple layers, forming papillations or lining papillary fibrous fronds. In the more central portion of the tumor, cells may be anaplastic or may form glandular structures. In the classic bronchioloalveolar carcinoma the bronchioles and alveolar septa are lined by proliferating neoplastic columnar epithelial cells that invaginate to form intraalveolar papillary processes (Fig. 4-4). These tumors may be indistinguishable from tumors metastatic to the lung from extrathoracic sites. In the majority of peripheral tumors there is a combination of glandular and papillary processes (Fig. 4-5). Such tumors in the kidney, ovary, thyroid, uterus, or colon are termed papillary adenocarcinomas. This term seems appropriate in the lung; it suggests maturity and differentiation of the neoplasm rather than histogenesis. There is a growing consensus that the majority of tumors with this papillary differentiation are, in fact, peripheral and bronchiolar in origin.

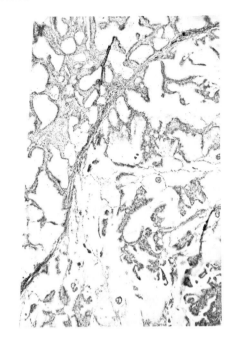

Fig. 4-4. Bronchioloalveolar carcinoma (H&E, × 50).

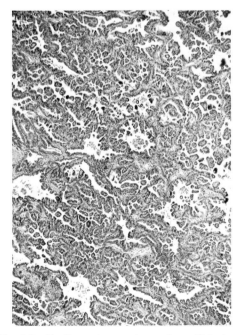

Fig. 4-5. Papillary adenocarcinoma (bronchioloalveolar carcinoma) (H&E, × 25).

In well-differentiated nonpapillary adenocarcinomas of the lung, neoplastic cuboidal or columnar cells proliferate to form relatively uniform glandular or acinar structures supported by a fibrous stroma. Nuclei may be enlarged, irregular, and vesicular with prominent nucleoli. The cytoplasm may contain mucin vacuoles. Mitoses are readily identifiable. In moderately differentiated tumor the cells may be arranged in nests or irregular lobules, may form small acini or glands, or may be arranged in a cribriform pattern. Nuclei are pleomorphic, and the stroma may be desmoplastic. Poorly differentiated tumors are composed of anaplastic cells with enlarged variable vesicular nuclei, prominent nucleoli, and abundant cytoplasm. Cytoplasm may contain mucin or clear vacuoles. Cells are arranged in small cords, nests, or sheets with central zones of necrosis. Distinct acinar formation is identifiable. The presence of mucin vacuoles alone is not sufficient to include a tumor in this category in either the WHO or WP-L classification.

In bronchiolopapillary forms of adenocarcinoma cuboidal to columnar epithelial cells proliferate to form glandular or alveolar structures, as was described above. In many areas the alveolar septa provide the framework for the growth of these cells. Elsewhere, a fibrous stroma supports the cells. In the well-differentiated variety the cells are columnar in type; they may contain glycogen or mucin and may have basally located, relatively uniform vesicular nuclei. Mitoses may be difficult to identify. In less well-differentiated types there is more marked nuclear atypism, and giant or multinucleated cells may be present. Acidophilic nuclear inclusions may be identified. Numerous atypical mitotic figures may be seen. Psammoma bodies are identified in 5–15 percent of these tumors.[61] These bodies represent calcified secretions or concretions. They are encrusted with iron and are similar to those formed in papillary tumors of the thyroid and ovary.

Adenocarcinomas of the lung are most frequently diagnosed by needle or surgical lung biopsy or by regional lymph node biopsy. Bronchial biopsies are less frequently diagnostic; when positive, diagnoses are often based on collections of neoplastic cells of indeterminate type plugging bronchial lymphatics or invading the adjoining submucous tissues. Such tumors cannot be distinguished from metastatic lesions.[54] Sputum and bronchial washings or brushings offer a somewhat better mechanism for obtaining diagnostic material. The identification of desquamated papillary cell clusters in cytologic specimens assures accuracy in cell typing. With improvement in fiberoptic bronchoscopic techniques and equipment it is anticipated that only a few small subpleural lesions should remain undiagnosed prior to exploratory thoracotomy.

Adenocarcinomas, when moderately differentiated to well differentiated, whether glandular or papillary in type, tend to invade regional lymph nodes and pleura. Of 30 patients with adenocarcinoma who died within 1 month of curative surgical resection, 13 (43 percent) had metastases to the adrenal glands, central nervous system, abdominal lymph nodes, bone, or alternate lung.[50] In the Washington, D.C., VAH autopsy study,[47] of 110 patients with adenocarcinoma, the mediastinal lymph nodes were involved in 80 percent, the pleura and alternate lung, in 60 percent, the adrenals in 50 percent, the liver in 41 percent, the central nervous system in 37 percent, the bones in 36 percent, and the kidneys and abdominal lymph nodes in 23 percent. The tumor was restricted to the thorax in only 18 percent. Auerbach reported relatively similar percentages, except that the central nervous system was involved in 47 percent, the bone in 44 percent, and the pleura in only 30 percent.[46]

An attempt was made to distinguish differences in behavior of papillary versus glandular lung tumors in the Washington, D.C., VAH autopsy study.[47] No distinction could be made. However, in 10 of 33 NCI-VA protocol patients with poorly differentiated adenocarcinoma, only 1 of 10 had tumor restricted to the thorax.[47] The regional lymph nodes and pleura were involved in 9 of the 10 cases, the alternate lung and liver in 7 cases, and the cardiovascular system, adrenals, bones, and central nervous system in 6 cases. In spite of this small number of tumors, there is little doubt that poorly differentiated tumors behave more adversely and metastasize more widely and frequently than the better-differentiated subtypes.

LARGE CELL CARCINOMA

Large cell carcinomas are epithelial neoplasms that show no obvious evidence of maturation to form prickled squamous cells, acini, or glands (Fig. 4-6). The concept of such a tumor type is particularly important in understanding and interpreting biopsy or surgical lung specimens. The diagnosis does not preclude the possibility that in small distant foci recognizable attempts at differentiation, usually glandular, may be identified. The predominant anaplastic nature of the tumor overshadows feeble attempts at cell differentiation and probably fairly predicts the clinical course of the tumor.

Grossly these tumors tend to be peripheral and subpleural in location and tend to present as large, bulky, somewhat circumscribed masses with gray white, hemorrhagic, or necrotic cut surfaces. Cavitation may be present. The majority of tumors are unrelated to bronchi, except by contiguous growth. They tend to extend into and replace pulmonary parenchyma and invade the overlying pleura.

Microscopically, large cell tumors are a composite of all the anaplastic features described in the poorly differentiated epidermoid carcinomas and adenocarcinomas. In general they are composed of large polygonal, spindle, or oval cells with abundant cytoplasm and large irregular pleomorphic nuclei.Nucleoli are prominent. Occasional intranuclear acidophilic inclusions may be identified. Individual cells may have giant nuclei or may form syncytial multinucleated giant cells. Intracytoplasmic hyalin droplets, glycogen, or mucin may be present. In portions of the tumors, cells may have abundant clear, almost empty cytoplasm. Cells tend to be arranged in small nests, clusters, or stratifying sheets, or in individual cell pattern, supported by a vascular fibrous stroma. Plasma cells and lymphocytes may infiltrate the stroma. Tumors that stratify in the mode of transitional cell carcinomas of the urinary bladder or nasopharynx are included in this group. Such tumors are called poorly differentiated or undifferentiated epidermoid carcinomas by many pathologists. In other tumors, cells may elaborate intracellular mucin. Such tumors are frequently called poorly differentiated or anaplastic adenocarcinomas by some pathologists. Giant cell carcinomas (Fig. 4-7), so called because of the predominance of bizarre cells with giant nuclei and extraordinary quantities of cyoplasm, frequently show cytoplasmic phagocytic activity or contain mucin vacuoles in their cytoplasm.[62] Tumors predominantly composed of clear cells are unusual. Giant cells and clear cells are frequently seen as components of adenocarcinomas, large cell carcinomas, and epidermoid carcinomas. Syncytial

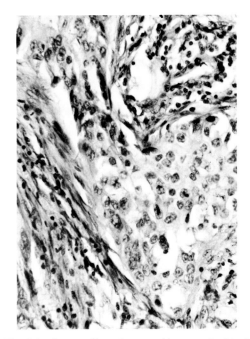

Fig. 4-6. Large cell carcinoma, without mucin (Mucicarmine, × 250).

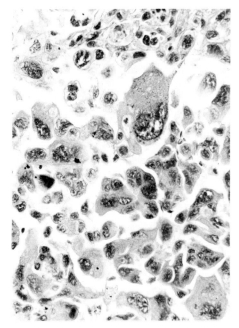

Fig. 4-7. Large cell carcinoma, giant cell subtype (H&E, × 250).

multinucleated giant cells are also occasionally seen in small cell carcinomas prior to treatment. Following therapy, these cells may be so numerous that the basic nature of the tumor may be overlooked.

Large cell carcinomas are most ·frequently diagnosed by needle or surgical lung biopsy or by regional lymph node biopsy. Diagnostic discrepancies occur in bronchial biopsies if representative portions of the tumor are not sampled. Thus a poorly differentiated adenocarcinoma or epidermoid carcinoma may be interpreted as a large cell tumor if only the anaplastic portions of the tumor have been biopsied. Sputum and bronchial washings or brushings of these tumors are frequently interpreted as adenocarcinomas because of the prominent irregular nucleoli present in neoplastic cells. It is possible that the cytopathologist offers more insight into the genesis and typing of this tumor than the tissue pathologist.

In a study of postoperative deaths,[56] 22 patients with large cell carcinoma died within 1 month of surgery. Only 3 of the 22 had evidence of persistent tumor, in spite of the bulky nature of the primary resected tumor. In all 3 patients there were multiple metastases to adrenals, kidneys, liver, and contralateral lung. Among 80 patients with large cell carcinoma studied in the Washington, D.C., VAH autopsy series,[47] 67 percent had tumors that invaded the pleura, while others had metastases: 59 percent in the adrenal glands, 48 percent to the liver, 34 percent to the alternate lung, 32 percent to the cardiovascular system (pericardium and/or heart), 30 percent to bones, 28 percent to kidneys, and 25 percent to the central nervous system. In Auerbach's autopsy series[46] the brain was involved in 49 percent, the adrenals in only 38 percent, and the pleura in 18 percent. In 11 of 18 NCI-VA protocol patients with anaplastic carcinoma the tumors had prominent giant cell components.[47] In 9 of the 11 patients the tumors invaded the pleura or metastasized to the adrenals; in 8 patients there were metastases to the mucosa or submucosa of the small bowel, in 7 patients there were metastases to the pericardium and/or myocardium, and in 6 patients there were metastases to the liver. The metastatic patterns in general resembled the behavior of the adenocarcinomas, except for the propensity to metastasize to the small bowel, which was seen most commonly in poorly differentiated epidermoid carcinomas.

BRONCHIAL CARCINOIDS

During the last century and in the early part of this century several bronchial gland tumors were described. Wessler and Rabin recognized their relatively benign course and favorable prognosis,[63] and Hamperl distinguished two varieties, carcinoids and cylindroids.[64] The majority were of the carcinoid variety; they had features similar to those of intestinal carcinoids, except that argyrophilic granules could not be demonstrated and mucin granules were identified in some.[65,66] In 1958 the carcinoid syndrome was first associated with these tumors,[67,68] and it has been estimated that 2–7 percent of patients with bronchial carcinoids have this syndrome.[69] Bensch et al.[70] demonstrated neurosecretory granules in bronchial carcinoids that were similar in appearance to those identified in intestinal carcinoids. These findings, along with the identification of K-type cells in human bronchial glands and bronchioles, appear to confirm their histogenesis.

Although these tumors can occur at virtually any age from the 1st to the 9th decade,[71,72] they are most frequently present in the 5th decades.[73] Thomas[74] quotes a 4:1 female–male ratio, but neither his series nor others[75,76] demonstrate a sex predilection. The vast majority of these tumors occur in the main, lobar, or segmental bronchi, with only 10–15 percent occurring in subsegmental and peripheral locations. There is a slight predilection for the lower lobes. They most commonly occur at bronchial bifurcations, and they vary from microscopic to over 10 cm in size.[77] Careful examination of the major bronchi at autopsy occasionally may reveal small 2-mm carcinoids at points of bronchial bifurcation.[78] The mucosa overlying the tumor is generally intact, or it may show squamous metaplasia, which explains the low diagnostic rate with exfoliative cytology.

Grossly the tumors tend to project as tongue-like processes into the bronchial lumina. In less than 10 percent of cases the lesions are wholly endobronchial. On reconstructing 9 cases, Goodner et al. demonstrated that in only 1 case was the tumor completely endobronchial, and in 6 cases 30–80 percent of the tumor bulk was outside of the bronchial wall, producing a dumbbell or iceberg configuration.[79] The tumors vary from grayish pink to red, depending on their vascularity, which if it is marked may cause excessive hemorrhage on biopsy.[80] A yellowish coloration appears to be related to positivity of a silver staining reaction.[65]

Microscopically carcinoids resemble the usual foregut variety, with cells arranged in a trabecular or ribbonlike pattern (Fig. 4-8). However, in some areas a mosaic pattern with solid nests of cells surrounded by a thin fibrovascular stroma is formed. Acinar formation and spindle cell variants may be identified. The neoplastic cells have round or ovoid nuclei with a well-defined nuclear membrane and a somewhat vesicular chromatin pattern. The cytoplasm is prominent, pale, eosinophilic, and granular, and there is a striking uniformity in cellular appearance (Fig. 4-9). Necrosis and hemorrhage are uncommon, and mitoses are rare. Small amounts of mucin may be seen. The argentaffine reaction is often negative. The supporting stroma is generally quite vascular, and it may undergo hyalinization as well as osseous or cartilaginous metaplasia.[81] Salyer et al. have stressed that peripheral carcinoids may show a greater degree of cellular pleomorphism with increased numbers of spindle cells and a more disorderly cellular arrangement.[82] A variation (the so-called oncocytoid type of tumor in which the cells are large and resemble the oxyphil cells of the parathyroid gland) has also been described.[83]

The incidence of regional metastases tends to be around 20–30 percent.[83–85] The most frequent sites of extrathoracic spread are liver and bone,[75] the latter being associated with osteoblastic or osteolytic bony lesions. Although the majority of bronchial carcinoids are considered to be of low-grade malignancy, with a reported 5-year survival rate ranging from 56 to 95 percent,[75,76] some cases have a relatively rapid course, with widespread metastases and death occurring within months. Five such highly malignant examples were mentioned by Turnbull et al., and histologically they resembled small cell carcinoma.[75] In the report by Salyer et al. a case of atypical carcinoid is described.[82] Such variants of pulmonary carcinoids, with a histologic appearance and clinical course intermediate between carcinoid and small cell carcinoma, have previously been described by Arrigoni et al.[86] The difficulty in differentiating bronchial carcinoids from small cell carcinoma of the lung in both biopsy and cytology specimens has been stressed by other investigators.[87,88] The distinction is most

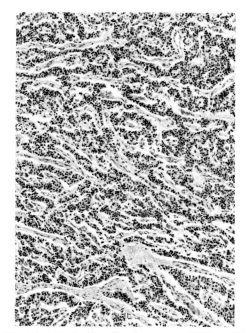

Fig. 4-8. Carcinoid, trabecular pattern (H&E, × 100).

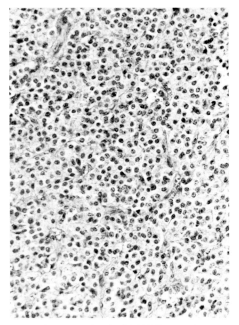

Fig. 4-9. Carcinoid (H&E, × 250).

readily based on the abundant cytoplasm of the carcinoids; in the absence of this as a predominant feature, it may be difficult if not impossible to distinguish the two by light-microscopic techniques.

MESOTHELIOMA

Mesotheliomas are derived from the lining tissues of serosal cavities. Over the years many names have been applied to these tumors, and there has been debate as to their very existence.[89] Klemperer and Rabin used the term mesothelioma.[90] Since then, a number of series of primary mesotheliomas have been reported.[91−105] Their occurrence at autopsy has varied from 0.018 to 0.77 percent.[92] The annual incidence of this tumor in Canada between 1966 and 1970 was 1.4 per million population.[106] In a review of 6406 autopsies performed between 1950 and 1967, Roberts found 20 cases (0.3 percent) of diffuse pleural mesothelioma.[102] Five of these tumors were identified in the first 9 years; 15 were diagnosed in the second 9-year period. Although this is a small number, it does suggest that the incidence of diffuse pleural mesotheliomas is increasing. There is a predominance of these tumors in males, and they have been described as occurring from the ages of 19 months to 92 years, with the majority occurring between 40 and 60 years.[101,107,108] The report of Wagner et al. associating mesothelioma with asbestos exposure has increased interest in this tumor.[109]

Stout proposed a classification of pleural mesotheliomas that divides them into solitary (localized) or diffuse forms, benign or malignant types, composed of epithelial or mesenchymal elements or an admixture of the two.[110] The localized form tends to be predominantly mesenchymal, with a gross and microscopic appearance resembling those of fibromas or fibrosarcomas. It is usually benign and may involve parietal or visceral pleura. Clagett et al. reported 24 cases; 6 were thought to arise from the parietal pleura and 18 from the visceral pleura.[103] These tumors may vary in size from 4 to 36 cm in diameter and may range in weight from 50 to 5,000 g. Grossly they tend to be encapsulated, circumscribed, or well demarcated, with a lobulated gray white to yellow gray fibrous cut surface.[104] Cyst formation, calcification, necrosis, and hemorrhage have

been described.[103,105] An unusual localized mesothelioma was reported by Yesner and Hurwitz[111] in which the tumor was essentially epithelial in nature, and its cut surface had a finely cobbled texture because of light gray and pink papillary projections. Foster and Ackerman reported 18 cases of localized pleural mesotheliomas.[104] Of 17 cases in which follow-up was available, only 2 had died. One had a "coronary," and the second had diffuse bilateral lung metastases. In the latter case there was no evidence of another primary, but no autopsy was performed. A third patient was terminally ill with disseminated renal cell carcinoma.

The diffuse form of mesothelioma generally behaves in a malignant fashion, and it was associated with asbestos exposure in 31 of 32 cases reported by Wagner et al.[109] Of 10 cases described by Godwin,[91] 9 died within 1.5 to 66 months, and a single patient was alive 4 years after the onset of his illness. In the report by Oels et al.,[100] of 37 cases with diffuse malignant mesothelioma, 28 patients died within 1 to 70 months of diagnosis. Five patients were alive with disease from 9 to 60 months from onset of symptoms, and 4 patients were lost to follow-up.

This form of mesothelioma grossly resembles a sheetlike growth of dense, firm, gray white to yellow gray tissue involving the parietal and/or visceral pleura. Caffrey and Lucido demonstrated, through whole lung sections, encasement of the lung, with growth along interlobar fissures by tumor.[112] The greatest pleural thickening is usually over the lower lobes and diaphragm. The cut surface of the tumor may show foci of cyst formation, hemorrhage, and/or necrosis. Invasion of the lung is generally superficial, but compression of the parenchyma may be marked. The tumor tends to infiltrate adjacent structures.

Mesothelial cells in tissue culture grow in both epithelial and mesenchymal fashion, which possibly may explain the morphology of this tumor. The epithelial cells are generally regular and uniform in appearance. Polygonal cells tend to form loosely adherent, varying-size medullary masses, while flattened to cuboidal epithelial cells may form tubular and glandular structures or line fibrous papillary stalks. The cytoplasm of mesothelial cells is fairly abundant; it is eosinophilic and slightly granular. Cytoplasmic vacuoles may be present. The nuclei have distinct membranes, and their outlines may be wrinkled or indented. The nuclear chromatin pattern is finely granular, and nucleoli are usually inconspicuous. In some cases the connective tissue proliferation is abundant, while in others it is sparse. In addition to the various epithelial patterns, there may be an associated proliferation of elongated cells with oval or spindle-shaped nuclei arranged in interwoven bundles. The nuclei are similar to those of the epithelial cells. Although either pattern may occur, the pure fibrous form is uncommon, and the mixed epithelial and fibrous patterns account for approximately 25–50 percent of cases.[108,114] This biphasic histology is diagnostically helpful (Figs. 4-10 and 4-11).

Histochemical analyses offer some assistance in diagnosis. Fine glycogen granules that are faintly positive to periodic acid Schiff (PAS) (which is removed by diastase) may be identified within the tumor cells. Hyaluronic acid has been identified in the pleural effusions of patients with mesothelioma, as well as within the tumor.[115–118] The presence of hyaluronic acid, particularly in and around epithelial cells, is compatible with (but not diagnostic of) this neoplasm,[108] since rapidly proliferating connective tissue also elaborates mucopolysaccharides. The identification of such material in the fibrous portion of the tumor is therefore meaningless. If strong mucicarminophilic material or PAS-positive material that is not removed by diastase is identified in the tumor, there is a strong likelihood that the neoplasm is a primary mucin-producing adenocarcinoma of the lung or a metastatic lesion from the breast, gastrointestinal tract, or pancreas.

There has been a prevailing opinion that malignant mesotheliomas do not metastasize beyond regional lymph nodes. It is possible that metastases occur more frequently than has been recognized. Whitwell and Rawcliffe reported that 50 percent of their autopsied cases showed lymph node metastases. In 15 of 33 cases distant metastatic nodules were identified, particularly in the liver and lung.[119] Metastases to bone, thyroid, brain, adrenals, and kidneys have been recorded.[91,94,102,120] The difficulty in distinguishing mesotheliomas from metastatic tumors or peripheral lung carcinomas must be stressed. The diagnosis of mesothelioma requires a thorough clinical workup to exclude these other tumors. Electron microscopic studies provide significant help in accurately diagnosing this tumor, and they may permit more frequent premortem diagnoses.

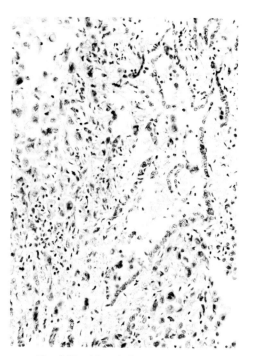

Fig. 4-10. Mesothelioma (H&E, × 200).

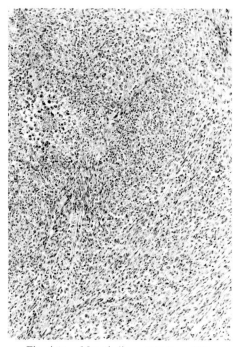

Fig. 4-11. Mesothelioma (H&E, × 100).

CONCLUSIONS

This chapter has attempted to stress the importance of embryology and histology in the development of the major types of lung cancer. The metaplastic potential of both bronchial and bronchiolar epithelium has been emphasized. Major exogenous and endogenous factors that induce these changes have been cited. Utilization of a WHO-oriented lung cancer classification assures some degree of uniformity in diagnoses and permits more meaningful evaluation of clinical data. The differentiated epidermoid, glandular, or papillary carcinomas and most small cell tumors offer few diagnostic problems in either tissue or cytology specimens. Poorly differentiated tumors, and some large and small cell malignancies, may by their very nature defy consistent diagnosis.

Because of the basic entodermal nature of lung tumors, it would be expected that the large majority of pulmonary malignancies would be adenocarcinomas. In fact, many anaplastic large cell carcinomas contain cytoplasmic organelles, suggesting their glandular origin. The adverse behavior of these tumors tends to support their separate classification.

Although this chapter has not discussed the role of the electron microscope, it is apparent that this tool will assume a critical role in the diagnosis of the various types of small cell carcinomas, carcinoids, and mesotheliomas. It may also provide insight and understanding of the morphogenesis of lung cancers of all cell types.

REFERENCES

1. Galofre M, Payne WS, Woolner LB, et al: Pathologic classification and surgical treatment of bronchogenic carcinoma. Surg Gynecol Obstet 119:51–61, 1964

2. Whitwell J: The histopathology of lung cancer in Liverpool; the specificity of the histologic cell type of lung cancer. Br J Cancer 15:440–459, 1961

3. Ratzer ER, Pool JL, Melamed MR: Pleural mesothelioma, clinical experience with thirty-seven patients. Am J Roentgenol Radium Ther Nucl Med 99:863–880, 1967

4. Moore KL: Embryology, The Developing Human. Philadelphia, WB Saunders, 1973, pp 167–173

5. Conen PE, Balis JO: Electron microscopy in the study of lung development, in Emery J (ed): Anatomy of the Developing Lung. London, Heinemann, 1969, chap 3

6. Cutz E, Conen PE: Endocrine-like cells in human fetal lungs: An electron microscopic study. Anat Rec 173:115–122, 1972

7. Soroken SP: The respiratory system, in Greep RO, Weiss L (eds): Histology (ed 3). New York, McGraw-Hill, 1973, pp 675–712

8. Terzakis JA, Sommers SC, Andersson, B: Neurosecretory appearing cells of human segmental bronchi. Lab Invest 26:127–132, 1972

9. Bensch KG, Corrin B, Pariente R, et al: Oat-cell carcinoma of the lung; its origin and relationship to bronchial carcinoid. Cancer 22:1163–1172, 1968

10. Tateishi R: Distribution of argyrophil cells in adult human lungs. Arch Pathol 96:198–202, 1973

11. Bolanch RP: The neurocristopathies; a unifying concept of disease arising in neural crest maldevelopment. Hum Pathol 5:409–429, 1974

12. Horai T, Nishihara H, Tateishi R, et al: Oat-cell carcinoma of the lung simultaneously producing ACTH and serotonin. J Clin Endocrinol Metab 37:212–219, 1973

13. Bensch KG, Gordon GB, Miller LR: Studies on the bronchial counterpart of the Kulchitsky (argentaffin) cell and innervation of bronchial glands. J Ultrastruct Res 12:668–686, 1965

14. Gmelich JT, Bensch KG, Liebow AA: Cells of Kulchitsky type in bronchioles and their relation to the origin of peripheral carcinoid tumor. Lab Invest 17:88–98, 1967

15. Nagaishi C: Pulmonary pleura, in: Functional Anatomy and Histology of the Lung. Tokyo, Igaku Shoin, 1972, pp 254–261

16. Macholda F: Bronchogenic carcinoma; study of growth and evolutionary dynamics of bronchogenic carcinoma; its significance for early diagnosis. Acta Univ Carol [Med] (Praha) [Suppl] 41:39–62, 1970

17. Auerbach O, Gere JB, Pawlowski JM, et al: Carcinoma in situ and early invasive carcinoma occurring in the tracheobronchial tree in cases of bronchial carcinoma. J Thorac Surg 34:298–307, 1957

18. Harris CC, Kaufman DG, Sporn MB, et al: Histogenesis of squamous metaplasia and squamous cell carcinoma of the respiratory epithelium in an animal model. Cancer Chemother Rep 3:43–54, 1973

19. Valaitis JN, McGrew EA, Chomet B, et al: Bron-

chogenic carcinoma in situ in asymptomatic high-risk population of smokers. J Thorac Cardiovasc Surg 57:325–332, 1969

20. Auerbach O, Stout, AP, Hammond, EG, et al: Changes in bronchial epithelium in relation to cigarette smoking and in relation to lung cancer. N Engl J Med 265:253–269, 1961

21. Kotin P, Falk HL: The role and action of environmental agents in the pathogenesis of lung cancer. Cancer 12:147–163, 1959

22. Hueper WC: Role of occupational and environmental air pollutants in production of respiratory cancers. Arch Pathol 63:427–450, 1957

23. Spencer H: Pathology of the Lung (ed 2). London, Pergamon, 1968, pp 778–863

24. Stoloff IL, Kanofsky P, Magilner L: The risk of lung cancer in males with bullous disease of the lung. Arch Environ Health 22:163–167, 1971

25. Berkheiser SW: Bronchiolar proliferation and metaplasia associated with bronchiectasis, pulmonary infarcts and anthracosis. Cancer 12:449–508, 1959

26. Sommers SC: Host factors in fatal human lung cancer. Arch Pathol 65:104–111, 1958

27. Kreus KE, Hakama M, Saxen E: Association of pulmonary tuberculosis and carcinoma of the lung. Scand J Respir Dis 51:276–289, 1970

28. Saccomanno G, Archer, VE, Auerbach O, et al: Histologic types of lung cancer among uranium miners. Cancer 27:515–523, 1971

29. Woolner LB: Atlas of Peripheral Lung Tumors. Chicago, American Society of Clinical Pathologists, 1969

30. Meyer EC, Liebow AA: Relationship of interstitial pneumonia honey-combing and atypical epithelial proliferation to cancer of the lung. Cancer 18:322–350, 1965

31. Batsakis JG, Johnson, HA: Generalized scleroderma involving lungs and liver with pulmonary adenocarcinoma. Arch Pathol 69:633–638, 1960

32. Moolten SE: Scar cancer of lung complicating rheumatoid lung disease. Mt Sinai J Med 40:736–743. 1973

33. Brincker H, Wilbek E: The incidence of malignant tumours in patients with respiratory sarcoidosis. Br J Cancer 29:247–251, 1974

34. Carroll R: The influence of lung scars on primary lung cancer. J Pathol Bacteriol 83:293–297, 1962

35. Berkheiser SE: The significance of bronchiolar atypia and lung cancer. Cancer 18:516–521, 1965

36. Berkheiser SW: Bronchiolar proliferation and metaplasia associated with thromboembolism; a pathological and experimental study. Cancer 16:205–211, 1963

37. Whitwell F: Tumourlets of the lung. J Pathol Bacteriol 70:529–541, 1955

38. Kreyburg L: Histological Typing of Lung Tumors. Geneva, World Health Organization, 1967

39. Yesner R, Gerstl B, Auerbach O: Application of the World Health Organization classification of lung carcinoma to biopsy material. Ann Thorac Surg 1:33–49, 1965

40. Matthews MD: Morphologic classification of bronchogenic carcinoma. Cancer Chemother Rep 3:229–302, 1973

41. Mountain CF, Carr DT, Anderson WAD: A system for the clinical staging of lung cancer. Am J Roentgenol Radium Ther Nucl Med 120:130–138, 1974

42. Feinstein AR, Gilfman NA, Yesner, R: The diverse effects of histopathology on manifestations and outcome of lung cancer. Chest 66:225–229, 1974

43. Matthews MJ, et al: manuscript in preparation

44. Hinson KFW, Miller, AB, Tall R: An assessment of the World Health Organization classification of the histologic typing of lung tumors applied to biopsy and resected material. Cancer 35:399–405, 1975

45. Matthews MJ: unpublished observations

46. Auerbach O, Garfinkel L, Parks UR: Histologic type of lung cancer in relation to smoking habits, year of diagnosis and sites of metastases. Chest 67:382–387, 1975

47. Matthews MJ: Problems in morphology and behavior of bronchopulmonary malignant disease, in Israel L, Chahanian P (eds): Lung Cancer, Facts, Problems and Prospects. New York, Academic, 1976, chap 2

48. Paulson DL: Superior sulcus tumors, results of combined therapy. NY State J Med 71:2050–2057, 1971

49. Salsali M, Clifton EE: Superior vena cava obstruction with lung cancer. Ann Thorac Surg 6:439–442, 1968

50. Matthews, MJ, Kanhouwa S, Pickren J, et al: Frequency of residual and metastatic tumors in patients undergoing curative surgical resection for lung cancer. Cancer Chemother Rep 3:63–68, 1973

51. Kato Y, Ferguson TB, Bennett DE, et al: Oat-cell carcinoma of the lung, a review of 138 cases. Cancer 23:517–524, 1964

52. Azzopardi JG: Oat-cell carcinoma of the bronchus. J Pathol Bacteriol 78:513–519, 1960

53. Shimosato H: personal communication

54. Rosenblatt MB, Lisa JR, Trinidad S: Pitfalls in the clinical and histological diagnosis of bronchogenic carcinoma. Dis Chest 49:396–404, 1966

55. DeLarue ND, Anderson W, Sanders D, et al: Bronchioloalveolar carcinoma, a reappraisal after 24 years. Cancer 29:90–97, 1972

56. Bennett DE, Sasser WF: Bronchiolar carcinoma,

a valid clinicopathologic entity. Cancer 23:876–887, 1969

57. Lisa JR, Trinidad S, Rosenblatt MB: Site of origin and histogenesis and cytostructure of bronchogenic carcinoma. Am J Clin Pathol 44:375–384, 1965

58. Liebow AA: Bronchioloalveolar carcinoma, in Dock W, Snapper I (eds): Advances in Internal Medicine X. Chicago, Year Book, 1960, pp 329–358

59. Campobasso O: The characteristics of peripheral lung tumors that suggest their bronchioloalveolar origin. Br J Cancer 22:655–662, 1969

60. Babolini G: The pleural form of primary cancer of the lung. Dis Chest 29:314–323, 1956

61. Unterman DH, Reingold IM: The occurrence of psammoma bodies in papillary adenocarcinoma of the lung. Am J Clin Pathol 57:297–302, 1972

62. Friedberg, EC: Giant cell carcinoma of the lung. Cancer 18:259–264, 1965

63. Wessler H, Rabin CB: Benign tumors of the bronchus. Am J Med Sci 183:164–180, 1932

64. Hamperl W: Über gutartige bronchial tumoren (Cylindroma und Carcinoide). Virchows Arch [Pathol Anat] 300:46–88, 1937; cited by Weiss L, Ingram M: Cancer 14:161–178, 1961

65. Williams ED, Azzopardi JG: Tumours of the lung and the carcinoid syndrome. Thorax 15:30–36, 1960

66. Holly, SW: Bronchial adenomas. Milit Surg 99:528–554, 1946

67. Stanford WR, Davis JE, Gunter JU, et al: Bronchial adenoma (carcinoid type) with solitary metastasis and associated functioning carcinoid syndrome. South Med J 51:449–454, 1958

68. Warner RRP, Southren AL: Carcinoid syndrome produced by metastasizing bronchial adenoma. Am J Med 24:903–914, 1958

69. Ricci C, Patrassi N, Massa R, et al: Carcinoid syndrome in bronchial adenoma. Am J Surg 126:671–677, 1973

70. Bensch K, Miller L, Gordon G: Fine structural and biochemical studies on the bronchial carcinoid adenoma and its precursor. Am J Pathol 46:30a, 1964 (abstract)

71. Cookson PJ: Delayed osteoblastic metastasis from a childhood bronchial carcinoid tumor. Hum Pathol 5:493–496, 1974

72. Baldwin JN, Grimes OF: Bronchial adenomas. Surg Gynecol Obstet 124:813–818, 1967

73. Carlens E, Wiklund T, Bergstrand A: Bronchial adenoma. Report of 70 cases and critical analysis of literature. Acta Chir Scand [Suppl] 185:1–55, 1954

74. Thomas CP: Benign tumours of the lung. Lancet 1:1–7, 1954

75. Turnbull AD, Huvos AG, Goodner JT, et al: The malignant potential of bronchial adenoma. Ann Thorac Surg 14:453–464, 1972

76. Markel SF, Abell MR, Haight C, et al: Neoplasms of bronchus commonly designated as adenomas. Cancer 17:590–608, 1964

77. Toole AL, Stern H: Carcinoid and adenoid cystic carcinoma of the bronchus. Ann Thorac Surg 13:63–81, 1972

78. Spencer H: Pathology of the Lung (ed 2). London: Pergamon, 1968, p 871

79. Goodner JT, Berg JW, Watson WL: The nonbenign nature of bronchial carcinoids and cylindromas. Cancer 14:539–546, 1961

80. Liebow AA: Tumors of the lower respiratory tract, in: Atlas of Tumor Pathology. Washington, DC, National Research Council, 1952, sect V, fasc 17, p 31

81. Thomas CP, Morgan AD: Ossifying bronchial adenoma. Thorax 13: 286–293, 1958

82. Salyer, DC, Salyer WR, Eggleston JC: Bronchial carcinoid tumors. Cancer 36:1522–1537, 1975

83. Stout AP: Cellular origin of bronchial adenoma. Arch Pathol 35:803–807, 1943

84. Zellos S: Bronchial adenoma. Thorax 17:61–68, 1962

85. Donahue JK, Weichert RF, Oshsner JC: Bronchial adenoma. Ann Surg 167:873–885, 1968

86. Arrigoni MG, Woolner LB, Bernatz PE: Atypical carcinoid tumors of the lung. J Thorac Cardiovasc Surg 64:413–421, 1972

87. O'Grady WP, McDivitt RW, Holman C, et al: Bronchial Adenoma. Arch Surg 101:558–561, 1970

88. Kyriakos M, Rockroff DS: Brush biopsy of bronchial carcinoid—a source of cytologic error. Acta Cytol 16:261–268, 1972

89. Robertson HE: "Endothelioma" of the pleura. J Cancer Res 8:317–375, 1924

90. Klemperer P, Rabin CB: Primary neoplasms of the pleura. Arch Pathol 11:385–412, 1931

91. Godwin MC: Primary mesotheliomas. Cancer 10:298–319, 1957

92. McCaughey WTE: Primary tumours of the pleura. J Pathol Bacteriol 76:517–529, 1958

93. Knappmann J: Beobachtungen an 251 obduzierten Mesotheliomfallen in Hamburg (1958–1968). Pneumonologie 148:60–65, 1972

94. Urschel HC, Paulson DL: Mesotheliomas of the pleura. Ann Thorac Surg 1:559–574, 1965

95. Ehrenhaft JL, Sensenig DM, Lawrence MS: Mesotheliomas of the pleura. J Thorac Cardiovasc Surg 40:393–409, 1960

96. Tobiassen G: Mesotheliomas. Acta Pathol Microbiol Scand [Suppl] 105:198–218, 1955

97. Poulsen T, Sorensen B: Pleural mesothelioma. Acta Radiol [Suppl] (Stockh) 188:216–223, 1959

98. Hourihane DO: A biopsy series of mesothelioma-

ta and attempts to identify asbestos within some of the tumors. Ann NY Acad Sci 132:647–673, 1965

99. Ratzer ER, Pool JL, Melamed MR: Pleural mesotheliomas. Am J Roentgenol Radium Ther Nucl Med 99:863–888, 1967

100. Oels HC, Harrison EG Jr, Carr DT, et al: Diffuse malignant mesothelioma of the pleura: A review of 37 cases. Chest 60:564–570, 1971

101. Semb G: Diffuse malignant pleural mesothelioma. A clinicopathological study of 10 fatal cases. Acta Chir Scand 126:78–91, 1968

102. Roberts GH: Diffuse pleural mesothelioma: A clinical and pathological study. Br J Dis Chest 64:201–211, 1970

103. Clagett OT, McDonald JR, Schmidt HW: Localized fibrous mesothelioma of the pleura. J Thorac Surg 24:213–230, 1952

104. Foster EA, Ackerman LV: Localized mesotheliomas of the pleura. Am J Clin Pathol 34:349–364, 1960

105. Stout AP, Himadi GM: Solitary (localized) mesothelioma of the pleura. Ann Surg 133:50–64, 1951

106. McDonald AD, McDonald JC: Epidemiologic surveillance of mesothelioma in Canada. Can Med Assoc J 109:359–362, 1973

107. Reals WJ, Russum BC, Egan WJ: Mesothelioma of pleura in a child. Am J Dis Child 80:85–90, 1950

108. Churg J, Selikoff I: Geographic pathology of pleural mesothelioma, in Liebow AA, Smith DE (eds): The Lung. Baltimore, Williams & Wilkins, 1968, pp 284–297

109. Wagner JC, Sleggs CA, Marchand P: Diffuse pleural mesothelioma and asbestos exposure in the northwestern Cape Province. Br J Ind Med 17:260–271, 1960

110. Stout AP: Mesotheliomas of the pleura and peritoneum. J Tenn Med Assoc 44:409–411, 1951

111. Yesner R, Hurwitz A: Localized pleural mesothelioma of epithelial type. J Thorac Surg 26:325–329, 1953

112. Caffrey PR, Lucido JL: The clinical and pathologic aspects of pleural mesotheliomas. Surgery 49:690–695, 1961

113. Maximow A: Über das Mesothel (Deckzellen der serösen Häute) und die Zellen der serosen Exsudate. Arch Exp Zellforsch 4:1–42, 1927

114. Magner D: Malignant mesothelial tumors—histologic type and asbestos exposure. N Engl J Med 287:570–571, 1972

115. Meyer K, Chaffee E: Hyaluronic acid in the pleural fluid associated with a malignant tumor involving the pleura and peritoneum. J Biol Chem 133:83–91, 1940

116. Motomiya M, Endo M, Arai H, et al: Biochemical characterization of hyaluronic acid from a case of benign localized pleural mesothelioma. Am Rev Respir Dis 111:775–780, 1975

117. Arai H, Endo M, Sasai Y, et al: Histochemical demonstration of hyaluronic acid in a case of pleural mesothelioma. Am Rev Respir Dis 111:699–702, 1975

118. Wagner JC, Munday DE, Harrington JS: Histochemical demonstration of hyaluronic acid in pleural mesotheliomas. J Pathol Bacteriol 84:73–78, 1962

119. Whitwell F, Rawcliffe RM: Diffuse malignant pleural mesothelioma and asbestos exposure. Thorax 26:6–22, 1972

120. Laurini RN: Diffuse pleural mesothelioma with distant bone metastasis. Acta Pathol Microbiol Scand (Section A) 82:296–298, 1974

Bruce Mackay
Barbara M. Osborne
Roma A. Wilson

5
Ultrastructure of Lung Neoplasms

Electron microscopy can play a valuable role complementary to the role of conventional light microscopy in the diagnosis of human lung neoplasms, but its contribution will vary with the tumor type. Well-differentiated squamous carcinomas and adenocarcinomas are readily identified from their light-microscopic histology, but an undifferentiated small cell carcinoma, with its peculiar proneness to artifactual cytologic distortion and its propensity for presenting in metastatic locations, may present a problem in differential diagnosis that can only be resolved by electron microscopy. The clinical relevance of ultrastructural studies of lung neoplasms is not confined to diagnostic situations. The cytologic detail that is revealed with excellent tissue preservation and high-resolution micrographs illuminates light-microscopic histology and provides a sounder basis for morphologic classification of human lung neoplasms than can be provided by light microscopy alone. Greatest benefit is derived from a close correlation of routine light-micro-

scopic procedures, including histochemistry, with electron microscopy. In turn, precision in the diagnosis and classification of lung neoplasms enhances the significance of clinical evaluations of biologic behavior and therapeutic response.

In this chapter the fine structural features of lung tumors are briefly described, following the main subdivisions of the classification that Drs. Matthews and Gordon have described and that has been adopted by the Working Party for Therapy of Lung Cancer (see Chapter 4). Personal observations are based on a study of over 100 lung tumors. Each lung tumor resected at the M. D. Anderson Hospital is studied by electron microscopy using tissue obtained promptly following surgical excision. An attraction of electron microscopy is the fact that a very small amount of tissue is adequate, provided that it is representative and is properly preserved. Our practice is to expose a fresh-cut surface of the tumor, avoiding areas of hemorrhage and necrosis, and use a clean scalpel blade or razor blade to slice a small wedge of tumor not more than 1 mm in thickness. The tissue is promptly placed in 2 percent glutaraldehyde solution, a supply of which is always available in previously prepared specimen bottles both in the frozen section laboratory and in the electron microscopy laboratory. Where tissue cannot be obtained by surgical excision or open biopsy, a needle biopsy may prove adequate, provided that

This study was supported by Grants NCI ICM 33737 and NCI CA 05831.

We wish to acknowledge the participation of Dr. M. Mandavia in the earliest phase of this study. The technical assistance of Mrs. Joyce Cox and Miss Diana Garza has been invaluable. We are particularly grateful to Dr. C. F. Mountain for his interest and cooperation.

representative tumor is obtained without crushing the artifact. When no other tissue is available, formalin-fixed tumor can be used, but its adequacy depends on the quality of the initial fixation and is consequently variable. Tissue is processed in routine fashion and embedded in Epon, and 1-μ sections stained with methylene blue are viewed by light microscopy prior to the cutting of thin sections for electron microscopy.

SQUAMOUS CARCINOMA

The better-differentiated tumors in this group are readily identified from their light-microscopic histology, and squamous carcinomas that are overall poorly differentiated may contain areas where so-called intercellular bridge formation and/or keratinization can be identified. Where these features cannot be recognized, the distinc-

tion from a poorly differentiated squamous carcinoma may be difficult or impossible by light microscopy.

Figure 5-1 illustrates a small region of a bronchogenic squamous carcinoma in which the tumor is well differentiated. Adjacent tumor cells are united by frequent prominent desmosomes with associated bundles of tonofilaments. It was the illusion of cytoplasmic continuity at these sites that led to the misnomer *intercellular bridges*. When keratin is present within the cytoplasm it is preferentially deposited on the tonofilament bundles, where it appears as relatively homogeneous osmiophilic zones in electron micrographs. As squamous carcinomas dedifferentiate, desmosomes become smaller and less frequent, and tonofilament bundles are correspondingly diminished in number and prominence. Keratin is not usually identified in the poorly differentiated squamous carcinomas.

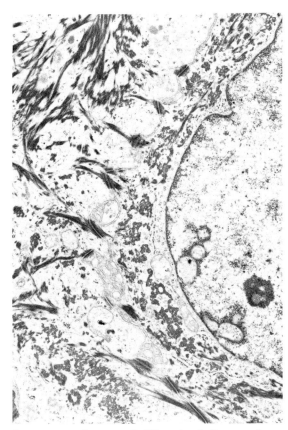

Fig. 5-1. Squamous carcinoma, well differentiated. Tumor cells are united by numerous large desmosomes with prominent tonofilament bundles (×15,000).

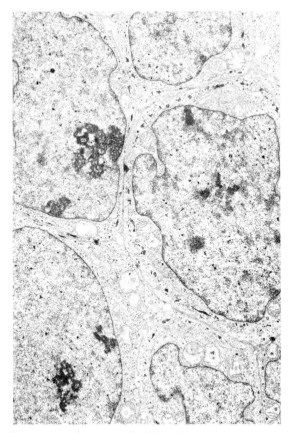

Fig. 5-2. Squamous carcinoma, poorly differentiated. The membranes of adjacent cells are closely apposed, but attempts at acinar formation are not evident and desmosomes are relatively few and small with inconspicuous tonofilament bundles (×8400).

Figure 5-2 illustrates the fine structural features of a rather poorly differentiated zone of a squamous carcinoma. The regions illustrated in Figs. 5-1 and 5-2 were almost contiguous in the same thin section, thus demonstrating that variations in differentiation can occur within a small area of a single neoplasm. In Fig. 5-2 the cell membranes of adjacent cells are closely apposed and are joined by scattered small desmosomes. With increasing dedifferentiation a squamous carcinoma can become indistinguishable from a poorly differentiated bronchogenic adenocarcinoma. Because of variations in differentiation that can occur throughout a tumor, it may be helpful to examine several different areas by electron microscopy rather than base an assessment on a single sampling. In this way, occasional squamous carcinomas will be found to contain foci with features of an adenocarcinoma. The

tumor illustrated in Figs. 5-1 and 5-2 contained areas in which acinar formation could be identified by electron microscopy.

ADENOCARCINOMA

The basic morphologic difference between squamous carcinoma and adenocarcinoma is the tendency of the latter to form acinar structures. As seen by electron microscopy, features of adenocarcinoma cells that will be present in varying degrees, depending on the degree of differentiation of the tumor, include microvilli projecting into the acinar lumen, tight junctions where apposed cell membranes border the lumen, small desmosomes with short tonofilament bundles uniting the lateral surfaces of the cells, and a tendency toward complex infoldings of the apposed lateral cell membranes. Microvilli on the sides of the cells can be seen in Fig. 5-3. A basal lumina may partially or completely invest groups of cells. Acinar lumina may be reduced to small spaces or cleftlike gaps between tumor cells, and microvilli may be infrequent. The latter are not of themselves a reliable criterion for adenocarcinoma since they may be observed at the periphery of loosely packed cells of squamous carcinoma. However, the presence of tight junctions adjacent to acinar spaces is a useful diagnostic feature.

Cytoplasmic components are of limited value in diagnosing adenocarcinomas by electron microscopy, since cytoplasmic polarity is obscured or lost with distortion of acinar formation. Aggregates of secretory material are easily recognized, but identification may depend on the experience of the microscopist, since their

appearance can vary with differing preparatory procedures.

Drs. Matthews and Gordon have discussed the so-called bronchioalveolar form of bronchogenic adenocarcinoma. In an attempt to elucidate the fine structural features of this tumor type and ascertain their specificity, we selected from a group of 40 lung adenocarcinomas 12 tumors that by light microscopy had features suggesting that they might be bronchioloalveolar neoplasms, including a papillary configuration and a tendency for extension of tumor cells along the stroma of distal air spaces. Electron microscopy inevitably revealed the basic ultrastructure of adenocarcinoma that has already been described, but attention was focused on features that might be shared by this group of tumors and that might serve to distinguish them from other adenocarcinomas and possibly throw light on their histogenesis. It

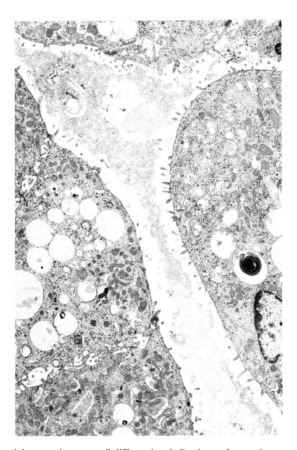

Fig. 5-3. Adenocarcinoma, well differentiated. Portions of several tumor cells are shown bordering an irregularly shaped acinar lumen. Apical microvilli are variable in number, and some lateral microvilli can be seen. Terminal bars and scattered small desmosomes unite adjacent cells. Some cytoplasmic mucin is present ($\times$5400).

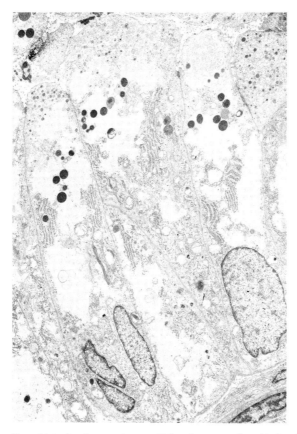

Fig. 5-4. Bronchioloalveolar carcinoma. Tall columnar cells with basal nuclei, extensive cytoplasmic glycogen (clear areas), and in the apical cytoplasm, electron-dense granules and aggregates of mucin. A few short stubby microvilli can be seen on the apical surfaces of the tumor cells at the upper edge of the illustration (×4200).

was readily apparent that the tumors were not identical. Two were mucin-producing adenocarcinomas, while a third showed no cytoplasmic differentiation. Among the remaining nine, some similarities could be recognized, and the cells of the tumor shown in Fig. 5-4 typify their ultrastructure. The tall columnar tumor cells possessed basal nuclei and closely apposed lateral cell surfaces with scanty and inconspicuous desmosomes. Terminal bars were invariably present. Microvilli projected from the apical cell surface, and they were generally short and flat-topped, with slender central filaments that extended downward into the apical cell cytoplasm. A single cilium projected from the apical surface of one cell in one of the tumors. Within the cytoplasm a Golgi complex was present, and endoplasmic reticulum bearing ribosomes was aggregated into stacks of short parallel cisternae. Extensive pools of glycogen occupied considerable portions of the

cell. In the apical cytoplasm, aggregates of mucin droplets could frequently be observed, together with osmiophilic dense granules limited by a closely apposed unit membrane. Lamellar bodies similar to those of type II pneumocytes were observed only ocasionally in these tumor cells.

Since the cytoplasmic features that have been described were confined to adenocarcinomas that by light microscopy were suspected to be of the bronchioloalveolar variety, the electron microscopic findings support specificity of this particular entity. However, it must be emphasized that the features were by no means constant throughout the group. It would appear, therefore, that light microscopy alone is inadequate for identification of tumors of this type. It further seems that the features described indicate a line of differentiation that may be manifested in varying degrees, with the extent being ascertainable only by electron microscopic study of the tumor cells.

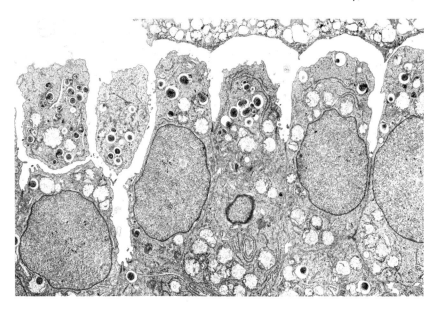

Fig. 5-5. Hyperplastic type II pneumocytes from the periphery of a broncioloalveolar carcinoma. The nuclei appear cytologically benign. Lamellar bodies can be seen in the apical cytoplasm (×5800).

As Kuhn[1] points out, early ultrastructural studies of bronchioloalveolar carcinomas had suggested that the cell of origin was the type II pneumocyte. This conclusion was based on observation of cells containing lamellar inclusions identical to the surfactant precursors of type II pneumocytes. Undoubtedly, cells with this morphology can be observed at the periphery of bronchioloalveolar carcinomas (Fig. 5-5), but the scarcity of lamellar bodies in the cytoplasm of cytologically neoplastic cells within the tumors argues against this hypothesis.[1,2] Tall columnar cells with apical microvilli and no cilia, containing relatively large osmiophilic granules in the apical cytoplasm, resemble the nonciliated bronchiolar (Clara) cells, and there would appear to be no good evidence that the tumors are of pure alveolar derivation. The cells in Fig. 5-5 are probably hyperplastic type II pneumocytes proliferating in the immediate vicinity of the tumor. In view of the common embryonic derivation of cells of the peripheral bronchial and alveolar epithelium, it is possible that different lines of differentiation could be manifested within a tumor arising from the bronchiolar epithelium. This would account for the occasional occurrence of lamellar bodies in the tumor cells and for the presence of mucin in company with the morphologic features of nonciliated bronchiolar cells. The subject is ably discussed by Bedrossian et al.[2]

SMALL CELL CARCINOMA

By light microscopy small cell carcinomas may be seen to be composed of monotonously similar cells that may on occasion exhibit architectural arrangements such as a cribriform pattern but that more often form solid sheets. Areas of necrosis and artifactual distortion are frequent. In the WHO classification an attempt is made to subdivide small cell carcinomas into groups based on the shapes of the cells: fusiform, polygonal, lymphocytelike. In the WP-L classification two groups are recognized: lymphocytelike or oat cell (type 21) and the so-called intermediate cell (type 22).

In order to determine whether a relationship existed between these frequently rather subtle variations in the light microscopic appearance of oat cell carcinomas and their fine structure, we carried out a light microscopic and electron microscopic study of 30 cases. Our hopes of establishing a meaningful subgrouping that could be consistently duplicated were thwarted by our inability to agree on which tumors were type 21 and which were type 22 in the WP-L classification by light microscopy. In the electron microscopic studies of these tumors it was not possible to relate the light microscopic appearance to any specific fine structural variations within the group.

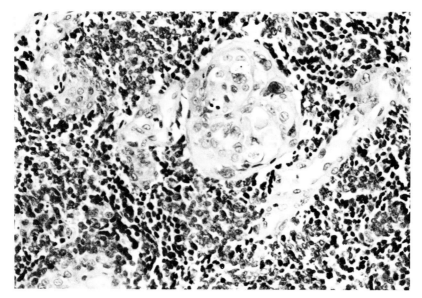

Fig. 5-6. Light micrograph of a small cell carcinoma that contained numerous foci of squamous differentiation. Fine structural features of this tumor are illustrated in Figs. 5-7 and 5-8 (×200).

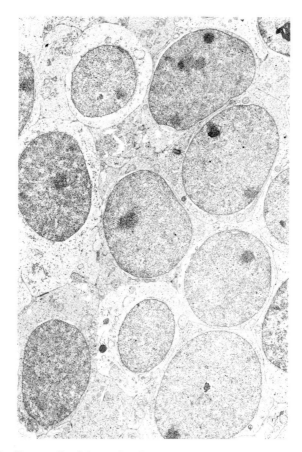

Fig. 5-7. Tumor cells of the small cell carcinoma shown in Fig. 5-6. The cells are monotonously similar, with scanty cytoplasm (×4000).

77

The small cell carcinoma illustrated in Fig. 5-6 consists predominantly of lymphocytelike cells whose fine structure is shown in Fig. 5-7. Nuclei are either round or ovoid, with fine, diffuse chromatin and inconspicuous nucleoli. Cytoplasm is scanty, with sparse organelles. The cell membranes of adjacent cells are closely apposed, without infoldings or surface specializations such as microvilli. Desmosomes are infrequent and minute, frequently being confined to small thickenings of the cell membranes without associated tonofilaments. Only an occasional cell contains a few small secretory granules of the type discussed below. An interesting feature of this tumor is the presence of numerous foci of squamous differentiation, and with the electron microscope the cells within these regions show typical squa-

mous features, including numerous prominent desmosomes and keratin (Fig. 5-8). Smaller desmosomes of the type seen between the oat cells also unite them to the squamous cells, thus arguing for differentiation of the squamous cells from the small cells of the tumor.

In small cell carcinomas in which the cells are elongated rather than ovoid, as in the tumor just described, we have not observed fine structural differences. Occasionally an undifferentiated bronchogenic carcinoma may be composed of cells that are distinctly larger than those of most oat cell carcinomas, but the fine structure is similar and the differentiating features of adenocarcinoma are lacking; we have considered such tumors variants of small cell carcinoma.

Discussion of the histogenesis of small cell

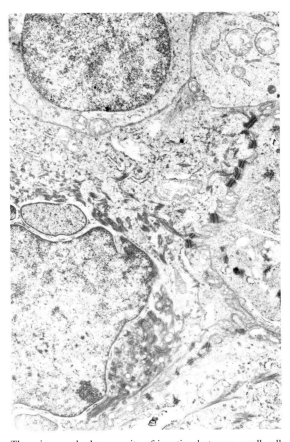

Fig. 5-8. The micrograph shows a site of junction between small cells and squamous cells from the small cell carcinoma in Fig. 5-6. Adjacent squamous cells are united by large desmosomes with prominent tonofilament bundles, characteristic of squamous carcinomas (×15,200).

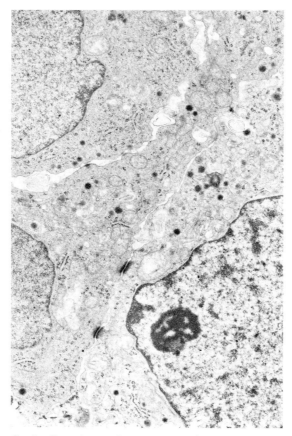

Fig. 5-9. Small cell carcinoma; desmosomes can be seen. The cytoplasm of one cell extends into a pseudopodlike process. Small membrane-bound cytoplasmic granules are present in small numbers in the tumor cell cytoplasm (×19,200).

bronchogenic carcinoma has focused on the observation that the cytoplasm of many of the cells of these tumors contains small secretory granules that are membrane-limited and rarely are more than 170 mμ in diameter. Bensch et al.[3] argued that their presence indicates a relationship between oat cell carcinoma and bronchial carcinoid and that the two might be malignant and locally malignant tumors, respectively, derived from the Kulchitsky cells normally found throughout the bronchial tree. Hattori et al.[4] provided support for this thesis by demonstrating that serotonin levels were elevated in some patients with small cell carcinomas. It appears probable that some small cell bronchogenic carcinomas are indeed derived from Kulchitsky cells of the bronchial epithelium. On the other hand, many small cell carcinomas contain only small numbers of secretory granules, and in our experi-

ence it is rare to encounter a small cell carcinoma containing granules as large or as numerous as those of bronchial carcinoid tumors. It might seem feasible to suggest that this is a consequence of dedifferentiation, but similar instances are rare (if, indeed, they occur at all) within the gastrointestinal tract, a common site of carcinoid tumors. We would agree with Hattori et al.[4] that the cytoplasmic granules in oat cell carcinomas are frequently within pseudopodlike cytoplasmic processes (Fig. 5-9). This is a common feature of neuroectodermal cells. Weichert[5] has suggested that neuroectodermal cells from the embryonic gastrointestinal tract could be carried outward in the developing lung bud and subsequently could participate in neoplastic proliferations, thereby accounting for ectopic hormone production by bronchogenic neoplasms. It would seem reasonable at the present time to suppose that the variations in the light microscopic and electron microscopic morphology of small cell bronchogenic carcinomas might be accounted for by their derivation from different cell types present within the bronchial tree. Further elucidation of these normal cell types and correlation with cells of the small cell carcinomas are required to clarify the situation, and additional ultrastructural studies of hormone-producing lung neoplasms would be welcome. The presence of numerous foci of squamous differentiation in the tumor illustrated in Figs. 5-6, 5-7, and 5-8 suggests that it may have arisen from bronchial reserve cells.

LARGE CELL CARCINOMA

The designation large cell carcinoma is used for epithelial neoplasms that show no discernible evidence of maturation by light microscopy, and cell size would appear to be the primary differentiating feature between tumors in this group and the small cell carcinomas. By electron microscopy some large cell carcinomas show feeble attempts at adenocarcinomatous differentiation, such as small aggregates of microvilli or mucin production. Two subgroups of the large cell carcinomas in the WP-L classification are designated giant cell and clear cell carcinomas. In our experience, areas of pleomorphic cells are not infrequent within bronchogenic adenocarcinomas, while zones of tumor cells having clear cytoplasm in light microscopic sections are relatively common and often extensive in adenocarcinomas and even on occasion in squamous carcinomas.

In pleomorphic zones of adenocarcinoma the cells do not show any specific ultrastructural features, although we have observed two cases in which there was profusion of cytoplasmic organelles, a nonspecific finding shared by giant cells in bone and soft tissue neoplasms. In general, ultrastructural observations support the thesis that pleomorphic carcinomas are poorly differentiated adenocarcinomas.[6]

Clear cells in bronchogenic tumors present a variety of fine structural appearances. Quantities of mucin, lipid, and glycogen may each be responsible for clear cytoplasm by light microscopy, but some clear cells do not contain demonstrable aggregates of secretory material, and electron microscopy reveals only a paucity of organelles. Baker and Soifer[7] found an abundance of free and membrane-bound glycogen in the benign clear cell tumor of the lung that they studied, while Hoch et al.[8] observed intracytoplasmic filaments in their case, prompting them to suggest smooth muscle or pericyte origin.

BRONCHIAL CARCINOID TUMOR

Bronchial carcinoid tumors are derived from the serotonin-producing cells of the bronchial epithelium. The tumor cells exhibit little pleomorphism and are usually spherical with a centrally located nucleus. Adjacent cells are generally closely apposed, with few interdigitations of the cell membranes but with obvious desmosomes possessing short tonofilaments. The cytoplasm contains the usual organelles, often with considerable numbers of mitochondria, but more significant is the presence of numerous small electron-dense membrane-bound granules that represent cytoplasmic accumulation of the secretory product or its precursor (Fig. 5-10). The granules may vary in number from one bronchial carcinoid tumor to another. In carcinoid tumors of the gastrointestinal tract the secretory granules are usually more numerous; they tend to be larger and may display considerable pleomorphism. As is the case with other endocrine neoplasms, cells of bronchial carcinoids frequently are closely adjacent to capillaries (Fig. 5-10). Salyer et al.[9] have recently described differences in the light microscopic appearance of central (mainstem and segmental bronchial) and peripheral bronchial carcinoids. They report that the central lesions are composed of fairly uniform cells, which contrasts with the more disorderly arrangement and pleomorphic tendency in peripheral neoplasms. They suggest that the peripheral carcinoids resemble to some degree primary chemodectomas, and they emphasize the need to distinguish between the two neoplasms. In this connection, the case illustrated in Fig. 5-11 may be relevant. The tumor was confined to three small adjacent foci within the lung. By light microscopy the tumor was seen to bear some resemblance to a carcinoid, but many cells were spindle-shaped. With the electron microscope the tumor cells were observed to be elongated and often angular,

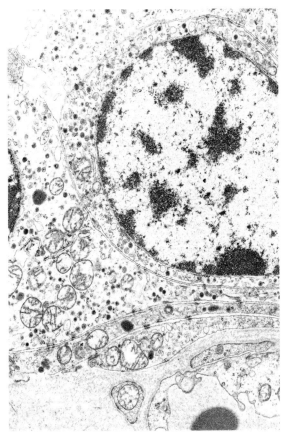

Fig. 5-10. Bronchial carcinoid. Cytoplasmic secretory granules are more numerous than those of the majority of small cell carcinomas. The intimate relationship of the tumor cells to a capillary can be seen (×16,800).

and occasional cells had electron-dense cytoplasm. The cytoplasmic granules were more variable in diameter and the cytoplasm was less electron-dense than in carcinoid tumors of the lung that we have studied, and the ultrastructure was reminiscent of a chemodectoma.[10] It is probable that several different cell types of neural crest derivation are present within the normal lung, and presumably each has neoplastic potential. Pearse et al.[11] have suggested the term "apudoma" for neoplasms of this group in order to emphasize their common properties of peptide and amine production, but obviously it would be preferable to be able to distinguish each neoplasm according to the specific cell from which it arose. There are undoubtedly neurosensory cells within the lungs about which we presently have little detailed information.[12,13]

MESOTHELIOMA

Drs. Matthews and Gordon have commented on the difficulties that may be associated with the diagnosis of this neoplasm as it involves the pleura. Although few electron microscopic observations on human mesotheliomas have been published, [14,15] it appears that the better-differentiated cases can be distinguished from adenocarcinomas by electron microscopy. Figure 5-12 shows portions of adjacent cells from a pleural mesothelioma and illustrates a profusion of long sinuous microvilli projecting from free surfaces of the tumor cells. The desmosomes in mesotheliomas are usually conspicuous, but tonofilament bundles may not be obvious. The cytoplasm is not unusual. Cell membranes of adjacent cells often separate to produce small

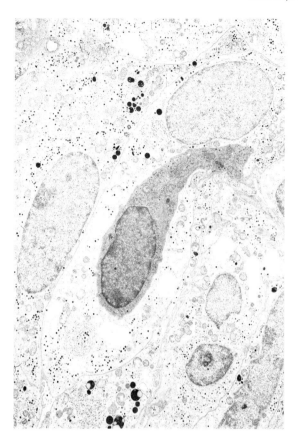

Fig. 5-11. Three small, closely adjacent tumor nodules were removed by wedge resection from the lung of a 52-year-old female patient where they had been detected as an incidental finding on routine chest x-ray. The tumor cells are elongated and often angular, and occasional cells have contrasting electron-dense cytoplasm. Cytoplasmic secretory granules are numerous and more variable in caliber than those of bronchial carcinoid tumors or small cell carcinomas. The largest cytoplasmic dense bodies are probably lysosomes. (×5100).

pseudoacinar spaces, and similar secondary channels may be seen in the adenomatoid tumor,[16] a benign neoplasm thought to be of mesothelial derivation. We have observed identical features in peritoneal mesotheliomas. With decreasing differentiation the morphologic differences between mesotheliomas and adenocarcinomas become blurred. In the so-called fibrous mesothelioma, where the tumor cells are seen to be spindle-shaped by light microscopy, the cytoplasm contains numerous distended sacs of rough-surfaced endoplasmic reticulum, and microvilli and prominent desmosomes are absent, which suggests that these tumors arise from underlying fibroblasts rather than from the surface mesothelial cells.

CONCLUSIONS

While the information obtained from ultrastructural studies of lung tumors has proved interesting and useful, more extensive work is needed to solve some of the persisting problems. The histogenesis and subclassification of the undifferentiated bronchogenic carcinomas are in particular need of clarification. Primary adenocarcinomas of the lung display a spectrum of histologic appearances that reflect their derivation and differentiation, and coexistence of a squamous element can occur; it is hoped that a correlated clinical and pathologic approach with the organization and depth of the Working Party Study will

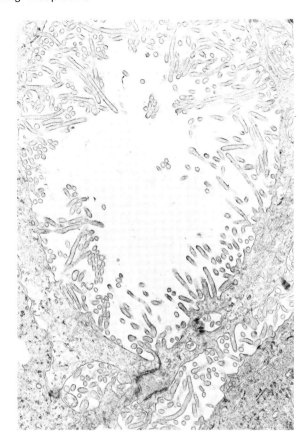

Fig. 5-12. Mesothelioma. The tumor was forming a plaquelike layer on the visceral pleura. The electron micrograph demonstrates the profusion of long sinuous micro-villi that extend from the free surfaces of the tumor cells (×16,000).

in time reveal the significance of these morphologic findings and their relevance to biologic behavior and response to therapy. The extent to which it may be possible to distinguish between primary and metastatic adenocarcinomas in the lung using electron microscopy has yet to be determined, although it can be anticipated that

this will be feasible in some instances and not in others. Using appropriate techniques it is possible to achieve good preservation of the fine structure of tumor cells in sputum and pleural effusions, and the diagnostic potential of electron microscopy using these easily obtained specimens and fine needle aspiration biopsies merits investigation.

REFERENCES

1. Kuhn C: Fine structure of bronchiolo-alveolar cell carcinoma. Cancer 30:1107–1118, 1972
2. Bedrossian CWM, Weilbaecher DG, Bentinck DG, et al: Ultrastructure of human bronchiolar alveolar cell carcinoma. Cancer 36:1399–1413, 1975
3. Bensch KG, Corrin B, Pariente R, et al: Oat cell carcinoma of the lung, its origin and relationship to bronchial carcinoid. Cancer 22:1163–1172, 1968
4. Hattori S, Matsuda M, Tateishi R, et al: Oat-cell carcinoma of the lung. Clinical and morphological studies in relation to its histogenesis. Cancer 30:1014–1024, 1972
5. Weichert WF: The neuroectodermal origin of peptide secreting endocrine glands. Am J Med 49:232–241, 1970
6. Razzuk MA, Lynn JA, Kingsley WB, et al: Giant cell carcinoma of the lung. J Thorac Cardiovasc Surg 59:574–580, 1970

7. Becker NH, Soifer I: Benign clear cell tumor (sugar tumor) of the lung. Cancer 27:712–719, 1971

8. Hoch WS, Patchefsky AS, Takeda M, et al: Benign clear cell tumor of the lung. An ultrastructural study. Cancer 33:1328–1336, 1974

9. Salyer DC, Salyer WR, Eggleston JC: Bronchial carcinoid tumors. Cancer 36:1522–1537, 1975

10. Glenner GG, Grimley PM: Tumors of the extra-adrenal paraganglion system (including chemoreceptors), in: Atlas of Tumor Pathology, second series, fasicle 9. Washington, DC, AFIP, 1974

11. Pearse AGE: The cytochemistry and ultrastructure of polypeptide hormone producing cells of the APUD series and the embryologic, physiologic and pathologic implications of the concept. J. Histochem Cytochem 17:303–313, 1969

12. Lauweryns JM, Cokelaere M, Theunynck P, et al: Neuroepithelioid bodies in mammalian respiratory mucosa: Light optical, histochemical and ultrastructural studies. Chest [Suppl] 65:22S–29S, 1974

13. Sorokin SP: The respiratory system, in Greep RO, Weiss L (eds): Histology (ed 3). New York, McGraw-Hill, 1973, pp 661–712

14. Wang NS: Electron microscopy in the diagnosis of pleural mesotheliomas. Cancer 31:1046–1054, 1973

15. Davis JMG: Ultrastructure of human mesotheliomas. J Natl Cancer Inst 52:1715–1719, 1974

16. Mackay B, Bennington MD, Skoglund RW: The adenomatoid tumor: Fine structural evidence for a mesothelial origin. Cancer 27:109–115, 1971

Martin H. Cohen

6
Signs and Symptoms of Bronchogenic Carcinoma

The natural history of lung cancer encompasses three stages: a period of months to years during which increasing degrees of cellular atypia are noted on sputum cytologic examination,[1] a period of variable duration characterized by progression of cytologic atypia to carcinoma in situ, and finally a period of clinically evident disease. Only during this latter phase does one note signs and symptoms related to local, regional, or systemic dissemination of the tumor or to development of systemic paraneoplastic symptoms unrelated to tumor location.

While studies are going on in an attempt to diagnose patients during the carcinoma in situ stage of illness (see Chapter 8), the vast majority of newly diagnosed patients are detected because of the finding of an abnormality on chest roentgenogram or because of the development of a new or worsening clinical symptom or sign.[2] In these individuals prompt recognition of either roentgen or clinical findings may lead to complete surgical resection of the tumor. In other patients certain symptoms or physical findings may represent potential medical or surgical emergencies, and early recognition is necessary for optimal care. Other symptoms and signs, depending on their duration and nature, may have prognostic importance or may determine the appropriate therapeutic strategy.[2-6] These various aspects of

patient symptomatology will be considered below for each of the major histologic subtypes of bronchogenic carcinoma, including epidermoid carcinoma, small cell (including oat cell) carcinoma, adenocarcinoma, and large cell anaplastic carcinoma.

Signs and symptoms in the lung cancer patient depend on the location and size of the primary tumor and on the metastatic potential of the neoplasm to regional sites (hilar and mediastinal nodes) or to distant sites. The relative frequencies of these various types of spread are indicated in Table 6-1. While the majority of bronchogenic carcinomas arise in peripheral bronchi,[7-8] by the time of clinical presentation epidermoid carcinoma and small cell anaplastic carcinoma have generally extended centrally. In these cell types bronchoscopy often reveals fungating lesions in mainstem, lobar, or proximal segmental bronchi. In contrast, adenocarcinoma generally remains peripheral and is identified less often on bronchoscopy.[9] Large cell anaplastic carcinoma is also often located peripherally, but it tends to form larger tumor masses than does adenocarcinoma.[19] Table 6-2 summarizes roentgenologic findings by histologic cell type at presentation. For a more detailed discussion of roentgenologic manifestations see Chapter 10.

Table 6-1
Origin of Symptoms and Signs in Patients with Bronchogenic Carcinoma

Histologic Cell Type	Primary Tumor	Intrathoracic Spread	Distant Metastases
Epidermoid	+++	++	+
Large cell anaplastic	+++	++	+
Small cell anaplastic	++	++	+++
Adenocarcinoma	+	+	+++

+, occasionally; ++, frequently; +++, very frequently.

PRIMARY TUMOR SYMPTOMS AND SIGNS

The symptom complexes associated with centrally and peripherally located lung tumors are different (Table 6-3). Thus epidermoid carcinoma and small cell anaplastic carcinoma, as representatives of centrally located tumors, generally present with cough, hemoptysis, wheezing, dyspnea related to loss of lung volume, or chest pain related to involvement of mediastinal structures or perivascular or peribronchial nerves.[12,20,21] By contrast, adenocarcinoma and to a lesser extent large cell anaplastic carcinoma generally present as peripheral lesions with cough, chest pain secondary to involvement of parietal pleura or chest wall, pleural effusion, or dyspnea on a restrictive basis. Cough and sputum production may be prominent in the bronchioloalveolar variant of adenocarcinoma.[22]

Less frequently seen symptom complexes related to the primary tumor include acute febrile and toxic illnesses resulting from lung abscesses developing in necrotic tumor cavities, which are usually seen with epidermoid and large cell anaplastic carcinoma,[20] and the superior sulcus or

Table 6-2
Roentgenologic Findings at Presentation

	Percentage with Finding			
	Epidermoid Carcinoma	Small Cell Anaplastic	Adeno-carcinoma	Large Cell Anaplastic
T Factor				
Nodule ≤ 4 cm	14	21	46	18
> 4 cm	18	8	26	41
Peripheral location	29	26	65	61
Central location	64	74	5	42
Atelectasis	23	31	2	14
Pneumonitis	13	21	14	24
Cavitation	5	0	3	4
Pleural and/or chest wall	3	5	14	2
N Factor				
Hilar adenopathy	38	61	19	32
Mediastinal adenopathy	5	14	9	10
Number of patients	338–585	114–252	135–301	97
References	10–12	13–14	15–18	19

T = primary tumor; N = regional lymph nodes.

The numbers of patients for the various parameters listed varied because information was not available in the cited reports on each of the parameters in all patients. The range listed indicates the minimum and maximum numbers of patients used in computing the percentages.

Table 6-3
Local Tumor Symptoms

Symptoms Secondary to Central and Endobronchial Tumor Growth	Symptoms Secondary to Peripheral Tumor Growth
Cough	Pain (pleural or chest wall)
Dyspnea–obstructive	Cough
Chest pain	Dyspnea–restrictive
Hemoptysis	
Wheeze or stridor	
Pneumonic (fever, productive cough)	

Pancoast syndrome. The latter is associated with epidermoid carcinoma most frequently and with adenocarcinoma and large cell anaplastic carcinoma less frequently. In the Pancoast syndrome a tumor growing in the apex of the lung may by local extension early in the course of illness involve the first thoracic and eighth cervical nerves, yielding characteristic pain in the shoulder and the ulnar-nerve-innervated portion of the arm.[23-25] Further local growth may result in erosion of the first and second ribs, and paravertebral tumor extension with sympathetic nerve involvement may lead to the development of Horner's syndrome.[23-25] The patient who presents in a physician's office in obvious pain, supporting the elbow of his affected arm, and who on examination is also found to have Horner's syndrome needs little further evaluation to diagnose a superior sulcus tumor.[26]

In working up a patient's primary tumor, one must answer the following questions: (1) What is the histologic subtype of the tumor? (2) Is there any bronchial obstruction that might require immediate radiation therapy to provide drainage of distal infection? (3) If infection is present, what are the causative organisms? (4) What is the patient's physiologic status in terms of cardiopulmonary function and other organ system function in case surgery becomes the indicated treatment modality? Generally, histologic cell type may be established by cytology for well-differentiated and moderately well-differentiated tumors,[27] by bronchoscopy and biopsy for lesions accessible to available instruments, or by needle biopsy[28] or bronchial brushing under fluoroscopic guidance[29] for peripheral lesions. Generally, bronchoscopy will also answer the question of lobar or segmental obstruction. For diagnosis of infection, unless

one has available a specially designed multilumen bronchoscope,[30] the best procedure for bacteriologic evaluation of the lower respiratory tree is translaryngeal aspiration.[31] Washings from fiberoptic bronchoscopy are of no value in this regard because gross contamination of the washings by upper respiratory tract flora occurs almost universally.[32] Physiologic determinants of patient operability will be discussed in Chapter 14.

REGIONAL DISEASE SYMPTOMS AND SIGNS

Intrathoracic spread of bronchogenic carcinoma either by direct extension or by lymphatics may produce a variety of symptoms and signs, as listed in Table 6-4. Neurologic deficits from local spread are most commonly manifested as hoarseness caused by recurrent laryngeal nerve involve-

Table 6-4
Causes of Regional Disease Symptoms

Nerve entrapment
  Recurrent laryngeal nerve
    Hoarseness
  Phrenic nerve
    Hemidiaphragm elevation with dyspnea
Vascular obstruction
  Superior vena cava syndrome
Pericardial or cardiac extension
  Tamponade
  Arrhythmia
  Cardiac failure
Mediastinal extension
  Esophageal compression with dysphagia
  Lymphatic obstruction with pleural effusion

ment. Hoarseness is more common with tumors in the left lung than in the right lung, since the left recurrent laryngeal nerve has a greater intrathoracic course than the right, i.e., the left recurrent laryngeal loops around the aortic arch at the level of the carina, while the right loops around the subclavian artery in the root of the neck.

Involvement of the phrenic nerve results in paralysis of the diaphragm. Either the right or left phrenic nerve may be involved, with characteristic radiologic findings of elevation of the hemidiaphragm and paradoxic motion or respiration or sniffing. Decreased, absent, or paradoxic diaphragmatic excursion during respiration with accompanying decrease in vital capacity[33] may contribute significantly to the dyspnea observed in such patients.

The principal vascular syndrome associated with extension of bronchogenic carcinoma into the mediastinum is superior vena caval syndrome. The superior vena cava, formed by the junction of the innominate veins, runs downward to the heart along the right sternal border and is thus more likely to be obstructed by right-sided lung lesions. Just before entering the pericardial sac the superior vena cava is joined by the azygos vein, and the clinical picture that one sees with superior vena caval obstruction depends on whether the obstruction is proximal or distal to this venous junction. Small cell bronchogenic carcinoma is the cell type most frequently associated with this complication, with epidermoid carcinoma as the second most frequent cause.[34] Clinically, with obstruction above the junction of inferior vena cava and azygos vein, one notes distension of arm and neck veins, suffusion and/or edema of the face, neck, and arms, and the presence of dilated tortuous collateral vessels on the upper chest and back. Confirmation of diagnosis can be made by demonstrating elevated venous pressure in an arm with normal venous pressure in the lower extremities.[35]

Obstruction of the vena cava proximal to the junction of the azygos vein causes a more severe clinical picture, with more extensive collateral circulation along the anterior and posterior abdominal walls to reach the systemic circulation via collaterals to the inferior vena cava. In this setting the direction of blood flow in abdominal collaterals is generally downward.[36]

Irrespective of the level of obstruction, tumor compression or invasion of the vena cava leads to venous stasis and secondary thrombus formation. Thus one cannot generally determine the extent of tumor involvement by angiographic studies. Therapy for this complication may have to include anticoagulants and/or fibrinolytic agents in addition to antineoplastic therapy (see Chapter 18).

Pericardial involvement by bronchogenic carcinoma may constitute a medical emergency, with death resulting from cardiac tamponade. The two most common presentations of pericardial involvement are sudden onset of an arrhythmia (generally sinus tachycardia or atrial fibrillation) or recognition of increasing cardiac diameter on chest x-ray with or without symptoms of congestive heart failure. Associated physical findings are those of pericarditis in general, and they may include paradoxic pulse, distant heart sounds, pericardial friction rub, cardiac percussion dullness lateral to the apex impulse, Kussmaul's sign (distension of cervical veins during inspiration), and Ewart's sign (percussion dullness and bronchial breathing beneath the angle of the left scapula). Diagnosis of pericardial effusion may be established by echocardiography or carbon dioxide angiography.

Dysphagia in a patient with bronchogenic carcinoma generally results from compression and/or invasion of the esophagus. Recently, however, dysphagia has also been noted to be a manifestation of recurrent laryngeal nerve paralysis.[37] The anatomic basis for this association is the fact that the recurrent laryngeal nerve in part innervates the cricoid muscles and the proximal esophagus. Dysphagia occurs for both solids and liquids, and aspiration is a serious problem; at times pharyngoesophageal myotomy is necessary for relief of symptoms.[37]

METASTATIC SYMPTOMS AND SIGNS

Metastatic involvement, and hence the frequency of metastatic symptoms, varies with histologic cell type; it is most prevalent with small cell carcinoma, followed by adenocarcinoma, large cell anaplastic carcinoma, and epidermoid carcinoma. Nearly every organ and tissue in the body may be a site for metastatic disease; thus the number and variety of metastatic symptoms are innumerable. In this discussion only one metastatic symptom (which often represents a medical and surgical emergency) will be discussed: epidural spinal cord compression. A typical presentation is the patient with known small cell carcinoma who after a variable period of symptomatic back pain (which may be localized or radicular in pattern) develops other neurologic abnormalities consisting of sensory or motor impairment or loss of normal bladder and bowel function.[38,39] Bone x-rays and scans frequently show vertebral involvement or destruction by tumor. The pathogenesis of the resultant neurologic deficit is extradural cord compression by the tumor or by a collapsed vertebrae or as a result of spinal vascular occlusion by the metastatic lesion. Careful follow-up must be made for all patients with bronchogenic carcinoma who have new back pain. With development of neurological signs, myelography is necessary to localize the level of the obstruction. In the case of complete block, additional contrast material injected into the cisterna magna will define the upper limits of the lesion and determine whether there are multiple levels of involvement. Therapy may require either decompressive laminectomy with postoperative radiation therapy or radiation therapy alone, with the choice of treatment being dependent on the radiosensitivity of the tumor and the acuteness with which the neurologic deficit develops.[40,41]

PARANEOPLASTIC SYNDROMES

Extrapulmonary nonendocrine manifestations of lung cancer are indicated in Table 6-5. Coagulation disorders present important clinical problems in lung cancer patients,[42] as in patients with other malignancies. For purposes of discussion one can classify coagulation disorders on the basis of whether their clinical presentation is predominantly as venous or arterial thrombosis or whether bleeding dominates the clinical picture. Venous thrombi may be multiple and migratory. The characteristics of the syndrome of migratory venous thrombophlebitis include the occurrence of thrombophlebitis in patients in whom there were no obvious predisposing causes (i.e., patients were not in postoperative status; patients had no evidence of cardiac disease; patients were not bedridden; there was no preexisting venous stasis). Second, thrombosis often occurs in an unusual distribution involving arm veins, the inferior vena cava, and the jugular venous system, in addition to the leg veins. Other characteristics are

the migratory pattern of thrombosis and the involvement of two or more different venous sites simultaneously. In lung cancer there is no difference in incidence of this syndrome by cell type. In one series the average time between onset of phlebitis and histologic proof of malignancy was 4 months. From the therapeutic viewpoint the thrombophlebitis is resistant to anticoagulants, especially coumarin-type drugs, and is best treated with heparin.

Arterial thrombosis generally presents as nonbacterial thrombotic endocarditis. This disorder is characterized by the presence of sterile verrucose lesions on left-sided heart valves. The clinical presentation is often as emboli to the brain, although systemic arterial embolization is usually found concomitantly. Frequent systemic sites of emboli include the spleen, kidneys, and

Table 6-5

Extrapulmonary Nonendocrine Manifestations of Bronchogenic Carcinoma

Coagulation disorders
  Thrombotic manifestations
    Migratory thrombophlebitis
    Nonbacterial thrombotic endocarditis
  Hemorrhagic manifestations
    Disseminated intravascular coagulation
      Microangiopathic hemolytic anemia
      Thrombotic thrombocytopenic purpura
Osseous
  Hypertrophic osteoarthropathy
Cutaneous and connective tissue
  Acanthosis nigricans
  Dermatomyositis
  Tylosis (hyperkeratosis palmaris et plantaris)
  Scleroderma
Neurologic
  Neuropathies
    Cortical cerebellar degeneration
    Peripheral neuropathies, sensory and
      sensorimotor
    Encephalopathy
  Myopathy
    Myositis
    Myasthenia-like
Miscellaneous
  Anorexia
  Weight loss
  Fever
  Weakness
  Fatigue

heart.[43,45] With cerebral embolization the onset of neurologic symptoms may be abrupt or insidious, with development of either focal neurologic deficits or diffuse abnormalities such as confusion, disorientation, generalized seizures, or disturbances in consciousness. Pathologically one sees occlusion of both large and small vessels of the brain.[45]

Patients with nonbacterial thrombotic endocarditis are generally afebrile if there is not other predisposing cause for fever. Only about one-third of patients have cardiac murmurs, which are generally systolic and unchanging in quality. Diagnosis during life is difficult and is generally made only when there is evidence of systemic embolization.

Bleeding disorders in lung cancer may be secondary to low-grade chronic disseminated intravascular coagulation (DIC). The mechanism of activation of coagulation in lung cancer is complex, as it is in cancer in general, and it may reflect release of thromboplastic substances from tumor or normal tissue,[46] vascular damage, or thrombocytosis and/or increased platelet adhesiveness.[47,48] Clinically the patient may present with ecchymosis, hematoma, or other bleeding manifestations. Abnormalities in blood coagulation studies reflect the rate at which intravascular coagulation is occurring, as well as the effects of secondary activation of the fibrinolytic system.[49] Less common bleeding abnormalities are a clinical picture compatible with microangiopathic hemolytic anemia with schistocytes present in the peripheral blood and fibrin thrombi in small blood vessels[50,51] or a clinical picture of thrombotic thrombocytopenic purpura.[50]

Hypertrophic pulmonary osteoarthropathy (HPO) is a clinical syndrome having two dominant features: (1) clubbing of the fingers and toes and (2) periostitis of the long bones. Diagnosis is established by demonstrating ossifying periostitis on bone x-rays. Symptoms include pain, tenderness, and swelling over affected bones, which may include the distal ends of the tibia, fibula, humerus, radius, and ulna. In addition to the bone symptoms, there may be an associated polyarthritis similar clinically to rheumatoid arthritis.[52,53] In HPO the synovial fluid is noninflammatory in character, and there is a good mucin clot. Generally, patients can date the onset of this syndrome fairly accurately, and it may precede by several months the overt appearance of the neoplasm.

Osteoarthropathy occurs in up to 12 percent of patients with adenocarcinoma of the lung and a lesser percentage of patients with other histologic types;[12] it is least frequent in patients with small cell carcinoma. The etiology of this syndrome is unclear, although estrogens,[54] growth hormone,[55] and neurologic innervation[56] have been implicated. Case reports attest to a response of hypertrophic osteoarthropathy to surgical treatment of the primary tumor[53,57] or to vagotomy.[56]

Concerning dermatologic manifestations, there is some specificity of cutaneous lesions relative to cell type of bronchogenic carcinoma. Thus acanthosis nigricans and scleroderma are usually associated with adenocarcinoma of the lung,[58-60] while tylosis (hyperkeratosis palmaris et plantaris) is associated with squamous cell carcinoma.[61] Dermatomyositis shows no clear relationship with histologic subtype.

Acanthosis nigricans is characterized by symmetric epidermoid thickening (hyperkeratosis and acanthosis) and hyperpigmentation usually involving the axillae but also other flexural surfaces and occasionally extending to involve the oral mucous membranes and the palms and soles.[58] The appearance of acanthosis nigricans may precede, coincide with, or follow the appearance of the lung tumor. It should be emphasized, however, that acanthosis nigricans is not necessarily premalignant, as a variety of benign conditions are associated with its development.[62] In this regard the age of the patient may be important, since benign causes are usually manifest at a younger age. If an individual above the age of 50 years develops acanthosis nigricans it must be viewed with suspicion.[62]

Of the diseases generally classified as collagen-vascular, dermatomyositis is the entity most often associated with malignancy. Dermatomyositis associated with internal malignancy accounts for 15 to 20 percent of all patients with dermatomyositis, with the percentage increasing among patients who develop dermatomyositis beyond the age of 40 years.[63-65] Prominent clinical features include muscle weakness (pelvic girdle greater than shoulder muscles) and a skin rash consisting of an erythematous facial rash frequently in a butterfly distribution with a lilac-colored "heliotrope" around the eyes. Useful laboratory tests for diagnosis or serial follow-up in this condition include electromyography, muscle biopsy, and serum enzymes, including SGOT,

SGPT, and aldolase. Serum creatinine phospho-kinase (CPK) is unpredictably elevated in this disease and cannot be relied on as a measure of disease activity.[63] While corticosteroids are useful in the management of dermatomyositis unassociated with malignancy, they are relatively ineffective when malignancy is present. Surgical removal of tumor may lead to clearing of dermatomyositis.

In contrast to dermatomyositis, scleroderma is only rarely associated with lung malignancy. Tomkin, in a literature review in 1959,[66] noted 16 cases of bronchogenic adenocarcinoma or a bronchioloalveolar carcinoma developing in patients with long-standing scleroderma and associated pulmonary fibrosis. Recently, single case reports of bronchogenic small cell carcinoma and epidermoid carcinoma developing in patients with pulmonary involvement by scleroderma have appeared.[66,67] One probably should screen all patients with scleroderma who have pulmonary fibrosis at regular intervals to detect early bronchogenic carcinoma.

Neurologic paraneoplastic syndromes present extreme difficulties in staging patients. In addition, they represent a source of major disability and discomfort for the patient. In one series 16 percent of lung cancer patients had evidence of neuromuscular dysfunction.[68] Manifestations may relate to the central nervous system or to peripheral nerves or muscle. Helpful clinically in pointing to a nonmetastatic origin of the neurologic symptoms is the fact that usually several different neurologic deficits are present in the same patient, e.g., cerebellar findings with a peripheral neuropathy or myopathy, etc.[69] Another helpful differential point is that neurologic deficits are usually symmetric.

Cerebral encephalopathy is characterized by varying degrees of dementia, psychosis, or organic brain syndrome. The electroencephalogram is often slow, and there may be a moderate pleocytosis in the spinal fluid.[70] One must in all cases rule out treatable causes of central nervous system dysfunction such as hypoglycemia, hypercalcemia, and other electrolyte abnormalities.

Cortical cerebellar degeneration is characterized by acute or subacute onset. Both the upper and lower extremities are affected bilaterally, resulting in difficulties in walking and in the use of the upper extremities. Intention tremor, dysarthria, and vertigo may be severe, but nystagmus

is relatively uncommon. Pathologically one sees degeneration of cerebellar Purkinje cells.[71,72] There is often accompanying degeneration of brainstem nuclei.[70]

Peripheral neuropathies generally also present in acute or subacute fashion. Neuropathies may be sensory or combined sensorimotor. Pure motor neuropathies do not occur, although there are suggestions that there might be an increased incidence of amyotrophic lateral sclerosis, with its characteristic upper and lower motor neuron signs in cancer patients.[73] Clinically one generally notes pain and paresthesias of the extremities, with decrease of deep tendon reflexes. With progression, sensory loss and ataxia occur. If motor fibers are also involved, muscle weakness and wasting accompany the sensory changes.[74,75] Examination of the cerebrospinal fluid may reveal elevated protein and pleocytosis. Occasionally one sees patients with unusual isolated sensory neuritides. Thus patients may present with paresthesias in the distribution of a single nerve, such as a branch of the trigeminal or a single nerve to the extremities. As with other neuropathies, the basis for these findings is obscure.

Carcinomatous myopathies may be divided into myositis (primary degeneration of muscle fibers) and myasthenia-like syndrome (primary defect in neuromuscular transmission). The latter is seen in patients with small cell carcinoma, the former with all cell types of bronchogenic carcinoma.[57,71,76,77] In both cases proximal muscles are involved, with symptoms of weakness of the thigh and pelvic girdle muscles being most prominent. The myasthenic syndrome may be differentiated from myasthenia gravis by characteristic electromyographic changes showing paradoxic increases in action potentials after a few seconds of exercise, by the absence of deep tendon reflexes, by a poor response to neostigmine, and by a favorable response to calcium and guanidine.[76-80]

Occurrences of anorexia, weight loss, fever, weakness, and fatigue are common to many types of cancer. Consideration of the pathogenesis of these findings is beyond the scope of this discussion, although some interesting hypotheses have been proposed by Nathanson and Hall.[81]

With regard to the association between symptoms and prognosis, Feinstein[3] has developed clinical symptomatic staging in lung cancer and has shown that prognosis is related to clinical symptoms. In his studies the best survival is seen in patients who are asymptomatic at presentation, with the next best survival being in those who have symptoms referable to the primary tumor of over 6 months duration.[2,3] Subsequently, Senior and Adamson applied Feinstein's symptom classification to their patient material with similar results.[5] Furthermore, Zelen has looked at the performance status of the patient as a prognostic variable in the randomized trials carried out by the Veterans Administration Lung Study Group in patients with both limited and extensive bronchogenic carcinoma.[6] In both groups the patients with better performance status consistently survived longer than patients disabled to a greater or lesser extent by their disease. As in the other series listed above, the presence of metastatic symptoms, especially those related to central nervous system or liver involvement, adversely affected prognosis.[6] Each of the above studies indicates the need for patient stratification in the conduct of therapeutic trials (see Chapter 20).

This review of the signs and symptoms of bronchogenic carcinoma is presented, in part, in the hope that early suspicion, rapid diagnosis, and prompt treatment of complications resulting from local tumor growth and mediastinal spread and distant metastases will improve the overall outlook for patients with bronchogenic carcinoma. In this regard, recognition of the various extrapulmonary nonendocrine manifestations of this tumor is especially important, since these manifestations may precede the appearance of a lesion on chest x-ray and may thus allow for early definitive surgical treatment.

REFERENCES

1. Saccomanno G, Archer VE, Auerbach O, et al: Development of carcinoma of the lung as reflected in exfoliated cells. Cancer 33:256–270, 1974
2. Carbone PP, Frost JK, Feinstein AR, et al: Lung cancer: Perspective and prospects. Ann Intern Med 73:1003–1024, 1970
3. Feinstein AR: Symptomatic patterns, biologic behavior and prognosis in cancer of the lung. Ann Intern Med 61:27–43, 1964
4. Feinstein AR: A new staging system for cancer and reappraisal of "early" treatment and cure by radical surgery. N Engl J Med 279:747–753, 1968
5. Senior RM, Adamson JS: Survival in patients with lung cancer. Arch Intern Med 125:975–980, 1970
6. Zelen M: Keynote address on biostatistics and data retrieval. Cancer Chemother Rep 4:31–43, 1973
7. Weiss W, Boucot KR: The Philadelphia pulmonary neoplasm research project. Early roentgenographic appearance of bronchogenic carcinoma. Arch Intern Med 134:306–311, 1974
8. Benfield JR, Juillard GJF, Piltch YH, et al: Current and future concepts of lung cancer. Ann Intern Med 83:93–106, 1975
9. Feinstein AR, Gelfman NA, Yesner R: The diverse effects of histopathology on manifestations and outcome of lung cancer. Chest 66:225–229, 1974
10. Carlisle JC, McDonald JR, Harrington SW: Bronchogenic squamous cell carcinoma. J Thorac Surg 22:74–82, 1951
11. Byrd RB, Miller WE, Carr DT, et al: The roentgenographic appearance of squamous cell carcinoma of the bronchus. Mayo Clin Proc 43:327–332, 1968
12. Green N, Kurohara SS, George FW, et al: The biologic behavior of lung cancer according to histologic type. Radiol Clin Biol 41:160–170, 1972
13. Kato Y, Ferguson TB, Bennett DE, et al: Oat cell carcinoma of the lung. Cancer 23:517–524, 1969
14. Byrd RB, Miller WE, Carr DT, et al: Roentgenographic appearance of small cell carcinoma of the bronchus. Mayo Clin Proc 43:337–341, 1968
15. Bennett DE, Sasser WF, Ferguson TB: Adenocarcinoma of the lung in men. Cancer 23:431–439, 1969
16. Lehar TJ, Carr DT, Miller WE, et al: Roentgenographic appearance of bronchogenic adenocarcinoma. Am Rev Respir Dis 96:245–247, 1967
17. DeLarue NC, Anderson W, Sanders D, et al: Bronchioloalveolar carcinoma. A reappraisal after 24 years. Cancer 29:90–97, 1972
18. Bennett DE, Sasser WF: Bronchiolar carcinoma. A valid clinical entity? Cancer 24:876–887, 1969
19. Byrd RB, Miller WE, Carr DT, et al: Roentgenographic appearance of large cell carcinoma of the bronchus. Mayo Clin Proc 43:333–336, 1968
20. Cohen MH: Signs and symptoms of bronchogenic carcinoma. Semin Oncol 1:183–189, 1974
21. Matthews MJ: Morphology of lung cancer. Semin Oncol 1:175–182, 1974
22. Ludington LG, Verska JJ, Howard T, et al: Bron-

chiolar carcinoma (alveolar cell). Another great imitator. A review of 41 cases. Chest 61:622–628, 1972

23. Pancoast HK: Superior pulmonary sulcus tumor. JAMA 99:1391–1396, 1932

24. Paulson DL: Superior sulcus tumors. Results of combined therapy. NY State J Med 71:2050–2052, 1971

25. Doehner GA, Marcus SS, Wolff WI: Pancoast's tumor. Five-year survival after combined radiotherapy and surgery. NY State J Med 67:2378–2380, 1967

26. Shaw RR, Paulson DL, Kee RL: Treatment of superior sulcus tumor by irradiation followed by resection. Ann Surg 154:29–40, 1961

27. Lukeman JM: Reliability of cytologic diagnosis in cancer of the lung. Cancer Chemother Rep 4:79–93, 1973

28. Landman S, Burgener FA, Lim GHK: Comparison of bronchial brushing and percutaneous needle aspiration biopsy in the diagnosis of malignant lung lesions. Radiology 115:275–278, 1975

29. Ujiki GT, Shields TW: Newer trends in the diagnosis and treatment of bronchogenic carcinoma. Surg Clin North Am 51:183–193, 1971

30. Laurenzi GA, Potter RT, Kass EH: Bacteriologic flora of the lower respiratory tract. N Engl J Med 265:1273–1278, 1961

31. Pecora DV: A comparison of transtracheal aspiration with other methods of determining the bacterial flora of the lower respiratory tract. N Engl J Med 269:664–666, 1963

32. Fossieck BE, Parker RH, Cohen MH: unpublished observations

33. Alexander C: Diaphragm movements and the diagnosis of diaphragmatic paralysis. Clin Radiol 17:79–83, 1966

34. Salsali M, Cliffton EE: Superior vana caval obstruction with lung cancer. Ann Thorac Surg 6:437–442, 1968

35. Lokich JJ, Goodman R: Superior vena cava syndrome. Clinical management. JAMA 231:58–61, 1975

36. Rubin P, Hicks GL: Biassociation of superior vena caval obstruction and spinal cord compression. NY State J Med 73:2176–2182, 1973

37. Henderson RD, Boszko A, Van Nostrand AWP: Pharyngoesophageal dysphagia and recurrent laryngeal nerve palsy. J Thorac Cardiovasc Surg 68:507–512, 1974

38. Bansal S, Brady LW, Olsen A, et al: The treatment of metastatic spinal cord tumors. JAMA 202:126–128, 1967

39. Mones RJ, Dozier D, Berrett A: Analysis of medical treatment of malignant extradural spinal cord tumors. Cancer 19:1842–1853, 1966

40. Rubin P, Mayer E, Poulter C: Extradural spinal cord compression by tumor. Part II. High daily dose experience without laminectomy. Radiology 93:1248–1260, 1969

41. White WA, Patterson RH, Bergland RM: Role of surgery in the treatment of spinal cord compression by metastatic neoplasm. Cancer 27:558–561, 1971

42. Byrd RB, Divertie MB, Spittell JA: Bronchogenic carcinoma and thromboembolic disease. JAMA 202:1019–1022, 1967

43. Reagan TJ, Okazaki H: The thrombotic syndrome associated with carcinoma. Arch Neurol 31:390–395, 1974

44. Bryan CS: Nonbacterial thrombotic endocarditis with malignant tumors. Am J Med 46:787–793, 1969

45. MacDonald RA, Robbins SL: The significance of nonbacterial thrombotic endocarditis. Autopsy and clinical study of 78 patients. Ann Intern Med 46:255–273, 1957

46. Holyoke ED, Frank AL, Weiss L: Tumor thromboplastin activity in vitro. Int J Cancer 9:259–263, 1972

47. Silvis SE, Turkbas N, Doscherholmen A: Thrombocytosis in patients with lung cancer. JAMA 211:1852–1853, 1970

48. Moolten SE, Vroman L, Vroman GMS, et al: Role of blood platelets in thromboembolism. Arch Intern Med 84:667–710, 1949

49. Colman RW, Robboy SJ, Minna JD: Disseminated intravascular coagulation (DIC): An approach. Am J Med 52:679–689, 1972

50. Goodnight SH: Bleeding and intravascular clotting in malignancy: A review. Ann NY Acad Sci 230:271–288, 1974

51. Mersky C: Pathogenesis and treatment of altered blood coagulability in patients with malignant tumors. Ann NY Acad Sci 230:289–293, 1974

52. Greenfield GB, Schorsch HA, Shkolnik A: The various roentgen appearance of pulmonary hypertrophic osteoarthropathy. Am J Roentgenol Radium Ther Nucl Med 101:927–931, 1967

53. LeRoux BT: Bronchial carcinoma with hypertrophic pulmonary osteoarthropathy. S Afr Med J 42:1074–1075, 1968

54. Jao JY, Barlow JJ, Krant MJ: Pulmonary hypertrophic osteoarthropathy, spider angiomata and estrogen hypersecretion in neoplasms. Ann Intern Med 70:581–584, 1969

55. Ennis GC, Cameron DP, Burger HG: On the aetiology of hypertrophic pulmonary osteoarthropathy in bronchogenic carcinoma: Lack of relationship to elevated growth hormone levels. Aust NZ J Med 3:157–161, 1973

56. Carroll KB, Doyle L: A common factor in hypertrophic osteoarthropathy. Thorax 29:262–264, 1974

57. Knowles JH, Smith LH: Extrapulmonary manifestation of bronchogenic carcinoma. N Engl J Med 262:505–510, 1960

58. Ellenbogen BK: Acanthosis nigricans associated with bronchial carcinoma. Report of 2 cases. Br J Dermatol 61:251–254, 1949

59. Jonsson SM, Houser JM: Scleroderma (progressive systemic sclerosis) associated with cancer of lung: Brief review and report of a case. N Engl J Med 255:413–416, 1956

60. Ezzo JA, Davis DK: Progressive systemic scleroses (scleroderma) with adenocarcinoma of the lung. Report of a case. Dis Chest 47:235–237, 1956

61. Schwindt WD, Bernhardt LC, Johnson SAM: Tylosis and intrathoracic neoplasms. Chest 57:590–591, 1970

62. Brown J, Winkelmann RK: Acanthosis nigricans: A study of 90 cases. Medicine 47:33–51, 1968

63. Pearson CM: Polymyositis. Ann Rev Med 17:63–82, 1966

64. Shy GM, Silverstein I: A study of the effects upon the motor unit by remote malignancy. Brain 38:515–529, 1965

65. Shy GM: The late onset of myopathy. A clinical pathologic study of 131 patients. World Neurol 3:149–158, 1962

66. Tomkin GH: Systemic sclerosis associated with carcinoma of the lung. Br J Dermatol 81:213–216, 1969

67. Haqqani MT, Holti G: Systemic sclerosis with pulmonary fibrosis and oat cell carcinoma. Acta Derm Venereol (Stockh) 53:369–374, 1974

68. Croft PB, Wilkinson M: Carcinomatous neuromyopathy: Its incidence in patients with carcinoma of the lung and breast. Lancet 1:184–188, 1965

69. Tyler HR: Paraneoplastic syndromes of nerve, muscle and neuromuscular junction. Ann NY Acad Sci 230:348–357, 1974

70. Joynt RS: The brain's uneasy peace with tumors. Ann NY Acad Sci 230:342–347, 1974

71. Morton DL, Itabashi HH, Grimes OF: Nonmetastatic neurological complications of bronchogenic carcinoma. The carcinomatous myopathies. J Thorac Cardiovasc Surg 51:14–29, 1966

72. Sealy WC: Nonmetastatic extrapulmonary manifestations of bronchogenic carcinoma. Surgery 68:906–913, 1970

73. Norris FH Jr, Engel WK: Carcinomatous amyotrophic lateral sclerosis, in Brain WR, Norris FH Jr (eds): The Remote Effects of Cancer on the Nervous System. New York, Grune & Stratton, 1965

74. Overholt BF, Green RA: Bronchogenic carcinoma and peripheral neuromyopathies. Postgrad Med 40:13–22, 1966

75. Kennedy JH: Extrapulmonary effects of cancer of the lung and pleura. J Thorac Cardiovasc Surg 61:514–529, 1971

76. Trojaborg W, Frantzen E, Anderson I: Peripheral neuropathy and myopathy associated with carcinoma of the lung. Brain 92:71–82, 1969

77. Kennedy JH, Coyne N, Khairallah P: Carcinomatous neuroendocrinopathy associated with cancer of the lung. J Thorac Cardiovasc Surg 57:276–283, 1969

78. Eaton LM, Lambert EH: Electromyography and electrical stimulation of nerves in diseases of the motor unit. Observations of myasthenic syndrome associated with malignant tumors. JAMA 163:1117–1124, 1957

79. Greene JG, Divertie MB, Brown AL, et al: Small cell carcinoma of the lung. Observation on four patients including one with a myasthenic syndrome. Arch Intern Med 122:333–340, 1968

80. Corbett JJ, Gordon EE, Becker GH: Myasthenic syndrome as the sole manifestation of cancer. Arch Phys Med Rehabil 50:86–90, 1969

81. Nathanson L, Hall TC: Lung tumors: How they produce their syndromes. Ann NY Acad Sci 230:367–377, 1974

Yener S. Erozan
John K. Frost

7

Cytopathologic Diagnosis of Lung Cancer

A definitive confirming diagnosis of lung cancer by microscopic examination is indicated before therapy whenever possible. In clinically suspected cancer of the lung, histologic confirmation usually is available; at times, cytologic confirmation must suffice. In the earlier and more curable stages of lung cancer, however, detection and diagnosis may depend entirely on the use of the most efficient methods of cytologic microscopic examination. Since these "early" lung cancers are commonly occult and do not produce any detectable clinical or radiologic signs, clinical cytopathology is frequently the only method by which detection, diagnosis, and even localization can be accomplished.[1-6]

Optimum cytologic sampling techniques may differ for the clinically manifest and the clinically occult cancers, as well as for tumor types and locations. In all of these categories, however, cytopathology provides a simple convenient method for sampling large areas of the respiratory tract and, by using proper techniques, virtually all of its mucous membranes.

This work was supported in part by National Cancer Institute Contract NIH 69-2172.

METHODS

There are many cytopathologic techniques available for examination of the respiratory tract, but some are especially valuable for obtaining diagnostic cellular specimens from individuals with lung cancer. These include spontaneous cough, sputum induction, tracheobronchial instrumentation, percutaneous transthoracic needle aspiration, and pleural or pericardial tap.

Spontaneous Cough

Spontaneous cough produces the most accessible and generally valuable pulmonary material for cytologic examination. However, its yield in the diagnosis of lung cancer varies greatly and depends on certain key factors, including method of sputum production, time of day the specimen is obtained, number of samples examined, type of neoplasm, and location of the lesion. The majority of symptomatic patients are able to produce satisfactory spontaneous cough samples following proper instruction.

EARLY MORNING SPUTUM

The most valuable specimen for routine cellular examination, the early morning sputum, yields the best samples of deep pulmonary material from all lung fields. Optimal yield results from a series of separate sputum samples collected on 5 consecutive days. The patient is instructed how to produce a deep cough, with deep inhalation and forceful expiration using his diaphragm. Clearing of the nose and throat and rinsing of the mouth are desirable before collection in order to decrease contamination and dilution of the deep sputum. A Petri dish or clear plastic container is an ideal receptacle for these samples. Unfixed sputum should be transported to the laboratory promptly, but it can be kept at room temperature a few hours without damaging the cells. For several reasons, fresh samples are preferred: diagnostic and morphologic representative cells can be selected for smears (i.e., blood flecks, nonpurulent and nonsalival material); unfixed cells lie flatter and thinner and have better diagnostic morphology; the remaining material can be concentrated (by mucolysis and filtering or by Saccomanno technique) for enrichment of the significant cell component.

When a considerable time lapse between collection of the sputum and processing in the laboratory is expected, fixation is imperative. The best method to date has been described by Saccomanno et al.;[7] it uses 50 percent ethyl alcohol with 2 percent Carbowax for fixation, followed by blending and smearing. In this way, when the more satisfactory fresh procurement is not possible, one can collect early morning sputum specimens singly or pool a series of three or five morning specimens.

PULMONARY OBSTRUCTION

The cytologic examination may be negative, even in the presence of a large bronchogenic carcinoma, because of obstruction of the involved bronchus with additional closure by inflammation and mucosal edema, or tenacious and inspissated mucus in the more peripheral airways associated with production of Curschmann's spirals and obstruction to flow. In these patients a 5-day course of broad-spectrum antibiotics, bronchodilators, and expectorates is given to reduce the obstruction and increase the pulmonary flow. On the third day of therapy a new series of five consecutive early morning sputa is started. The result is a 7-day procedure that allows the obstruction to be cleared sufficiently to obtain a satisfactory cytologic specimen.[8]

PERCUSSION OR VIBRATION OF CHEST WALL

Percussion or vibration maneuvers, either manual or mechanical (ITI Mechanical Percussor, model T1), can be employed in conjunction with spontaneous cough or with special techniques such as postural drainage[9] or aerosol induction.[10] In some cases this combination of techniques yields more satisfactory diagnostic material.

POSTBRONCHOSCOPIC SPUTUM

Sputum brought up during the first 2 hr or so after bronchoscopy and on the following morning is frequently of great diagnostic value. As the first secretions are frequently the best, collection is routinely begun immediately after the bronchoscope is removed, or as the patient regains consciousness, and is continued for 2 hr. The following early morning sputum is also collected, and it often contains valuable deep diagnostic material.

Induced Sputum

For patients who cannot produce satisfactory sputum samples, or for those who cannot expectorate any pulmonary secretions at all, induction can be a significant help. Various methods have been described[11-14] utilizing tap water, hypertonic or hypotonic saline, or additives such as mucolytic agents, propylene glycol, or SO_2.[15] These enable the patient to bring up tenacious secretions already produced but adhering to the air passages.

An *aerosol lavage* has been devised for use when these methods fail or when there are virtually no secretions (for example, asymptomatic screenees). The aim is to produce a gentle, nonirritating, cleansing aerosol to lavage the total respiratory network from the alveoli and terminal bronchioles outward through the major bronchi. A tissue culture balanced salt solution (Hanks' BSS) is aerosolized by ultrasonic nebulizers to deliver a high volume of mist containing a large percentage of droplets less than $5~\mu$ that enters the alveoli and lavages the passages on its return outward. Twenty-five minutes of aerosolization during gentle normal breathing have been found to be optimum. The material is processed by cell spreads, filtering (Millipore, Nuclepore, or Gelman), or Saccomanno technique.[7]

Early morning sputum the day following induction frequently contains large quantities of Curschmann's spirals and diagnostically valuable deep material previously blocked and unobtainable.

Tracheobronchial Instrumentation

MATERIAL COLLECTED THROUGH
A BRONCHOSCOPE

Numerous types of cellular samples (aspirations, washings, brushings, curettings) aid in the diagnosis and localization of lung tumors, especially the small, peripheral, occult, or early lesions. Proper techniques have been described in detail.[6,16] Extreme care must be taken to obtain adequate samples that have not been contaminated from other areas. In very peripheral tumors that are visible on x-ray, fluoroscopic guidance of the fiberbronchoscope may assist visual guidance in obtaining diagnostic cellular brushings. Filter and cellular spread preparations are made from the material obtained.

MATERIAL COLLECTED BY BRUSH
UNDER FLUOROSCOPY

This procedure has been successfully employed in peripheral lesions that are visible by x-ray and can be reached by a catheter-protected brush directed under television fluoroscopy.[17-19] Because significant morphologic destruction results from unavoidable air drying while cellular spreads are being made directly from the brush, it is preferable to rinse the brush in a BSS (i.e., Hanks') and prepare a cellular filter therefrom.

Transthoracic Needle Aspiration

The roentgen-guided percutaneous aspiration biopsy technique for the diagnosis of intrathoracic cancer has been described and its effectiveness documented in the recent literature.[20-23] Some cell spreads can be made directly from material collected in the syringe and fixed immediately in 95 percent alcohol for Papanicolaou staining, while others can be air dried for Wright or Giemsa stain. In addition, the syringe and needle should be rinsed with a BSS (i.e., Hanks'), and filter preparations should be made. We prefer to collect all of the material from the syringe and needle in Hanks' BSS rather than make direct smears. When larger-caliber needles are used, gross tissue fragments are separated for tissue processing, and filter preparations and cell spreads are prepared from the remaining material.

Pleural and Pericardial Tap

Lung tumors sometimes first present clinically as involvement of pleura or pericardium by direct or lymphatic extension. In these instances cytopathology can be of great value in establishing the diagnosis.[24-29] Proper collection techniques and processing play a major role in obtaining optimal results. Material should be collected in a bottle containing at least 3 U of heparin for each milliliter of fluid to be aspirated. The bottle is gently agitated as the specimen is added and is sent to the laboratory as soon as possible. If delay is unavoidable, the material should either be refrigerated or fixed by adding an equal amount of 95 percent ethyl alcohol. A combination of cytologic preparations (smears, filters, and cell blocks) provides optimal use of cellular material for routine (Papanicolaou, H&E) and special (i.e., PAS, mucicarmine) stains.

RESULTS AND DISCUSSION

Early Occult Versus Classical Clinical Lung Cancer

Because pulmonary carcinoma can be detected effectively in its early occult stage (in situ or early invasive) by cytologic examination of the sputum,[1-6] this method has a definitive place in screening populations at high risk of developing bronchogenic carcinoma (i.e., male, heavy smoker, over 45 years of age). Carefully designed and coordinated screening studies employing cytologic and x-ray examinations are under way at the Johns Hopkins Medical Institutions, the Mayo Clinic, and the Memorial Hospital for Cancer and Allied Diseases in an attempt to determine whether such detection of bronchogenic carcinoma in asymptomatic individuals will increase the cure rate of this disease.

The early occult lung cancer is to be found chiefly in apparently healthy *screenees*. In con-

Table 7-1
Evaluation of a Sputum Examination in Asymptomatic
Healthy Workers

	Number of Screenees	Satisfactory [No.] %	
One examination (consisting of multiple subspecimens):			
High-risk chemical workers	660	635	96.2
Smokers in low-risk industry	692	687	99.3
All workers	1,352	1,322	97.8
One subspecimen:			
Cough, spontaneous	263	121	46.0
Aerosolization, 25 min	263	247	93.9
Cough, 5 early mornings after aerosolization	220	190	86.4

trast, the classical clinical tumor today is a more advanced lesion that is mainly present in ambulatory or hospitalized *patients*. Again, the proper collection techniques are essential in both types to obtain optimal results.

In persons who are able to raise sputum spontaneously, the series of early morning samples is preferable. In individuals who cannot produce satisfactory specimens, it is necessary to induce sputum. Induction techniques using hypertonic saline aerosol vary widely in their effectiveness.[11-14,30-32] When used on hospital or clinic patients these methods produce satisfactory deep sputum specimens in 82–99 percent;[12,30,31] however, when used on asymptomatic screenees, the reported efficacy drops to 81–86 percent.[12,30]

Utilizing the ultrasonic physiologic aerosol described earlier, our asymptomatic screenees (not patients of a hospital or clinic) have produced 93.9 percent satisfactory specimens (Table 7-1). One examination of multiple sputum subspecimens obtained by various cytopathologic techniques including aerosol from 1,352 apparently healthy and actively employed screenees who were not patients of either a hospital or a clinic revealed a satisfactory specimen from 97.8 percent. Six hundred sixty of these screenees, workers in a chemical plant, produced 96.2 percent satisfactory sputum specimens, even though many were young and were not smokers; 99.3 percent of the 692 apparently healthy, cigarette-smoker screenees over 45 years of age produced satisfactory sputum specimens.

When the subspecimens were evaluated separately and blindly, the effect of multiplicity of samples and the differing efficacy of various techniques became apparent. Of the subspecimens produced by spontaneous coughing for 5 min after detailed instruction for deep cough, only 46.0 percent were satisfactory (Table 7-1). The combined early morning samples obtained by the screenees for the 5 days following the visit yielded 86.4 percent satisfactory samples. However, a single specimen produced the day of the visit during 25 min of aerosolization with ultrasonically nebulized Hanks' BSS yielded 93.9 percent satisfactory specimens.

Diagnostic Accuracy

With experienced personnel using multiple, combined proper techniques, 70–90 percent of all lung cancers can be diagnosed by cytologic examination alone.[22,33-35] The diagnostic yield is affected by several factors.

ROLE OF COLLECTION AND
PROCESSING TECHNIQUES

Sputum. Proper collection methods and processing are essential to obtain a representative cell sample. Early morning sputum provides the best specimen for a deep sampling of the lung. Sputum samples collected during other times in the day, in the physician's office or on the wards, for example, are usually less satisfactory, as they tend to produce more shallow material and to represent more patchy sampling of pulmonary areas. Use of the special techniques described earlier increases the diagnostic rate in obstructive conditions and among patients who are not able to produce sputum. Induction methods provide good sampling of the peripheral bronchial airways and increase diagnostic yield.[31,32] Antibiotics, postural drainage, and chest percussion[9,10] all increase the diagnostic accuracy of sputum examination in properly chosen cases.

The disparity in positive cytologic results reported in the literature is partly due to a broad and inconsistent interpretation of the term positive. That is, in the literature positive cytology does not necessarily imply the definitive cytopathologic diagnosis of cancer. Some authors include suspicious, inconclusive, or atypical cytologic findings as positive, giving a higher sensitivity, but lower specificity, and consequently more false positives. Numerical classifications add to the confusion.

Taking these differences into consideration and attempting to evaluate reports in the literature objectively, the overall cytologic *diagnosis* of lung cancer by sputum examination alone appears to be 60–75 percent.[8,33,34,36–40] Detection, which includes such categories as suspicious, inconclusive, and atypical, appears to reach 95 percent of proven lung cancer.

Bronchoscopy. Aspirations and washings obtained through the conventional rigid bronchoscope yield 70–90 percent cytologic detection in clinically suspicious, centrally located lesions.[34,37,41,42] The diagnostic yield of this technique for cancers in all areas of the lung, however, is lower than that obtained by examination of a series of five sputum specimens.[36,38,43] Proper bronchoscopic cuffing for bronchial occlusion and a specially designed lavage aspirating catheter (LAC) carefully used by a bronchoscopist experienced with the technique[6] produce selective cellular samples that can be most valuable in lateralizing and localizing occult tumors.

For lesions outside the central hilar region the flexible fiberoptic bronchoscope of Ikeda[44] represents a significant breakthrough technique for localization of the early occult lesion.[45] It allows examination of the upper and lateral lobes and the more peripheral smaller bronchi in all regions. Results in occult lesions when this fiber-

bronchoscope is used are far better than those for the rigid bronchoscope,[16,45–48] since in addition to being able to see around corners and into the smaller subsegmental bronchi, localized cellular washings and direct cell sampling by brush and currette are possible. Twenty-one occult, radiologically negative, cytologically positive tumors from 17 patients have been localized by this method.[49]

Transthoracic needle aspiration. Transthoracic needle aspiration is usually employed when other methods (i.e., sputum, bronchoscopy, television-guided brushing) have failed to provide a microscopic diagnosis. This method usually provides a definitive cytologic diagnosis in 80–90 percent of cancer cases. Failure of the method can be usually attributed to (1) inadequate cellular sample, (2) aspiration of the necrotic center of the tumor, or (3) aspiration of the inflammatory area surrounding the neoplasm. Complications are negligible when thin needles are used,[20,23] and only 2 neoplastic implants have been reported in 3,000 aspirations, about half of which were proven to be from malignant neoplasms.[22]

Pleural and pericardial tap. Peripheral and advanced primary carcinomas, as well as secondary carcinomas of the lung, often involve the pleura and can be diagnosed cytologically. Yields of cytopathologic diagnosis ranging from 33 percent[50] to 87 percent[29] have been reported. The low rates, in some instances, can be attributed to inclusion of all tumor cases with pleural effusion in the series whether or not there is firm evidence of pleural involvement. The use of proper collection and processing techniques, on the other hand, substantially increases diagnostic accuracy.

In two separate series studied at the Johns Hopkins Hospital, of 43 and 95 cases of malignant neoplasms involving pleura, 77 percent and 72 percent, respectively, were cytologically diagnosed by examination of pleural effusions.[27,28] A combination of cytology and closed needle biopsy of pleura provided the diagnosis in 90 percent of the cases in the latter series.[28] No misdiagnosis of cancer was made on either series. Mesothelial proliferation in some conditions can mimic cancer; examples are individual cell atypia in pulmonary infarct and papillary and pseudoacinar formations in collagen diseases. In addition, the pure lympocytic exudate of tuberculous effusions can

be mistaken for lymphocytic lymphoma or leukemia. Complete clinical information and a cautious
approach to the diagnosis of equivocal cellular
changes can prevent a misdiagnosis of cancer.
Repeat examinations, by providing freshly exfoliated cells and information about the evolution of
the disease, often help to establish the diagnosis.

NUMBER OF SPECIMENS EXAMINED

The value of multiple samples has been well
established.[36-38,50-52] One sputum sample should
not suffice for a cytologic examination for pulmonary cancer. For 197 patients with primary bronchogenic carcinoma seen at Johns Hopkins and
the University of Maryland between 1956 and
1959, the *detection* rate increased from 45 percent on the first sputum to 86 percent for three
sputum samples and to 95 percent for patients
from whom five sputum samples were examined.[8]
In this group a definitive cytopathologic *diagnosis* was established in 20 percent, 40 percent, and
56 percent of the cases when one, three, and five
sputum samples, respectively, were evaluated.
The lower sensitivity in the latter is due to higher
specificity, and no false cancer diagnoses were
rendered during this period when 1,014 specimens were examined.

In another group of 141 cases of histologically proven lung cancer in patients on whom a
definitive cytopathologic *diagnosis* was made on
sputum or bronchoscopic cytology,[13] only 42 percent had a cytopathologic diagnosis of cancer on
the first sample examined. This figure increased
to 73 percent for three samples and to 84 percent
for five sputum samples. Eighty-seven percent of
the cases were diagnosed when eight sputum
samples were examined.

Examination of multiple samples also
increases the effectiveness of bronchoscopic and
transthoracic needle aspiration techniques, as
well as pleural taps.[27,28]

LOCATION OF LESION

Centrally located lesions of the main and
lobar bronchi give higher diagnostic rates on sputum examination than do peripheral lesions.[34,36,38]
The latter can be diagnosed more effectively with
fiberoptic bronchoscopy,[45,48] brushing,[19] or
transthoracic needle aspiration[22] under television
control. The diagnostic yield for sputum examination and conventional rigid bronchoscopy is lower for carcinomas of the upper lobes than for

those located in the lower lobes.[34] Both areas can
be more effectively diagnosed when the fiberoptic
bronchoscope is used. The relationship between
the lesion and the bronchus also affects the diagnosis. Lesions involving the bronchial mucosa
are more easily diagnosed than those involving
only septae and submucosal stroma, and transthoracic needle biopsy is more effective in the
latter.

SIZE OF NEOPLASM

There is parallelism between the size of
peripheral neoplasms and the sputum cytologic
diagnostic rate.[34] On the other hand, when *centrally* located bronchial carcinomas increase in
size, the diagnostic rate decreases.[34,36] This
apparent paradox is attributable to (1) obstruction, which prevents the neoplastic cells from
appearing in the sputum, and (2) necrosis, which
renders the definitive cytologic diagnosis difficult
because of degenerative changes in the exfoliated
neoplastic cells. Size apparently does not significantly affect the diagnostic yield of either bronchoscopy[45] or transthoracic needle aspirations.[22]

TYPE OF NEOPLASM

The highest yield in the diagnosis of bronchogenic carcinoma by sputum examination[33,36,38]
is obtained for epidermoid carcinomas (67–85
percent); these are lesions that usually arise in the
surface bronchial epithelium and exfoliate into
bronchial secretions. They are clearly discernible
on microscopic examination. Small cell undifferentiated carcinomas give the next highest yield
(64–70 percent), while adenocarcinomas give the
lowest yield (54–57 percent) mainly because of
their usual peripheral location and their origin
beneath the surface. When other techniques fail,
television-guided brushing and transthoracic
needle aspiration can provide material for the
diagnosis of peripheral neoplasms that produce
radiologic shadows. The differential cytologic
diagnosis between poorly differentiated adenocarcinomas and benign alveolar proliferations or
reactive histiocytes (viral pneumonia, organizing
pneumonitis) can sometimes be very difficult. In
addition, localized bronchial adenomas, even
though centrally located, cannot be diagnosed by
sputum examination. Rarely, however, a metastasizing carcinoid will exfoliate cells into the sputum, and vigorous aspiration of an adenoma at
bronchoscopy can produce a diagnostic cellular
specimen.[54]

Accuracy of Cytopathologic Results

INTERPRETATION

In competent and experienced hands, false cancer diagnoses are minimal. If the positive category is used strictly to mean a definitive cytologic diagnosis of cancer,[55] false positive results do not usually exceed 1 percent.[8,20,22,33,36,56] The most common sources of false positive and false suspicious reports in pulmonary cytopathology are alveolar cell and histiocytic proliferation (i.e., organizing pneumonitis, infarct) and atypical squamous metaplasia (i.e., chronic irritations, bronchiectasis, chronic bronchitis, lung abscess). In pleural effusions the common cause of error is mesothelial cell proliferation overlying the healing pulmonary infarction.

It has been stated that "although there are various reasons and excuses which might explain false negative results, there is only one causative factor for the occurrence of false positive results: the misinterpretation of smears by the cytologist!"[33] Experience and the use of rigid criteria for a definitive diagnosis[55] prevent the majority of false cancer diagnoses. Further, it is extremely important for the pathologist to have all pertinent clinical information in order to avoid misinterpretation of certain morphologic changes.

ACCURACY OF CELL TYPING

The tissue type of tumor differentiation can be determined accurately from adequate cellular specimens.[40,57,58] Well-differentiated carcinomas, either epidermoid or adenocarcinoma, and small cell undifferentiated (oat cell) carcinomas are the most accurately diagnosed. On the other hand, poorly differentiated carcinomas and large cell undifferentiated carcinomas are both difficult to type. Again, the number of samples examined and the collection technique affect the accuracy of type identification. Sputum specimens are reported to be more accurate than bronchoscopic material, probably as a result of availability of multiple samples in the former.[58] Correlations of the cytopathologic and histopathologic diagnoses are given for sputum specimens (Table 7-2) and bronchoscopic material (Table 7-3) from 241 and 223 patients with primary lung carcinoma, respectively. Tissue diagnosis is based on biopsy, surgical, or autopsy material.

Evaluation based on cytopathologic diagnosis reveals that tissue correlation within the same general category was obtained in 98 percent of the well-differentiated or moderately differentiated epidermoid carcinomas (89 of 91) in sputum and in all of the same type carcinomas in bronchoscopic material, while 48 percent of the poorly differentiated epidermoid carcinomas by sputum cytopathology and 71 percent by bronchoscopic cytopathology were diagnosed as epidermoid carcinoma on tissue. Similarly, 96 percent of the well-differentiated or moderately well-differentiated adenocarcinomas on sputum cytopathology and 86 percent of the same type of cancers on bronchoscopic cytopathology were diagnosed as adenocarcinomas by histopathology, while 65 percent of the poorly differentiated adenocarcinomas in sputum and 47 percent in bronchoscopic material had histopathologic diagnoses of adenocarcinoma. Eighty-five percent of the cytopathologically diagnosed small cell undifferentiated carcinomas in sputum and all of those in bronchoscopic material had the same tissue diagnosis. Two of the four cytologically diagnosed large cell undifferentiated carcinomas in sputum and only one of the six in bronchoscopic material had correlating histopathologic diagnoses.

Evaluation based on tissue, on the other hand, reveals that well-differentiated or moderately differentiated epidermoid carcinomas were identified within the category of epidermoid carcinoma cytologically in 96 and 91 percent of cases in sputum and bronchoscopic material, respectively. The respective figures for well-differentiated or moderately differentiated adenocarcinomas were 97 and 90 percent. The degree of differentiation in cytologic samples, however, correlated less well with histopathology in both epidermoid carcinomas and adenocarcinomas, especially in bronchoscopic material. In sputum, 89 percent of well-differentiated or moderately differentiated epidermoid carcinomas and 72 percent of well-differentiated or moderately differentiated adenocarcinomas were diagnosed correctly. Corresponding figures for bronchoscopic material were 74 and 60 percent. Poorly differentiated epidermoid carcinomas and adenocarcinomas were diagnosed cytologically within their respective groups in 66 and 67 percent of cases in sputum and in 69 and 64 percent, respectively, in bronchoscopic material. The degree of differentiation in cytologic samples correlated poorly with histopathologic differentiation, especially for epidermoid carcinomas. Sixteen percent of epidermoid

Table 7-2
Typing of Neoplasms by Sputum Specimens (241 Cases)

| | Histopathology | | | | | | | | |
| | Epidermoid Ca. | | Adenoca. | | Small Cell Undiff. Ca. | Large Cell Undiff. Ca. | Adeno-epid. Ca. | Unclas-sified* | Total |
Cytopathology	Well or Mod. Diff.	Poorly Diff.	Well or Mod. Diff.	Poorly Diff.					
Epidermoid carcinoma									
Well or mod. diff.	73	16	—	—	—	—	—	2	91
Poorly diff.	6	5	—	5	1	1	1	4	23
Adenocarcinoma									
Well or mod. diff.	—	—	21†	3	—	—	—	1	25
Poorly diff.	—	3	7	15	1	3	2	3	34
Small cell undiff. carcinoma	—	—	—	1	34	—	1	4	40
Large cell undiff. carcinoma	—	—	—	1	—	2	—	1	4
Adenoepidermoid carcinoma	—	—	—	—	—	—	—	—	—
Unclassified	3	8	1	2	3	1	1	5	24
Total	82	32	29	27	39	7	5	20	241

*Only biopsies.
†Three bronchioloalveolar carcinomas are included in this group.

Table 7-3
Typing of Neoplasms by Bronchoscopic Specimens (223 Cases)

Cytopathology	Epidermoid Ca.		Adenoca.		Small Cell Undiff. Ca.	Large Cell Undiff. Ca.	Adeno-epid. Ca.	Unclassified*	Total
	Well or Mod. Diff.	Poorly Diff.	Well or Mod. Diff.	Poorly Diff.					
Epidermoid carcinoma									
Well or mod. diff.	58	19	—	—	—	—	—	—	77
Poorly diff.	13	17	—	3	2	3	1	3	42
Adenocarcinoma									
Well or mod. diff.	—	—	6†	—	—	—	—	1	7
Poorly diff.	2	5	3	14	1	4	1	6	36
Small cell undiff. carcinoma	—	—	—	—	31	—	—	—	31
Large cell undiff. carcinoma	—	3	—	—	—	1	—	2	6
Adenoepidermoid carcinoma	—	—	—	—	—	—	1	—	1
Unclassified	5	8	1	5	1	1	—	2	23
Total	78	52	10	22	35	9	3	14	223

*Only biopsies.
†Two bronchioloalveolar carcinomas included in this group.

carcinomas poorly differentiated in sputum and 33 percent in bronchoscopic material had the same histopathologic diagnosis, while 56 percent of adenocarcinomas poorly differentiated in sputum and 64 percent in bronchoscopic material were diagnosed as such by histopathology. However, correct assessment of the degree of differentiation is difficult on biopsies alone, especially in poorly differentiated tumors, and this difficulty also contributed to the poor correlation between histopathologic and cytopathologic diagnoses. Small cell undifferentiated carcinomas were diagnosed correctly by cytopathology in 87 percent of cases in sputum and in 89 percent in bronchoscopic material. Only 2 of 7 (29 percent) large cell carcinomas were diagnosed in sputum and 1 of 10 in bronchoscopic material. None of 5 adenoepidermoid carcinomas was identified in sputum; however, 1 of 3 adenoepidermoid carcinomas was correctly diagnosed in bronchoscopic material.

Transthoracic needle aspirations also allow high accuracy in cell typing, but poorly differentiated carcinomas again present a problem.

It is also possible to determine the type of the tumor accurately in pleural and pericardial effusions,[59,60] but the primary site of the tumor can be difficult to determine on a morphologic basis alone.[61] Adequate clinical information often helps to establish the diagnosis.[60,61] In some cases, examination of other material (sputum, bronchoscopic and needle aspiration material) is necessary to reach a specific diagnosis. This is especially true in the case of small cell undifferentiated carcinomas, since prostatic and breast carcinomas that have metastasized to serous cavities sometimes mimic these tumors in effusions.

SUMMARY

Clinical cytopathology is an effective means of microscopically diagnosing lung cancer in its early clinically occult stage and in its more classical, clinically manifest form. Cytologic examination of sputum is virtually the only method available today to detect and diagnose radiologically occult pulmonary cancer; furthermore, it can be of great assistance in its localization. It should thus play a key roll in screening segments of the population at high risk of developing lung cancer.

Factors for successful cytopathologic examination include properly chosen and properly carried out cytologic techniques and experienced, careful microscopic interpretation. Five early morning deep cough sputum specimens yield highest routine results with the classical, clinically manifest tumors. Materials from sputum induction, transbronchial instrumentation, television-guided brushing, and needle aspiration have proven of additional value in peripheral early or radiologically occult cancers. Tumor type can be determined cytologically with high accuracy, especially for the well-differentiated squamous cell carcinomas and adenocarcinomas and the small cell undifferentiated carcinomas.

REFERENCES

1. Melamed MR, Koss LG, Cliffton EE: Roentgenologically occult lung cancer diagnosed by cytology: Report of 12 cases. Cancer 16:1537–1551, 1963

2. Pearson FG, Thompson DW, Delarue NC: Experience with the cytologic detection, localization, and treatment of radiographically undemonstrable bronchial carcinoma. J Thorac Cardiovasc Surg 54:371–382, 1967

3. Meyer JA, Bechtold E, Jones DB: Positive sputum cytologic tests for five years before specific detection of bronchial carcinoma. J Thorac Cardiovasc Surg 57:318–324, 1969

4. Woolner LB, David E, Fontana RS, et al: In situ and early invasive bronchogenic carcinoma. Report of 28 cases with postoperative survival data. J Thorac Cardiovasc Surg 60:275–290, 1970

5. Grzybowski S, Coy P: Early diagnosis of carcinoma of the lung. Simultaneous screening with chest X-ray and sputum cytology. Cancer 25:113–120, 1970

6. Marsh BR, Frost JK, Erozan YS, et al: Occult bronchogenic carcinoma. Endoscopic localization and television documentation. Cancer 30:1348–1352, 1972

7. Saccomanno G, Saunders RP, Ellis H, et al: Concentration of carcinoma or atypical cells in sputum. Acta Cytol (Baltimore) 7:305–310, 1963

8. Frost JK: Manual of Second Postgraduate Institute for Pathologists in Clinical Cytopathology. Baltimore, Johns Hopkins, 1961, section 3

9. Tweeddale DN, Harbord RP, Nuzum CT, et al: A new technique to obtain sputum for cytologic

study: External percussion and vibration of the chest wall. Acta Cytol (Baltimore) 10:214–219, 1966

10. Masin F, Masin M: Sputum cytology (letter to the editor). Acta Cytol (Baltimore) 10:391, 1966

11. Barach AL, Beck GJ, Bickerman HA, et al: Physical methods simulating mechanisms of the human cough. J Appl Physiol 5:85–91, 1952

12. Bickerman HA, Sproul EE, Barach AL: An aerosol method of producing bronchial secretions in human subjects: A clinical technic for the detection of lung cancer. Dis Chest 33:347–362, 1958

13. Barach AL, Bickerman HA, Beck GJ, et al: Induced sputum as a diagnostic technique for cancer of the lungs and for mobilization of retained secretions. Arch Intern Med 106:230–236, 1960

14. Roberts TW, Pollak A, Howard R, et al: Tracheobronchial cytology utilizing an improved tussilator (cough machine). Acta Cytol (Baltimore) 7:174–179, 1963

15. Allan WB, Whittlesey P, Haroutunian LM, et al: The use of sulfur dioxide as a diagnostic aid in pulmonary cancer; preliminary report. Cancer 11:938, 1958

16. Marsh BR, Frost JK, Erozan YS, et al: Flexible fiberoptic bronchoscopy. Its place in the search for lung cancer. Ann Otol Rhinol Laryngol 82:757–764, 1973

17. Fennessy JJ: Bronchial brushing. Ann Otol Rhinol Laryngol 79:924–932, 1970

18. Hattori S, Matsuda M, Nishihara H, et al: Early diagnosis of small peripheral lung cancer—Cytologic diagnosis of very fresh cancer cells obtained by the TV-brushing technique. Acta Cytol (Baltimore) 15:460–467, 1971

19. Bibbo M, Fennessy JJ, Lu CT, et al: Bronchial brushing technique for the cytologic diagnosis of peripheral lung lesions. A preview of 693 cases. Acta Cytol (Baltimore) 17:245–251, 1973

20. Dahlgren S, Nordenstrom B: Transthoracic Needle Biopsy. Stockholm, Alqvist and Wiksell/Gebers Förlag AB, Chicago, Year Book, 1966

21. Dahlgren SE: Aspiration biopsy of intrathoracic tumours. Acta Pathol Microbiol Scand 70:566–576, 1967

22. Dahlgren SE, Lind B: Comparison between diagnostic results obtained by transthoracic needle biopsy and by sputum cytology. Acta Cytol (Baltimore) 16:53–58, 1972

23. Zelch JV, Lalli AF, McCormack LJ, et al: Aspiration biopsy in diagnosis of pulmonary nodule. Chest 63:149–152, 1973

24. Cardozo PL: A critical evaluation of 3,000 cytologic analyses of pleural fluid, ascitic fluid and pericardial fluid. Acta Cytol (Baltimore) 10:455–460, 1966

25. Johnson WD: The cytological diagnosis of cancer in serous effusions. Acta Cytol (Baltimore) 10:161–172, 1966

26. Jarvi OH, Kunnas RJ, Laitio MT, et al: The accuracy and significance of cytologic cancer diagnosis of pleural effusions (a followup study of 338 patients). Acta Cytol (Baltimore) 16:152–158, 1972

27. Light RW, Erozan YS, Ball WC Jr: Cells in pleural fluid: Their value in differential diagnosis. Arch Intern Med 132:854–860, 1973

28. Salyer WR, Eggleston JC, Erozan YS: Efficacy of pleural needle biopsy and pleural fluid cytopathology in the diagnosis of malignant neoplasm involving the pleura. Chest 67:536–539, 1975

29. Grunze H: The comparative diagnostic accuracy, efficiency and specificity of cytologic technics used in the diagnosis of malignant neoplasm in serous effusions of the pleural and pericardial cavities. Acta Cytol (Baltimore) 8:150–163, 1964

30. Rome DS, Olson KB: A direct comparison of natural and aerosol produced sputum collected from 776 asymptomatic men. Acta Cytol (Baltimore) 5:173–176, 1961

31. Brenner SA: Induced sputum cytodiagnosis as an aid in the detection of lung cancer. J Am Med Wom Assoc 18:705–710, 1963

32. Fontana RS, Carr DT, Woolner LB, et al: Value of induced sputum in cytologic diagnosis of lung cancer. JAMA 191:134–136, 1965

33. Grunze H: A critical review and evaluation of cytodiagnosis in chest diseases. Acta Cytol (Baltimore) 4:175–198, 1960

34. Umiker W: The current role of exfoliative cytopathology in the routine diagnosis of bronchogenic carcinoma. A five-year study of 152 consecutive, unselected cases. Dis Chest 40:154–159, 1961

35. Grunze H: Cytologic diagnosis of tumors of the chest. Acta Cytol (Baltimore) 17:148–159, 1973

36. Koss LG, Melamed MR, Goodner JT: Pulmonary cytology—A brief survey of diagnostic results from July 1st 1952 until December 31st 1960. Acta Cytol (Baltimore) 8:104–113, 1964

37. William S: The cytologic diagnosis of lung cancer. Med J Aust 48:233–236, 1961

38. Rosa UW, Prolla JC, Gastal ES: Cytology in diagnosis of cancer affecting the lung. Results in 1,000 consecutive patients. Chest 63:203–207, 1973

39. Sirtori C, Talamazzi F: Cytology in lung cancer and in heavy smokers. Acta Un Int Cancer 15:477–479, 1959

40. Lukeman JM: Reliability of cytologic diagnosis in cancer of the lung. Cancer Chemother Rep [Suppl] (Part 3) 4:79–93, 1973

41. McKay DG, Ware PF, Atwood DA, et al: Diagnosis of bronchogenic carcinoma by smears of bronchoscopic aspirations. Cancer 1:208–222, 1948

42. Herbut PA, Clerf LH: Bronchogenic carcinoma; diagnosis by cytologic study of bronchoscopically removed secretions. JAMA 130:1006–1012, 1946

43. Erozan YS, Frost JK: Cytopathologic diagnosis of cancer in pulmonary material: A critical histopathologic correlation. Acta Cytol (Baltimore) 14:560–565, 1970

44. Ikeda S, Yanai N, Ishikawa S: Flexible bronchofiberscope. Keio J Med 17:1–16, 1968

45. Marsh BR, Frost JK, Erozan YS, et al: Role of fiberoptic bronchoscopy in lung cancer. Semin Oncol 1:199–203, 1974

46. Ikeda S: Flexible bronchofiberscope. Ann Otol Rhinol Laryngol 79:916–923, 1970

47. Zavala DC, Richardson RH, Mukerjee PK, et al: Use of the bronchofiberscope for bronchial brush biopsy. Diagnostic results and comparison with other brushing techniques. Chest 63:889–892, 1973

48. Zavala DC: Diagnostic fiberoptic bronchoscopy: Techniques and results of biopsy in 600 patients. Chest 68:12–19, 1975

49. Marsh BR: Personal communication

50. Poppius H, Kokkola K: Diagnosis and differential diagnosis in tuberculous pleurisy. Scand J Respir Dis [Suppl] 63:105–110, 1968

51. Farber SM, Benioff MA, Frost JK, et al: Cytologic studies of sputum and bronchial secretions in primary carcinoma of the lung. Dis Chest 14:633–664, 1948

52. Russell WO, Neidhardt HW, Mountain CF, et al: Cytodiagnosis of lung cancer. A report of a four-year laboratory, clinical, and statistical study with a review of the literature on lung cancer and pulmonary cytology. Acta Cytol (Baltimore) 7:1–44, 1963

53. Carbone PP, Frost JK, Feinstein AR, et al: Lung cancer: Perspectives and prospects. Ann Intern Med 73:1003–1024, 1970

54. Pierson B: Cyto-diagnosis of bronchial adenoma in: Transactions of the Sixth Annual Meeting of the Inter-Society Cytology Council. 1958, pp 157–159

55. Frost JK: The Cell in Health and Disease. Basel, Karger, Baltimore, Williams & Wilkins, 1969

56. Umiker W: False positive reports in the cytologic diagnosis of lung cancer. Br J Cancer 11:391–397, 1957

57. Foot NC: The identification of types of pulmonary cancer in cytologic smears. Am J Pathol 28:963–983, 1952

58. Lange E, Hoeg K: Cytologic typing of lung cancer. Acta Cytol (Baltimore) 16:327–330, 1972

59. Luse SA, Reagan JW: A histocytological study of effusions. II. Effusions associated with malignant tumors. Cancer 7:1167–1181, 1954

60. Murphy WM, Ng ABP: Determination of primary site by examination of cancer cells in body fluids. Am J Clin Pathol 58:479–488, 1972

61. Foot NC: Identification of types and primary sites of metastatic tumors from exfoliated cells in serous fluids. Am J Pathol 30:661–677, 1954

Bernard R. Marsh
John K. Frost
Yener S. Erozan
Darryl Carter

8
Fiberbronchoscopy

In the diagnosis of bronchogenic carcinoma few studies have proved more valuable than endoscopic examination of the tracheobronchial tree. The advent of the flexible fiberbronchoscope has further enhanced the value of this study by allowing exploration of previously inaccessible segments. The remarkable features of this new instrument have captured the imagination of physicians everywhere, so that we now find ourselves asking what role remains for the open-tube instruments.

It is the purpose of this chapter to summarize current developments in fiberbronchoscopy for lung cancer diagnosis and to suggest when more traditional techniques may still be useful.

NATURE OF FLEXIBLE FIBERBRONCHOSCOPE

Flexible instruments may now be obtained from several manufacturers, each boasting some special feature. For purposes of lung cancer diagnosis, however, today's most practical instrument consists of a 5- to 6-mm-diameter flexible

shaft containing a glass fiber image bundle, an illumination bundle, a 2-mm lumen, and a mechanism for tip deflection. Various types of brushes, curets, and biopsy forceps provide the necessary means for retrieving specimens from nearly anywhere in the lung.

This equipment is far more expensive and delicate than standard bronchoscopic instruments. It does not tolerate rough handling nor abuse, but when properly cared for it provides long and reasonably trouble-free operation. Our first fiberscope, after 6 years of use, still functions well and has few broken fibers in the original bundle.

For maximum service we find it best to limit use of the instrument to a few qualified physicians, since repair bills seem to increase geometrically with the number of people using it. Even though they are seldom needed, a complete duplicate set of instruments should be available if a properly functioning instrument is to be available at all times. Repairs may require up to several weeks for completion, and if another instrument is not available, one may find himself in a dilemma.

Before investing in this equipment one should be acquainted not only with its proper use but also with some of the differences from traditional bronchoscopy.

Supported in part by National Cancer Institute Contract NIH 69-2172.

1. These investigations usually require more time than standard bronchoscopy. A more detailed study is often performed, and multiple specimens, a small suction channel, and a small lens tend to prolong the examination.
2. Considerable care is required in cleaning and sterilization; therefore this task should be assigned only to specially qualified personnel who thoroughly understand these details.
3. A single misadventure may require replacement of an entire image bundle, which is a very costly experience. Sufficient funds for maintenance should be allowed, and everyone having access to the equipment should be thoroughly trained.
4. Biopsy specimens are extremely small, requiring the cooperation and support of a highly competent pathology staff.
5. Complications such as hypoxia, pneumothorax, uncontrollable bleeding, and fever are potentially greater threats than during open-tube bronchoscopy. It is therefore recommended that these procedures be performed in an operating room or other suitably equipped area.

TECHNIQUES

Long experience has shown that standard endoscopic techniques allow successful documentation in slightly more than one-third of cases of clinical lung cancer.[1-5] Current fiberoptic methods, however, now provide diagnostic material in 70–90 percent of primary bronchogenic carcinomas.[6,7] Such impressive gains have led some to conclude that rigid instruments are now obsolete. Experienced endoscopists, however, will appreciate that these instruments are complementary, each having valuable features not shared by the other.

Since 1969 we have performed more than 2500 rigid and flexible bronchoscopic examinations. While we now use the flexible instrument in more than 90 percent of our procedures, we find the open-tube instrument still valuable for use in addition to, or instead of, the flexible equipment as the case demands.

The following guidelines suggest when each instrument may best be used. Continued development of flexible instruments with larger channels and forceps will doubtless enhance their value in areas where the open tube is now preferred.

INDICATIONS FOR OPEN-TUBE INSTRUMENT

1. Major airway problems. Better biopsy, foreign body, and aspirating capabilities recommend its use in these conditions: (a) Foreign body. (b) Broncholith. (c) Tracheobronchial stricture. (d) Carcinoid. (e) Massive hemoptysis. (f) Advanced malignancies involving the major bronchi. The open-tube instrument not only provides better biopsy capabilities but sometimes permits the removal of an obstructing tumor mass causing atelectasis. (g) Biopsy of the lobar spur or carina. Currently available microforceps are inadequate, but improvements in these instruments can be anticipated. (h) Transbronchial biopsy for diffuse lung disease. Larger specimens more frequently provide a diagnosis than when microforceps are used.[8,9]
2. Small children. Inadequate ventilation around the flexible instrument makes its use inadvisable in most.
3. Cases requiring differential cytology. A cuffed rigid bronchoscope may be required for reliable separation of secretions from the two lungs. This is not frequently necessary, but it may be useful in some patients with occult tumors.

INDICATIONS FOR FLEXIBLE INSTRUMENT

1. Mechanical problems involving the neck or jaws.
2. Hemoptysis (except massive). More precise localization is possible, and a significant percentage of tumors may be identified.[7]
3. Presence of thoracic aortic aneurysm.
4. Peripheral, upper lobe, or hilar tumors not involving a main bronchus.
5. X-ray negative lung cancer diagnosed by sputum cytology. Here the lesion is often less apparent, and a detailed study of the segments may be required. The brilliant image of rod-optics telescopes allows detection of some of these tumors; others require not only the deeper penetration of the fiberscope but also the magnification allowed by close approximation to the tumor area to identify the subtle changes of less-advanced disease in the segments.[6]

6. Transbronchial biopsy of peripheral lung lesions using fluoroscopic guidance. This may be especially helpful in the upper lobes where use of the rigid instrument is not only difficult but hazardous.

The flexible instrument may be passed into the tracheobronchial tree through any available orifice. The two most common are the transnasal and transorotracheal routes. Each has its proponents, although we prefer the latter in most cases.

The transnasal route may be useful in relatively brief examinations where aspiration of secretions and the acquisition of visual information are of principal interest. Its value is somewhat more limited where multiple brushing specimens are required for cytologic localization. In the presence of nasal infection or deformity it is best avoided.

The transorotracheal route allows the use of a large (9 to 10 mm) endotracheal tube through which the instrument may be passed while providing ample lumen for ventilation. The endotracheal tube may be inserted under local anesthesia by slipping it over the fiberscope, as described by Hodgkin et al.[10] This has one advantage in that it allows careful study of the larynx and trachea before the tube is passed. Others prefer to pass the tube using a laryngeal mirror for guidance, while some prefer direct laryngoscopy using an anesthesia laryngoscope. In any case, the presence of an orotracheal tube offers a number of advantages. Control of the airway is assured, allowing for assisted or controlled ventilation, if desired, and the use of supplemental oxygen or general anesthesia when indicated. The endotracheal tube allows for insertion and removal of the instrument as many times as necessary for specimen removal or lens cleaning without trauma to the upper respiratory tract. This may be especially important for curette and brush specimens, which are best dislodged before retrieving the instrument from the fiberscope.

The fiberscope may also be passed through the open-tube bronchoscope, but a compromised airway and technical inconvenience factors limit its uefulness to a brief examination.

X-RAY-VISIBLE TUMOR

Tumors located in the hilum usually demonstrate some visible abnormality in the major or

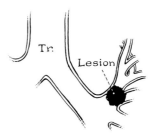

Fig. 8-1. Endobronchial tumor. Tr. is trachea.

segmental bronchi. This may assume different forms, but usually one of the following major types is observed:

1. If the lesion originates from a large bronchus it usually presents as a friable endobronchial mass and can be diagnosed by tissue biopsy or cytology specimen obtained by brushing (Fig. 8-1).
2. If the lesion originates in the periphery and has become large enough to involve the hilum, it more often presents as a bronchial stenosis (Fig. 8-2A–D). Endobronchial tumor, if present, is often limited to a peripheral bronchus and cannot be seen. Diagnostic material is frequently difficult to obtain, but the curette is especially valuable in reaching several peripheral bronchi, thus improving the chances of obtaining diagnostic material. Biopsy forceps are less often valuable in tumors presenting this way.

Tumors located outside the hilum are best approached with the use of fluoroscopy to guide the biopsy instruments into precisely the proper area. Frequently no endobronchial abnormality will be found, and choice of the proper bronchus may be impossible without fluoroscopy. Here again the curette and the brush are valuable in obtaining representative material, but biopsies are also useful. Considerable care should be exercised since hemorrhage and pneumothorax are potential complications of these procedures.[9,11]

RADIOLOGICALLY OCCULT TUMOR

Sputum cytology provides a means for identifying tumors not otherwise apparent. As greater use is made of this and other screening techniques, the bronchoscopist will be called on more frequently to localize the source of malignant cells in patients whose x-rays are unrevealing.

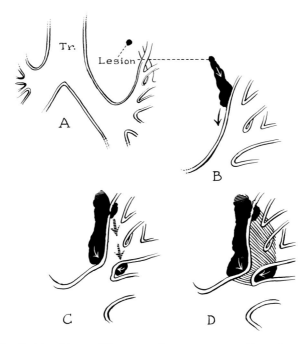

Fig. 8-2. Peripheral tumor (A); tumor adjacent to segmental bronchus (B); endobronchial tumor invasion and beginning bronchial stenosis (C); extensive extrabronchial tumor with marked stenosis (D).

The search for these tumors must include a careful examination of the oral cavity, nasopharynx, and larynx. Cells shed from these areas appear in the sputum and frequently cannot be differentiated from those originating in the lung. A recent study supports our observation that in head and neck tumors that shed malignant cells into the sputum, bronchoscopic cytology is usually negative.[12] Indeed, if malignant cells are found at bronchoscopy, a second primary lung tumor should be suspected.

The bronchial lesions in this group cover a spectrum from large, friable tumors to those with only a patch of in situ carcinoma hidden in a small subsegmental bronchus. The less extensive tumors require a detailed segment-by-segment fiberoptic study for discovery and evaluation. Early changes indicating tumor presence may be no more than slight mucosal roughening, friability, or slight thickening of a segmental or subsegmental spur. Much later in the natural history of this disease one may find an endobronchial mass with bronchial obstruction, ulceration, and fixation.

The considerable time required to complete a comprehensive study for occult disease frequent-ly necessitates the use of general anesthesia, which also provides the cough control needed for differential cytology. A 9-mm endotracheal tube with a **T** adapter is adequate for ventilation, and it allows freedom to carry out as detailed a study as necessary. A new endotracheal tube has recently been introduced to minimize resistance to gas flow, and it may further enhance the usefulness of this technique.[13]

Even though an advanced lesion may be found in a few moments, a careful search of both lungs may uncover evidence of multifocal disease. In 15 patients with occult primary bronchogenic carcinoma we found 4 with two or more noncontiguous bronchial lesions.

SPECIMENS

Specimens are obtained after completion of the entire visual search. This allows careful inspection of the bronchial mucosa after secretions have been aspirated and before mucosal changes and bleeding develop from the trauma of forceps or brush. If a gross lesion is found, it should be left until last to be brushed or biopsied.

This allows less chance for cross-contamination when searching for cytologic evidence of multifocal disease.

To obtain selective cytology specimens the instrument is first cleaned by aspirating a BSS through the channel, and a brush is inserted. The instrument is then placed in a lobar bronchus, where the brush is passed out of the instrument and into each segment for a thorough sampling of the lobe. The brush is then brought back to the end of the bronchoscope and both are carefully removed. The specimen is dislodged and the brush removed. The instrument channel is again rinsed, and a new brush is placed for the next lobe to be studied. This procedure is repeated until each lobe has been thoroughly studied and the specimens labeled according to lobe. This technique reduces the risk of cross-contamination and provides useful information regarding the presence or absence of multifocal disease. Such a detailed study may not be required in every case, but it is clearly indicated in the study of patients with inapparent tumors.

Following the brushing procedure, biopsies are obtained from all suspicious areas. If the tumor is present in a segmental bronchus, the curette is also used because the deeper cells obtained may be required for diagnosis. Multiple specimens greatly improve the diagnostic yield in these procedures and should be considered routine.

Repeated observations have shown that in situ carcinoma may extend from a small segmental lesion well into the lobar bronchus and even the main bronchus. Since these changes may be so slight as to escape the eye of the bronchoscopist, biopsies should be obtained from the lobar spur and carina to aid in determining safe bronchial margins[14] (Fig. 8-3A–D). Currently available microforceps are inadequate for this purpose, but as larger instrument channels are provided, better biopsy forceps will become available and one may not have to resort to rigid instruments to obtain these specimens. We have found a specially designed retrograde-introduced cup forcep particularly valuable, but this instrument is not generally available.[6]

For 3 days following the procedure, early morning sputum specimens should be submitted for postbronchial cytology studies. These are especially important and will frequently provide diagnostic information not obtained at bronchoscopy.

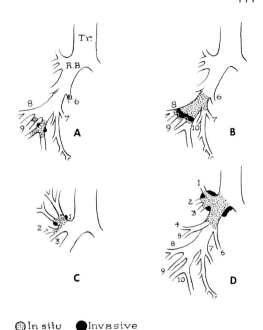

@In situ   ●Invasive

Fig. 8-3. Pathological findings on four resected tumors (A–D). The stippled areas indicate carcinoma in situ. Areas shown in solid black represent invasive disease; Tr. is trachea; R.B. is right main bronchus. Bronchial segments are identified as follows: numbers 1, 2, and 3 indicate apical, posterior, and anterior segments of upper lobe; 4 and 5 are lateral and medial segments of middle lobe; 6 is superior segment of lower lobe; 7 is medial basal; 8 is anterior basal; 9 is lateral basal; 10 is posterior basal. (Reproduced by permission from Marsh BR, Frost JK, Erozan YS, et al: Flexible fiberoptic bronchoscopy, its place in the search for lung cancer. Ann Otol Rhinol Laryngol 82:757–764, 1973.)

CONCLUSION AND OUTLOOK

The fiberbronchoscope has greatly extended our capabilities for diagnosis of lung cancer, especially the earlier segmental lesions. Yet we also often discover the disease in an advanced stage, when the present forms of therapy are inadequate.

More sophisticated methods are needed for detection of truly early tumors where no endobronchial abnormality can be found. Means to enhance detection of smaller, less-visible areas of in situ carcinoma are being studied.

As more effective and economical screening techniques are developed, these highly reliable localizing techniques will allow definitive therapy in truly early cancer.

REFERENCES

1. Ikeda S: Flexible bronchofiberscope. Ann Otol Rhinol Laryngol 79:916–923, 1970

2. Woolner LB, Anderson HA, Bernartz PE: Occult carcinoma of the bronchus: A study of 15 cases of in situ or early invasive bronchogenic carcinoma. Dis Chest 37:278–288, 1960

3. Bell JW: Positive sputum cytology and negative chest roentgenograms. Ann Thorac Surg 9:149–157, 1970

4. Bernstein L: Two thousand bronchoscopies in search of cancer. Ann Otol Rhinol Laryngol 76:242–249, 1967

5. Pearson FG, Thompson DW, DeLarue NC: Experience with the cytologic detection, localization and treatment of radiologically undemonstrated bronchial carcinoma. J Thorac Cardiovasc Surg 54:371–382, 1967

6. Marsh BR, Frost JK, Erozan YS, et al: Flexible fiberoptic bronchoscopy, its place in the search for lung cancer. Ann Otol Rhinol Laryngol 82:757–764, 1973

7. Zavala DC: Diagnostic fiberoptic bronchoscopy: Techniques and results of biopsy in 600 patients. Chest 68:12–19, 1975

8. Andersen H, Fontana R: Transbronchoscopic lung biopsy for diffuse pulmonary diseases: Techniques and results in 450 cases. Chest 62:125–128, 1972

9. Joyner LR, Scheinhorn DJ: Transbronchial forceps lung biopsy through the fiberoptic bronchoscope. Chest 67:532–535, 1975

10. Hodgkin JE, Rosenow EC, Stubbs SE: Oral introduction of the fiberoptic bronchoscope. Chest 68:88–90, 1975

11. Flick MR, Wasson K, Dunn LJ, et al: Fatal pulmonary hemorrhage after transbronchial lung biopsy through the fiberoptic bronchoscope. Am Rev Respir Dis 111:853–856, 1975

12. Dellon AL, Chu EW, Hall CA, et al: Cytology of bronchial washings. Arch Otolaryngol 101:465–466, 1975

13. Medical Engineering Corporation, 3037 Mt. Pleasant Street, Racine, Wisconsin

14. Marsh BR, Frost JK, Erozan YS, et al: Role of fiberoptic bronchoscopy in lung cancer. Semin Oncol 1:199–203, 1974

Edward M. Goldberg

9

Mediastinoscopy in Assessment of Lung Cancer

The management of lung carcinoma is a major undertaking; it requires the combined efforts of surgeon, radiotherapist, chemotherapist, and others involved in patient care. Although surgical treatment of lung carcinoma is often unsuccessful, at present only patients who have undergone surgical resection can expect long-term survival. Radiotherapy, although sometimes effective for local control, has a disappointing rate of cure; chemotherapy is likewise ineffectual at this time. Among the many reasons for therapeutic failure, of major significance are the innate biologic behavior of these tumors and the individual host resistance. To improve therapeutic results, early diagnosis and staging techniques are required so that appropriate treatment can be instituted.

Mediastinoscopy, a relatively new surgical endoscopic technique, is rapidly proving itself an indispensable diagnostic tool for examination of the upper chest cavity. Many problems in the diagnosis and prognosis of cancer of the chest can be solved by this safe and direct approach to the mediastinum. Mediastinoscopy should be considered not only for patients with lung cancer but also for those with suspected or known metastatic tumors of other organs before radical surgery or radiotherapy is attempted.

ORIGIN OF MEDIASTINAL TUMORS

The most common mediastinal tumor is metastatic carcinoma in the lymph glands from a primary pulmonary tumor. Less frequently the primary tumor may be mammary, esophageal, gastrointestinal, renal, or lymphatic; still less frequently it may involve the thymus or another mediastinal structure.

Upper mediastinal lymph nodes are very important in the diagnosis and prognosis of many malignant tumors of primary organs other than the lung. With pulmonary tumors, for example, metastasis from the lung to the mediastinum is frequently the first clinical sign of the primary growth. The mediastinal metastasis is often revealed by a routine roentgenogram showing a localized or generalized prominence of the mediastinum, a displacement of the esophagus, or a paralysis of the phrenic or recurrent laryngeal nerves or by bronchoscopy showing a widening of the tracheal carina.

DIAGNOSIS AND PROGNOSIS

Early Methods

Prior to the development of mediastinoscopy, information sufficient to provide a rational basis for therapy of lung cancer was not available with even the most exacting diagnostic techniques. Furthermore, the usual diagnostic procedures commonly failed to indicate the extent of metastasis—the most important determinant for successful intervention. Long-term survival of patients with bronchogenic carcinoma has been correlated with the extent of pulmonary lymph node involvement, and the Salzer classification is particularly useful in the staging of these metastases.[1] Nohl and Bergh have demonstrated that segmental and interlobar nodes do not appreciably influence the prognosis; on the other hand, involvement of mediastinal nodes is a very important factor in survival.[1-3] Separate studies by Nohl and by Bergh and Schersten reported 4-year survival rates of 42 and 49 percent, respectively, following pulmonary resection when the mediastinum was free of metastasis; but in both studies the survival rate fell below 10 percent when there was upper mediastinal metastasis.[2,3]

Contralateral spread of cancer to mediastinal nodes has been recognized for some time.[4-12] Mascagni first reported the crossing of lymphatics from the left main bronchus to the right paratracheal nodes in 1787.[5] Rouviere demonstrated in 1932 that nodes located at the tracheal bifurcation drained entirely into the right paratracheal chain, thus indicating that most of the drainage pathways from the nodes of the left lower lobe crossed over to the right paratracheal nodes.[10] In 1958 Cardier reported that crossover drainage occurs from left to right and from right to left. Crossover occurs not only at the level of the carinal nodes but also between right and left paratracheal nodes.[6] Thus tumor metastases may involve any of the following three chains: the anterior mediastinal (vascular) chain, the middle mestiastinal (paratracheal) chain, or the posterior mediastinal (esophageal) chain. The primary tumor may be in the ipsilateral or contralateral lung.

Scalene Node Biopsy

Biopsy of the scalene fat pad was formerly used to assess the operability of lung carcinoma, since the presence of tumor in the biopsy specimen was generally believed to preclude a successful resection of the primary lesion.[13] A negative biopsy, on the other hand, was considered a favorable sign. Nevertheless, in 1962 Reynders found that, despite negative scalene node biopsies in 223 patients, 107 (48 percent) had nonresectable lesions. The most frequent cause of nonresectability was invasive growth of the tumor or lymph node metastasis in the upper mediastinum.[14]

Thoracotomy

Exploratory thoracotomy was often considered necessary to provide tissue samples for diagnosis and to determine the extent of the disease. Kirklin and Gibbon and his associates collectively reported 1253 patients whose lung cancers were presumed operable. Of these, 558 (43 percent) were found unresectable at thoracotomy.[15,16] In 1962 Rodinov reported that thoracotomy revealed unresectable lesions in over 43 percent of 20,508 patients.[17] Thoracotomy itself is associated with a mortality rate of 10 percent and a morbidity rate as high as 20 percent.[14,17] Furthermore, this procedure provides an adequate evaluation only of the ipsilateral superior mediastinal nodes.

Gibbon, Bergh, Nohl, and Wurnig have shown that patients with cancers confined to the lung parenchyma have better prognoses than those with cancers extending outside the lung.[2,3,16,18] Several surgeons have recently advocated extended resection for certain locally advanced cases; however, this procedure has a high mortality rate, and very few patients survive for 3 years. In Bergh's series no patient was alive 5 years after resection, and no patient with extensive tumor and mediastinal lymph node involvement was alive after 1 year.[3]

Thus exploratory thoracotomy cannot be justified if a less hazardous technique is available to provide a histologic diagnosis and to determine resectability and curability. Excision of mediastinal nodes with thoracotomy may be more useful as a staging procedure, rather than as a therapeutic procedure.

Roentgenography

The use of highly refined rotentgenograms, including tomograms, arteriograms, and venograms, has improved assessment. But in significant numbers of patients roentgenography fails to identify metastases to upper mediastinal structures.

MEDIASTINOSCOPY

History

Mediastinoscopy originated in the techniques introduced by Harken in 1954 and Radner in 1955. Harken introduced cervicomediastinal exploration, in which a lighted laryngoscope exposed a limited area on one side of the mediastinum for tissue biopsy and diagnosis.[19] Radner approached the mediastinum through a suprasternal incision, exposed the trachea, and with blunt dissection entered the upper mediastinum.[20] He was thus able to remove accessible paratracheal lymph nodes. In 1959 Carlens developed a lighted instrument that enabled him to examine mediastinal structures; he called it a mediastinoscope.[21] Since that time mediastinoscopy has been used in many parts of the world, and the results of well over 35,000 cases have been reported.

Boyd reported that mediastinoscopy was positive in 28 percent of cases in which scalene node biopsy was negative.[22] DeLarue, in a comparative series of patients with lung cancer, found that 97 percent of cancers were resectable when mediastinoscopy was negative; however, only 58 percent were resectable when scalene node biopsy was negative.[23] Pearson reported that mediastinoscopy avoided unnecessary thoracotomy in 25 percent of his patients with lung cancer. He found superior mediastinal tumor metastases by mediastinoscopic examination in 31 percent of patients with lung cancer that were presumed to be operable by other diagnostic techniques.[24] Reynders reported that the proportion of tumors judged to be resectable rose from 60 to 90 percent with routine use of mediastinoscopy.[25] Nohl identified mediastinal metastases in 50 percent of patients with lung carcinoma; he found these metastases in 35 percent of patients with squamous cell carcinoma and in 75 percent of those with oat cell carcinoma.[2] A summary of 4983 cases of lung carcinoma reported by 28 authors revealed positive mediastinoscopic biopsies in 1854 (39 percent).[26] A survey by Bowlin revealed that only 12 percent of patients with lung carcinoma had scalene or supraclavicular node metastases.[27]

Obviously, preoperative assessment of patients with lung cancer has prevented unnecessary thoracotomy in a significant number of patients with local or distant metastases. In addition to the advantage of direct endoscopic visualization, the benefits of mediastinoscopy include the ability to palpate the involved structures and to biopsy the invasive tumor or the nodal metastases in the upper mediastinum on both sides of the trachea and the major bronchi. Although mediastinoscopy permits assessment and confirmation of histologic evidence of upper mediastinal spread, and so permits prediction of resectability, its limitations are obvious. Jepson analyzed 179 patients who had had negative mediastinoscopies and who subsequently underwent thoracotomy. Pulmonary resection was successful in 152 (83 percent) of these patients. In the remaining 27 patients (17 percent), thoracotomy demonstrated tumors that could not be resected. In 10 (6 percent) of these, nonresectability was related to involvement of the heart, the pericardium, or the great vessels; therefore these tumors were inaccessible to mediastinoscopy. In 17 (11 percent), however, the upper mediastinum was involved and should have been accessible to mediastinoscopy.[28]

Pearson reported 356 thoracotomies in patients with presumably operable lung cancer who had had negative mediastinoscopies. Resection was possible in 341 patients, for a resectability rate of 96 percent. Thoracotomy identified metastatic superior mediastinal tumor in 30 patients, indicating an 8 percent incidence of false negative mediastinoscopy. In 28 of these patients, metastatic tumor was present in the posterior subcarinal nodes, anterior mediastinal nodes, or subaortic nodes—locations inaccessible to the mediastinoscope. In all patients with anterior mediastinal metastases the primary tumor was in the left upper lobe or the left hilum. Only 2 patients had metastatic tumor in areas that should have been accessible at mediastinoscopy. As a result of these observations, Pearson has performed anterior mediastinotomy in the preoperative assessment of left upper lobe and left hilar tumors in which mediastinoscopy was negative. This procedure was performed under the same anesthetic with the mediastinoscopy incision open. The mediastinoscope was introduced through a 2-inch incision in the second intercostal space after palpation with fingers in both incisions.[29]

Apparently, resectability can reliably be predicted in over 83 percent of cases in which mediastinoscopy reveals no metastasis in the upper mediastinum.

A review of published data on the mortality and morbidity of mediastinoscopy in 7876 patients indicates a total of 3 deaths and 99 complications. The complications listed below represent a morbidity rate of 1.2 percent and a mortality of 0.038 percent.[26] The specific complications were as follows:

1. Bleeding from:
   a. innominate artery
   b. azygos vein
   c. bronchial artery
   d. pulmonary artery
2. Pneumonia
3. Hemothorax
4. Vocal cord paralysis
5. Perforation of esophagus
6. Mediastinal infection
7. Incision infection
8. Bradycardia
9. Myocardial infarction
10. Tumor seeding in suture line
11. Stroke
12. Air embolus

It is apparent that although mediastinoscopy is a relatively safe procedure it should be performed only with thorough knowledge of the anatomic relationships involved in and the possible complications of the procedure.

Anatomy

The two pleural cavities enclose the mediastinum. The parietal pleura comprises the lateral mediastinal walls; the sternum is the anterior wall, the vertebral column is the posteriour wall, and the diaphragm and the superior aperture of the thorax form the inferior wall. The mediastinum is further divided by planes. The superior and inferior mediastinum may be arbitrarily separated by a horizontal plane running from the sternal angle to the fourth vertebra. The anterior mediastinum is the area in front of the pericardium, and the posterior mediastinum is behind it.

Mediastinoscopy is primarily the examination of the superior or upper mediastinum with its anterior, middle, and posterior compartments. This, basically, is a paratracheal exploration, and the path of the trachea is critical. The trachea descends from the anterior cervical neck area and enters the thorax in an oblique plane, traversing posteriorly through the superior mediastinum and bifurcating at the posterior portion of the middle mediastinum.

For a mediastinoscopic examination the trachea is exposed through a small incision in the suprasternal fossa. This fossa is enclosed by the sternal attachments of the sternocleidomastoid muscles of the neck. Within it the inferior thyroid veins lie immediately in front of the trachea. In some individuals an arteria thyroidea ima also lies before the trachea; the root of the neck is directly connected with the superior mediastinum and the structures that lead into and from the chest.

Anterior mediastinum. The thymus, lying immediately behind the sternum, is the most anterior structure of the mediastinum. Next are the great venous structures. The bracheocephalic (innominate) veins and the superior vena cava lie anterior to the major arterial vessels, including aortic arch, innominate artery, and carotid artery. The one exception is the important azygos vein, which arises posteriorly and runs anteriorly to join the superior vena cava just above the right main upper lobe bronchus (Fig. 9-1).

Middle and posterior mediastinum. The middle compartment contains the trachea, the right and left main bronchi, the right upper lobe bronchus, the aortic arch, the innominate artery, the vagi, the left recurrent laryngeal nerve, the phrenic nerves, the heart and its pericardium, the arch of the azygos vein, and the pulmonary veins and arteries. The posterior compartment contains the esophagus, the thoracic duct, and the vertebral column (Fig. 9-2 and 9-3).

The trachea lies to the right of the midline and recedes from the sternum as it passes down from the neck into the upper mediastinum. The arteries lie between the trachea and the large veins. The innominate artery runs diagonally from the left of the trachea and ascends toward the right. The aorta arches in front of the tracheal bifurcation and lies to the left of the trachea with the left recurrent nerve. The mediastinal pleura and the right vagus nerve lie to the right of the trachea.

The tracheal bifurcation is located at the level of the fourth thoracic verbebra approximately 5 to 6 cm from the suprasternal notch. The right main bronchus is wider and shorter than the left. The left bronchus lies mainly under and in the

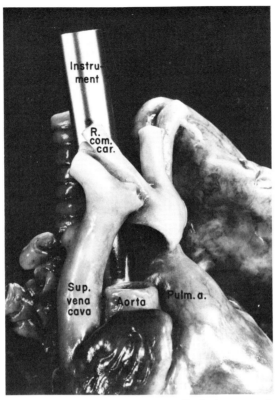

Fig. 9-1. Representation of relevant upper mediastinal anatomy from anterior view, with thymus removed. (Reproduced by permission from Goldberg EM, Glicksman AS, Kahn FR, et al: Mediastinoscopy for assessing mediastinal spread in clinical staging of carcinoma of the lung. Cancer 25:347–353, 1970.)

notch of the aortic arch. The right upper lobe bronchus is located 2.5 cm from the tracheal bifurcation; the left is about 5 cm from it The pulmonary arteries pass 2 to 3 cm under the tracheal bifurcation in front of both bronchi; the right artery lies below the upper lobe bronchus, and the left lies above it. Mediastinoscopy involves mainly the superior division of the right pulmonary artery. The azygos vein arches over the right main bronchus above the right upper lobe bronchus. Both vagi descend behind the main bronchi. The esophagus passes through the upper mediastinum from the neck and in its course follows an anteroposterior and lateral curvature. The curve in the neck is convex, toward the left, about 5 mm beyond the margin of the trachea. As it passes through the upper mediastinum it gradually returns to the midline. In the upper mediastinum the esophagus is positioned in back and to the left of the trachea to the limits of the tracheal bifurcation. The left main bronchus crosses in front of the esophagus under the aortic arch, which passes on its left side to form the bronchoaortic constriction. At the level of the right pulmonary artery the esophagus is separated anteriorly from the left atrium of the heart by the pericardium.

Recurrent laryngeal nerves. The left recurrent laryngeal nerve branches from the main trunk of the vagus, curves around the aortic arch and through the aortic notch, and passes upward in the groove between the left border of the trachea and the esophagus. Paralysis of the left vocal cord can indicate invasion of the left recurrent nerve and similar invasion of the left side of the trachea or the esophagus. The right recurrent laryngeal nerve branches from the main trunk of the vagus in front of the subclavian artery and curves behind it, passing upward and medial to the right common carotid artery in the groove between the trachea and esophagus (Fig. 9-4).

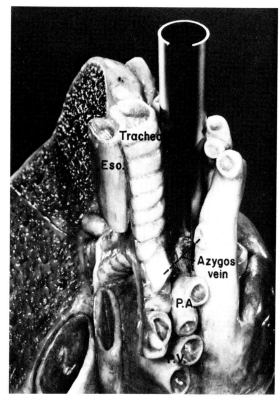

Fig. 9-2. Representation of relevant upper mediastinal anatomy from right lateral view. (Reproduced by permission from Goldberg EM, Glicksman AS, Kahn FR, et al: Mediastinoscopy for assessing mediastinal spread in clinical staging of carcinoma of the lung. Cancer 25:347–353, 1970.)

Connective tissue and fascia. The mediastinal pleura forms the lateral mediastinal borders with significant right and left border variations: on the right side it touches the innominate artery, the trachea, and the esophagus; on the left side it touches the aortic arch, the trachea, and the esophagus. The connective (loose areolar) tissue surrounds and connects all mediastinal organs. Its scanty blood supply comes from the pleural vessels. The mediastinal fascial layers are continuous from the neck. The perivisceral fascia encloses all compartments of the neck. Over the trachea it is called the pretracheal fascia and extends to the tracheal bifurcation and both main bronchi. The pretracheal fascia is an anatomic landmark to the mediastinoscopist, since its proper identification is critical to safe entry into the upper middle mediastinum. The only safe endoscopic route through the upper mediastinum is under the pretracheal fascia along the anterior surface of the trachea to its bifurcation.

Division of tracheobronchial tree. The validity of mediastinoscopy in limited paratracheal exploration lies in the centralization of peripheral pulmonary lymphatic flow to the pulmonary hilum and from there around the paratracheal area. The trachea branches into 23 bronchial dichotomies, which are numbered as follows: 1 to 16 are conductive bronchials; 17 to 22 are transition bronchials with increasing partial alveolation; 23 is the alveolar sac with the terminal alveoli. The lymphatic collecting system begins at the level of the respiratory bronchial or secondary lobule and drains to the third bronchial dichotomy and the site of the first node (the intersegmental nodes). The second node is the interlobar or hilar node, and the third is the mediastinal node around the trachea and its bifurcation.

Lymphatic drainage of lung. Nohl's modification of Rouviere's and Cardier's description

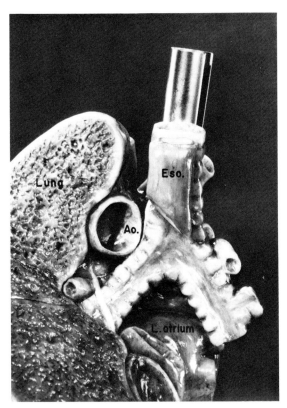

Fig. 9-3. Representation of relevant upper mediastinal anatomy from posterior view. (Reproduced by permission from Goldberg EM, Glicksman AS, Kahn FR, et al: Mediastinoscopy for assessing mediastinal spread in clinical staging of carcinoma of the lung. Cancer 25:347–353, 1970.)

of the right pulmonary lymphatic flow has the right upper lobe lymphatics drained by the right paratracheal nodes. The middle and lower lobes drain into the right paratracheal nodes via both the bifurcation nodes and the posterior esophageal nodes. In the left lung the lower lobe is drained by the bifurcation node to the left paratracheal and posterior nodes. This drainage also crosses to the contralateral right paratracheal area. The upper lobe drains into the left paratracheal or bifurcation nodes.[2] It should be noted that the normal lymphatic flow pattern is apt to vary with lymphatic blockage. The right paratracheal lymph nodes apparently drain all of the right lung and a major portion of the left lung. This is supported by clinical observation of predominant involvement of right paratracheal nodes in various types of intrathoracic disease.

Lymph nodes. The mediastinal lymph nodes also drain from the lymphatics of the neck,

the diaphragm, the anterior thoracic wall, and the abdominal cavity. All three lymphatic chains are probably connected; therefore metastasis can occur both vertically and horizontally. Other deviations in lymphatic metastasis can be related to anatomic variations and pathologic blocks that enhance collateral and retrograde flow. The superior mediastinal lymph nodes comprise the following groups: (1) anterior mediastinal or vascular, (2) middle mediastinal or peritracheobronchial, and (3) posterior mediastinal or esophageal. The anterior or vascular lymph nodes are located with the large vessels in the anterior and middle mediastinum. They can easily be palpated, but not dissected, by the mediastinoscopist.

The peritracheobronchial group includes the pretracheobronchial and paratracheobronchial lymph nodes, which are of primary importance in mediastinoscopy. They are located anterior and on both sides of the trachea and the main bronchi.

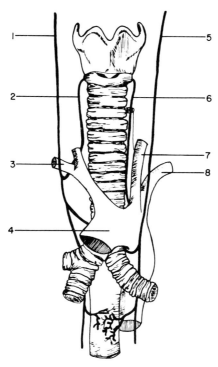

Fig. 9-4. Representation of relevant anatomy of vagi and recurrent laryngeal nerves: 1. Right vagus nerve. 2. Right recurrent laryngeal nerve. 3. Right subclavian artery. 4. Aortic arch. 5. Left vagus nerve. 6. Left recurrent pharyngeal nerve. 7. Left common carotid. 8. Left subclavian artery.

The pulmonary segmental and interlobar nodes drain to these nodes, which are continuous to the scalene nodes in the neck. The lymphatics of the trachea, the esophagus, and the thymus also drain into these nodes. The right chain apparently drains the right lung, the left lung's lower lobe, the trachea, the esophagus, and the thymus. The left paratracheal nodes drain the lymphatics from the left upper lobe, the trachea, and the esophagus. Crossover drainage can occur either from right to left or from left to right. The posterior or esophageal lymph nodes are behind the trachea in close relationship to the esophagus. Drainage is probably from the esophagus, the pericardium, and the lungs. These nodes are particularly important in esophageal carcinoma.

Technique

The instruments used for mediastinoscopy include a lighted fiberoptic mediastinoscope; a special curved retractor for safe introduction of the scope; a blunt-tipped suction tube for dissection, aspiration, and coagulation; a long needle for test puncture; and laryngeal biopsy forceps.

The mediastinoscope can be fixed with a chest stay brace so that both hands are free for dissection and biopsy. The Zeiss operative microscope is also used by some mediastinoscopists.

The procedure may be performed under either general endotracheal or local anesthesia. It is reasonable and appropriate to monitor the electrocardiogram continuously. The patient is placed with the head tilted slightly backward and rotated to the left. The neck is well extended to elevate the trachea. The surgeon stands at the head and the assistant to the right of the patient. A 2- to 4-cm transverse suprasternal notch incision is ideally placed below the thyroid isthmus (Fig. 9-5). Through this incision the strap muscles are separated along the midline to expose the anterior wall of the trachea. The only vascular structure that normally occurs immediately in front of the trachea is the inferior thyroid vein; however, approximately 10 percent of patients have an arteria thyroidea ima arising either from the innominate artery or the aortic arch in the superior mediastinum or from the right common carotid artery in the neck. The thyroid can, of course, also cover the trachea in the suprasternal area

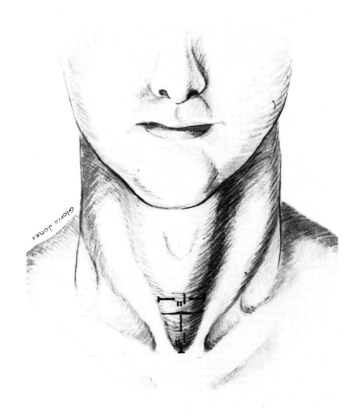

Fig. 9-5. Representation of topography of small (2–4-cm) transverse suprasternal notch incision. (Reproduced by permission from Goldberg EM, Shapiro CM, Glicksman AS: Mediastinoscopy for assessing mediastinal spread in clinical staging of lung carcinoma. Semin Oncol 1:205–215, 1974.)

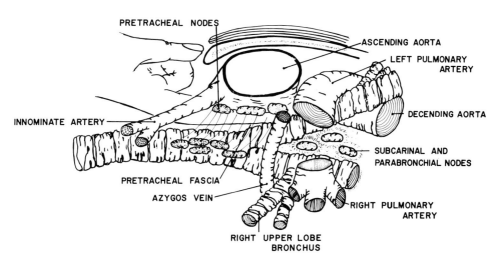

Fig. 9-6. Representation of relevant mediastinal anatomy as blunt digital dissection is carried down under pretracheal fascia.

and can frequently descend into the mediastinum. The pretracheal fascia is always opened inferior to the thyroid. A blunt digital dissection is made downward along the trachea posterior to the innominate artery and the aortic arch. The paratracheal area is palpated with the finger to detect nodes or tumor masses. The tissue is loose, permitting easy exposure of the entire trachea to its bifurcation. The surgeon must remember to keep the dissection behind the innominate artery and the aortic arch at all times (Fig. 9-6). The pretracheal fascia acts as a shield for the introduction of the mediastinoscope. The instrument is then introduced to visualize the trachea and paratracheal areas (Fig. 9-7), the carina, the right and left main bronchi, the right upper lobe bronchus, the innominate artery, the aortic arch, the right pulmonary artery, the azygous vein, the left recurrent nerve, and the esophagus from the neck to the level of the carina (Fig. 9-8). Tumor masses and lymph nodes are readily enucleated in entirety, or a specimen may be taken for biopsy. Specimens are excised at different areas as indicated and are always taken from both sides of the mediastinum whenever malignancy is suspected. A blind biopsy should never be taken; if any

doubt exists as to the site and nature of the tissue, a test puncture should be made. Bleeding during mediastinoscopy is minimal and easily controlled by cautery, silver clip, or hemostatic agents. Silver clips may also be used to identify the site of biopsy. The incision is closed primarily and without drainage.

Superior Vena Cava Obstructive Syndrome

Mediastinal metastasis produces a wide variety of symptoms and signs. Occasionally it obstructs the superior vena cava. The resulting symptoms, which are at first mild, reach their maximum with headache, cyanosis of the face, and edema of the eyelids. Distended veins appear in the root of the neck, and dyspnea and hemoptysis finally become evident as the obstruction involves the pulmonary veins (see Chapter 18). Idiopathic mediastinal fibrosis causes a similar progressive obstruction of the superior vena cava. Etiology has been causally or incidentally related to syphilis, tuberculosis, idiopathic fibrosis, histoplasmosis, and the drug Sansert.

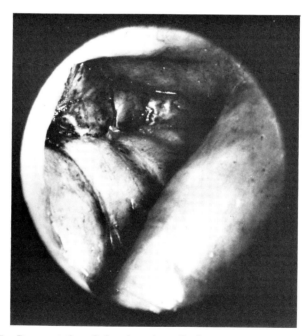

Fig. 9-7. Representation of view through mediastinoscope at level of innominate artery with left paratracheal lymph nodes. (Reproduced by permission from Goldberg EM, Glicksman AS, Kahn FR, et al: Mediastinoscopy for assessing mediastinal spread in clinical staging of carcinoma of the lung. Cancer 25:347–353, 1970.)

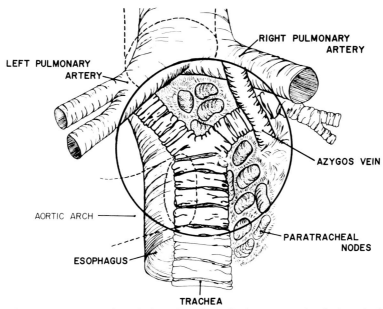

Fig. 9-8. Representation of view through mediastinoscope at level of tracheal bifurcation with subcarinal lymph nodes and right pulmonary artery and azygous vein.

With an accurate tissue diagnosis, appropriate therapy may begin promptly. This avoids such measures as "test doses" of radiotherapy or major thoracotomy. Random cervical or scalene node biopsy not only is a bloody procedure but also is usually unrewarding. Mediastinoscopy is both safe and effective in the assessment of patients with superior vena cava obstructive syndrome. However, certain technical precautions must be observed: (1) The head and trunk should be elevated to minimize the additive effect of gravity on venous hypertension. (2) Intravenous fluids should be administered through a vein of a lower extremity. (3) As the incision is carefully made, the subcutaneous dilated veins are best retracted rather than ligated and divided. (4) Dissection is extended down to the pretracheal fascia. Once this fascia is identified and opened, no further venous engorgement is encountered. (5) As digital dissection is extended down under the pretracheal fascia, the tumor is encountered promptly. Extensive dissection and exploration are not indicated. A biopsy is usually made without excessive bleeding.

Clearly, a clinical staging program based on a careful mediastinoscopic evaluation of the upper mediastinum would help to distinguish those patients who would benefit from surgery, radio-therapy, or chemotherapy from those patients for whom these treatments would be futile or even harmful.

STAGING OF LUNG CANCER

The International Union Against Cancer has recently stated:

> The immediate purpose of staging is to facilitate the accurate, concise description of the apparent extent of the disease in a way that can readily be communicated to others or reproduced by them. What is needed is simply an agreement on the recording of such precise information on the extent of the disease as to make possible the combination or recombination of cases according to any agreed plan.

Ideally, a staging technique should describe the primary site, the presence of cancerous nodes, their locations, and the presence or absence of metastasis. Such a technique would facilitate the assessment and comparison of various modes of treatment at various institutions. The following staging proposal is based on the histologic proof of tumor in the mediastinal lymph nodes; therefore it requires mediastinoscopy for a precise assessment of the upper mediastinum (see Chapter 12).

The diagnosis of lung carcinoma is considered established by any of the following: (1) biopsy of the pulmonary tumor, (2) collection of bronchial or sputum secretions with cytology indicating primary lung carcinoma, or (3) biopsy of a lymph node or an extrapulmonary site with metastatic growth in the presence of a chest mass and a histopathology indicating primary lung carcinoma. Other common sites of tumor origin, such as the gastrointestinal tract or prostate, must be excluded.

Proposed Classification

T, N, and M staging system. The classification of lung carcinoma suggested here is based on the T, N, and M system and utilizes conventional diagnostic procedures and mediastinoscopy. The position and extent of growth of the tumor should determine the T parameter.[30,31] This is in accord with the conclusions reached by Bignall and Moon, Nohl, Bergh, Cliffton and Nickson, and others.[2,3,32-34] Clinically it is not always possible to determine whether a lesion that involves the parietal pleura also extends beyond it. This is so with even the most exacting x-ray planography. However, medial lesions within reach of mediastinoscopy may be so delineated.

Nodal involvement within the mediastinum determines the N parameter. Nodes inferior to the right second division of the trachea are not considered mediastinal.[30,31] Mediastinal lymph node involvement may include any or all of the three chains (the anterior mediastinal, the posterior mediastinal, and the paratracheal) and is either ipsilateral, contralateral, or bilateral.

The presence of extrathoracic metastatic disease determines the M parameter and indicates evidence of disease in supraclavicular nodes, liver, bone, etc.

This classification gives no consideration to cell type and does not account for metastasis to the lower mediastinum or below the diaphragm. Generally it is customary to group together the combination of T, N, and M so that a reproducible assessment of the extent of disease can be made in sufficient numbers of patients to be useful for prognostic purposes.[30,31]

Histology. Tumor histology is arbitrarily divided into four broad categories: (1) well-differentiated squamous cell carcinoma; (2) poorly differentiated, undifferentiated, or anaplastic large cell carcinoma; (3) very undifferentiated small cell (oat cell) carcinoma; (4) adenocarcinoma.

Results with the classification system. In our series of 179 patients with lung cancer confirmed by thoracotomy, bronconscopy, or mediastinoscopy, 48 percent had positive biopsy findings with mediastinoscopy. The incidence of positive findings on mediastinoscopy depends on the method of patient selection; in patients with advanced disease the incidence of positive biopsy will presumably be high. In this series the incidence of upper mediastinal spread correlated better with the histologic characteristics than with the anatomic site and origin of the primary tumor.

Table 9-1
Lung Carcinoma Mediastinal Spread

Site	Number of Patients	Mediastinoscopy			
		Positive	*Ipsilateral*	*Contralateral*	*Bilateral*
Both lungs	179	86(48%)	35(41%)	8(9%)	43(50%)
Right lung	108	57(53%)	22(38%)	1(2%)	34(60%)
RUL	75	46(60%)	17(37%)	1(3%)	28(60%)
RLL	22	8(36%)	5(63%)	—	3(37%)
Multiple L	11	3(27%)	—	—	3(100%)
Left lung	71	29(40%)	13(45%)	7(24%)	9(31%)
LUL	48	20(42%)	9(45%)	6(30%)	5(25%)
LLL	16	4(25%)	2(50%)	1(25%)	1(25%)
Multiple L	7	5(71%)	2(40%)	—	3(60%)

Reproduced by permission from Goldberg EM, Glicksman AS, Kahn FR, et al: Mediastinoscopy for assessing mediastinal spread in clinical staging of carcinoma of the lung. Cancer 25:347–353, 1970.

Table 9-2
Lung Carcinoma Mediastinal Spread

Site	Number of Patients	Mediastinoscopy			
		Positive	*Ipsilateral*	*Contralateral*	*Bilateral*
Upper lobes	123	66(54%)	26(40%)	7(11%)	33(49%)
Right	75	46(60%)	17(37%)	1(3%)	28(60%)
Left	48	20(42%)	9(45%)	6(30%)	5(25%)
Lower lobes	38	12(32%)	7(58%)	1(9%)	4(33%)
Right	22	8(36%)	5(63%)	—	3(37%)
Left	16	4(25%)	2(50%)	1(25%)	1(25%)

Reproduced by permission from Goldberg EM, Glickman AS, Kahn FR, et al: Mediastinoscopy for assessing mediastinal spread in clinical staging of carcinoma of the lung. Cancer 25:347–353, 1970.

The relationship of mediastinal metastases to primary pulmonary tumors is shown in Table 9-1. Of 57 patients with mediastinal spread from right-sided tumors, only 1 had only contralateral nodes; but of 29 patients whose tumors originated on the left, 7 had only contralateral nodes.

The relationship of mediastinal metastases to primary lobar tumors is shown in Table 9-2. Although mediastinal spread occurred less frequently with lower lobe tumors, the distribution of the metastases was not significantly different. Surprisingly, 6 of 20 patients (30 percent) with mediastinal spread from the left upper lobes had only contralateral nodes.

The relationship between mediastinal lymph node involvement and tumor histology is shown in Table 9-3. Evidence of mediastinal lymph node metastases and the pattern of bilateral mediastinal node involvement were less evident in patients with well-differentiated squamous cell carcinoma than in those with all other types of tumors.

Of the patients with group 1 well-differentiated squamous cell carcinoma, almost three-fourths (73 percent) were classified in the lower stages. Of the patients with group 2 large cell, poorly differentiated, undifferentiated, or anaplastic carcinoma, more than three-fourths (76 percent) were classified in the higher stages. The small number of patients with group 3 small cell or oat cell carcinoma had staging distribution similar to that of group 2 patients. Fifty percent of patients with group 4 adenocarcinoma were classified in the higher stages. Obviously the degree of differentiation among the four histologic groups accurately corresponds with the stages in the proposed staging system, which indicates that the staging system validly represents a tumor's biologic character.

Table 9-3
Lung Carcinoma Mediastinal Spread

Pathology	Number of Patients	Mediastinoscopy			
		Positive	*Ipsilateral*	*Contralateral*	*Bilateral*
All cell types	179	86(48%)	35(41%)	8(9%)	43(50%)
Well-differentiated squamous cell	64	10(16%)	7(70%)	2(20%)	1(10%)
Large cell poorly differentiated, undifferentiated, anaplastic	74	47(68%)	17(36%)	6(13%)	24(51%)
Small cell undifferentiated (oat cell)	23	17(70%)	5(30%)	—	12(70%)
Adenocarcinoma	18	12(66%)	6(50%)	—	6(50%)

Reproduced by permission from Goldberg EM, Glicksman AS, Kahn FR, et al: Mediastinoscopy for assessing mediastinal spread in clinical staging of carcinoma of the lung. Cancer 25:347–353, 1970.

CONCLUSION

A most interesting aspect of this study was the correlation between mediastinal spread (both contralateral and bilateral) and the degree of differentiation in the tumor; metastasis was increasingly frequent as tumor differentiation was lost. It is important to note that lung carcinoma originating in any lobe may be spread to the contralateral mediastinal nodes. Furthermore, although ipsilateral upper mediastinal spread is still guardedly considered to be curable, contralateral spread absolutely precludes a curative resection. Consequently, biopsy should be performed from both sides of the upper mediastinum in all suspected and confirmed cases of lung cancer. Mediastinoscopic staging contributes significantly to the assessment of operability and prognosis, and it is equally important in patients in whom radiotherapy or chemotherapy is required either alone or with surgical treatment.

REFERENCES

1. Salzer G, Wenzl M, Jenny RH, et al: Das Bronchuscarcinom. Wein, Springer-Verlag, 1952
2. Nohl HC: The Spread of Carcinoma of the Bronchus. London, Lloyd-Luke, 1962
3. Bergh NP, Schersten T: Bronchogenic carcinoma: A follow-up study of a surgically treated series with special reference to the prognostic significance of lymph node metastases. Acta Chir Scand [Suppl] 1965, p 347
4. Weinberg JA: Identification of regional lymph nodes in the treatment of bronchogenic carcinoma. J Thorac Surg 22:517–526, 1951
5. Mascagni P: Vasorum lymphaticorum corporis humani historia et ichnographia. Senis 1787
6. Cardier G, Papamiltiades M, Cedard C: Les lymphatiques des bronches et des segments pulmonaires. Bronches 8:8–52, 1958
7. Ghon A: Der primare Lungenherd bei der Tuberkulose der Kinder. Berlin, Urban and Schwartzenberg, 1912
8. McCort JJ, Robbins LL: Roentgen diagnosis of intrathoracic lymph node metastases in carcinoma of the lung. Radiology 57:339–360, 1951
9. Most A: Die lymphgefasse der Lunge. Bibliotheca Medica (Abteil C) 16:21, 1908
10. Rouviere H: Anatomie des lymphatiques de l'homme. Paris, Masson et Cie, 1932
11. Steinert R: Untersuchungen des Lymphsystems der Lunge, zugleich ein Beitrag zur Frage der Topographic der bronchialen Lymphknoten. Beitr Klin Tuberk 68:497–510, 1928
12. Warren MF, Drinker CK: Flow of lymph from lungs of dog. Am J Physiol 136:207–221, 1942
13. Daniels AC: A method of biopsy useful in diagnosing certain intrathoracic disease. Dis Chest 16:360,1949
14. Reynders H: The value of mediastinoscopic study in ascertaining the inoperability of pulmonary carcinoma. J Int Coll Surg 39:597–610, 1963
15. Kirklin JW, McDonald JR, Clagett OF, et al: Bronchogenic carcinoma. Surg Gynecol Obstet 100:429, 1955
16. Gibbon JH, Templeton JY, Nealon TF: Factors which influence the long-term survival of patients with cancer of the lung. Ann Surg 145:637–643, 1957
17. Rodinov VV: Immediate and late results of exploratory thoracotomy for lung carcinoma. Vopr Onkol 8:12–18, 1962
18. Wurnig P: Zur Method der Beurteilung kurativer Erfolge der Carcinomchirurgie an Hand des Bronchuscarcinoms. Thoraxchirurgie 2:281–289, 1954
19. Harken DE, Black H, Claus R, et al: A simple cervico-mediastinal exploration for tissue diagnosis of intrathoracic disease. N Engl J Med 251:1041–1044, 1954
20. Radner S: Suprasternal node biopsy in lymph spreading intrathoracic disease. Acta Med Scand 152:413–415, 1955
21. Carlens E: Mediastinoscopy: A method for inspection and tissue biopsy in the superior mediastinum. Dis Chest 36:343–352, 1959
22. Boyd AD: Mediastinoscopy; comparison with scalene fat-pad biopsy. NH State J Med 7:445, 1971
23. DeLarue NC, Sanders DE, Silverberg SA: Complementary value of pulmonary angiography and mediastinoscopy in individualizing treatments for patients with lung cancer. Cancer 26:1370, 1970
24. Pearson FG, Kergin FG: Mediastinoscopy: A method of biopsy in the superior mediastinum. J Thorac Cardiovasc Surg 49:11, 1965
25. Reynders H: Mediastinoscopy in bronchogenic cancer. Dis Chest 45:605–612, 1964
26. Jepson O, Rahbek SH: Mediastinoscopy. Copenhagen, Munksgaard, 1970
27. Bowlin JW: Primary carcinoma of the lung; prevention, diagnosis and treatment. J Mass State Med Assoc 10:331, 1969
28. Jepson O: Mediastinoscopy. Copenhagen, Munksgaard, 1966

29. Pearson FG, Nelems JM, Henderson RD, et al: The role of mediastinoscopy in the selection of treatment for bronchial carcinoma with involvement of superior mediastinal lymph nodes. J Thorac Cardiovasc Surg 44:382–390, 1972

30. Goldberg EM, Glicksman AS, Kahn FR, et al: Mediastinoscopy for assessing mediastinal spread in clinical staging of carcinoma of the lung. Cancer 25:347–353, 1970

31. Goldberg EM, Shapiro CM, Glicksman AS: Mediastinoscopy for assessing mediastinal spread in clinical staging of lung carcinoma. Semin Oncol 1:205–215, 1974

32. Bignall JR, Moon AJ: Survival after lung resection for bronchial carcinoma. Thorax 10:183–190, 1955

33. Cliffton EE: The criteria for operability and resectability in lung cancer. JAMA 195:1031–1032, 1966

34. Nickson JJ, Cliffton EE, Selby H: Carcinoma of the lung. Am J Roentgenol Radium Ther Nucl Med 77:826–835, 1957

W. Eugene Miller

10
Roentgenographic Manifestations of Lung Cancer

EARLY LUNG CANCER

Early manifestations. The earliest roentgenographic features of lung carcinoma have been determined from studies of asymptomatic patients who had roentgenographic abnormalities that were retrospectively proved to be caused by lung carcinoma.[1] The roentgenographic manifestation of early lung cancer is very different from that of later disease. The earliest signs that are caused by the tumor depend on whether the tumor is centrally located near the hilus or is more peripheral. If the lesion is central the first appearance may be a slight hilar prominence (Fig. 10-1); if the lesion is peripheral a small nodule, usually with ill-defined margins, is seen.[2,3]

About half of the early carcinomas present as peripheral nodules: one-fourth of these have ill-defined margins (Fig. 10-2), and one-fourth are small, irregular, nonhomogeneous infiltrates. The latter may represent either a diffusely infiltrating tumor or a subsegmental atelectasis or pneumonitis secondary to a tumor obstructing a segmental or lobar bronchus (Fig. 10-3). Small nodules with sharply defined borders usually are granulomas, but these features are not reliable for benignancy because some carcinomas also have this appearance. Carcinomas as small as 3 mm in diameter have been detected, but only infrequently. Most early cancers are at least 1 cm in diameter when first detected. If the lesion is smaller than 1 cm the subtle roentgenographic densities are frequently overlooked (except in retrospect).[3,4]

The most impressive feature of many early peripheral tumors is their small, ill-defined, rather unimpressive appearance (Fig. 10-4), which can easily mislead the radiologist to consider inflammatory or nonmalignant diseases. Detection of central tumors also remains a problem. A subtle hilar mass obliterates the space between the pulmonary artery and the mediastinum (Fig. 10-1)—a sign that is significant but easily overlooked.[1]

Bronchographic manifestations. Bronchography is indicated in patients who have sputum that is positive for carcinoma but who have negative chest roentgenograms and negative whole lung tomograms. In most of these patients the tumors are found at bronchoscopy or fiberbronchoscopy and are biopsied, but if the tumor is not found, then bronchography is indicated. Bronchography, especially with the use of tantalum agents (still an investigational drug), has resulted in localization of these otherwise occult cancers.[5] Delayed films showing failure of tantalum clearance from the bronchus distal to the tumor have been especially helpful in early detection of these subtle cancers.[5]

Ikeda[6] prefers bronchography before endoscopy because the former provides a road map for

129

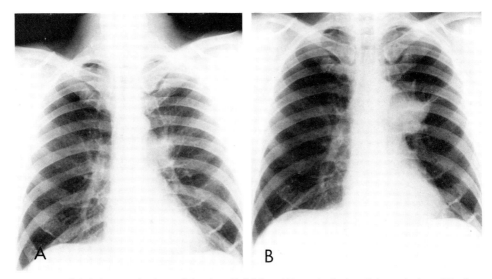

Fig. 10-1. Subtle increase in size and density of left hilum (A) overlooked until 4 months later (B) when a large hilar mass due to small cell undifferentiated bronchogenic carcinoma was noted.

fiberbronchoscopy and is helpful in locating suspicious tumor sites. In more advanced disease in which the chest roentgenogram is positive, endoscopy, including fluoroscopic-guided fiberbronchoscopy for localizing biopsy brushes to the site of peripheral lesions, has a high diagnostic yield. Thus in these cases we do not use bronchography. However, accurate diagnostic signs of lung carcinoma can be observed during conventional bronchography.[7,8] To be diagnostic, contrast medium (usually Dionosil) must fill the bronchus leading to the lesion. If carcinoma is present it may occlude the lumen (Fig. 10-5) or cause annular constriction, or it may be seen as an irregular mass of contrast medium giving a rat-tailed appearance because a small amount of contrast medium coats the irregular tumor surface.[6,7]

Roentgenographic screening manifestations. Many physicians accept the results of such widely publicized studies as the Philadelphia Pulmonary Neoplasm Research Project and conclude that screening programs using serial chest roentgenograms are of no value in the early detection of lung cancer. Only 6 of 94 patients with lung cancer detected by semiannual screening in the Philadelphia study survived 5 years.[9] However, that study included participants who were not at high risk, and only 15 percent were heavy smokers.[10]

Results of other studies, particularly those that have concentrated roentgenographic screen-

ing of the high-risk group (heavy-smoking older men), have been more encouraging for early diagnosis. Brett[11] found that the 5-year survival rate for patients with lung cancer who were examined at 6-month intervals was 23 percent, compared with 6 percent for the control series of patients who had lung cancer. Nash,[12] in a South London study of 6136 men, found results similar to Brett's. In both studies screening was done at 6-month intervals for a 4-year period.

Since no long-term controlled study has ever been made of the high-risk group of older male smokers by applying rigorous use of chest roentgenology and sputum cytology screening, we became interested in such a study in August 1971. This project, titled the Mayo Lung Project, is sponsored by the National Cancer Institute. Lung cancer screening programs of complementary design are being conducted at the Johns Hopkins University and at the Memorial Sloan–Kettering Cancer Center. The study groups are designated by the National Cancer Institute as the Early Lung Cancer Cooperative Group. The Mayo Lung Project has nearly completed recruitment of 10,000 high-risk male smokers, with half of these being chosen at random to be in the study group that is undergoing intensive study (pulmonary cytology, roentgenographic screening, and health questionnaires); the other half serve as controls. These patients in the control group are told that they are at high risk for developing lung cancer and therefore should obtain a sputum cytology

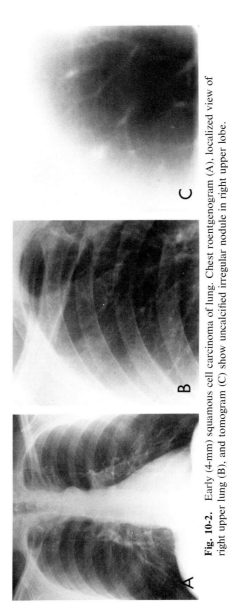

Fig. 10-2. Early (4-mm) squamous cell carcinoma of lung. Chest roentgenogram (A), localized view of right upper lung (B), and tomogram (C) show uncalcified irregular nodule in right upper lobe.

131

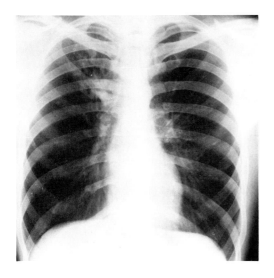

Fig. 10-3. Ill-defined infiltrate in right upper lobe, with ill-defined mass or infiltrate in suprahilar region (see Fig. 10-5).

and chest roentgenogram at least once a year, but they are not otherwise studied. In the Mayo Lung Project chest roentgenograms are obtained at 4-month intervals (the shortest interval for which patient cooperation is deemed possible) and are interpreted by two physicians (chest internists and radiologists) after initial interpretation in the radiology department. Follow-up films (postero-

anterior and lateral views), if done in the patient's home community, are mailed to the Mayo Lung Project. All initial and follow-up films undergo dual interpretation.

As of January 1975, 7027 patients have been screened. Of this group, 52 patients (0.9 percent) have had carcinomas detected on initial examination (prevalence cases), and 15 patients have had their lesions detected on follow-up examination (4.5/1000 per year incidence cases). Comparison of cytologic and roentgenologic detection methods demonstrates their complementary role in the diagnosis of early lung cancer.[13-15] Chest roentgenographic screening has detected more new cases on follow-up examination than has sputum cytology (9 cases detected by roentgenograms, 5 by sputum cytology, and 1 by both).

The prognosis of detected cases, based on predictions anticipated from disease stage (according to data from the American Joint Committee for Cancer Staging and associated survival rates based on cell type), should be between 30 and 40 percent for 5-year survival. This prediction is for patients with cancer detected on follow-up examination. Most of the newly detected tumors are small (less than 3 cm) peripheral tumors for which the prognosis is excellent (see Chapter 14).

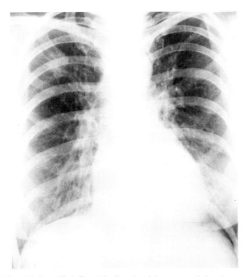

Fig. 10-4. Ill-defined lesion in right upper lobe due to adenocarcinoma.

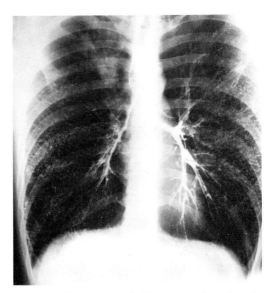

Fig. 10-5. Same case as in Fig. 10-3. Infiltrate in right upper lobe is obstructive pneumonitis due to squamous cell carcinoma occluding most of right upper lobe bronchus.

The value of this screening program will be determined by the fate of cases detected on follow-up studies (incidence cases). Results at this early stage must be interpreted with caution.

OPERABLE BRONCHOGENIC CARCINOMA

Roentgenographic abnormalities indicating more advanced but still operable lung cancer are more common than those indicating early cancer (Table 10-1). The most common roentgenologic features of lung cancer result from the tumor itself, although atelectasis or obstructive pneu-monitis caused by airway obstruction frequently occurs. It is often difficult to tell whether the roentgenographic feature is caused by the tumor itself or by secondary changes.[16] Although the exact site of origin of the lung lesion can be difficult to determine, 60 to 80 percent of lesions arise within the segmental level, and 20 to 40 percent arise at the main and lobar bronchial levels.[13]

Hilus enlargement or increased hilus density is also a frequent early sign of a bronchogenic carcinoma that either is in a mainstem bronchus or more frequently is due to hilar node metastasis from a more peripheral but less visible carcinoma. This finding is especially common with small cell carcinoma.

Table 10-1
Classification of Radiographic Abnormalities Associated with Bronchogenic Carcinoma

Region Involved	Type of Involvement
Hilus	1. Hilar prominence: slight enlargement of structures in hilar area without discrete mass
	2. Hilar mass: discrete mass limited to hilar area
	3. Perihilar mass: discrete mass limited to perihilar area with center within 4.0 cm of hilus
Pulmonary parenchyma	1. Small mass: single mass 4.0 cm or less in diameter within substance of lung, not necessarily with well-defined border
	2. Large mass: single mass greater than 4.0 cm in diameter within substance of lung, not necessarily with well-defined border
	3. Apical mass: single mass of any size limited to apex of lung
	4. Multiple masses: two or more masses of any diameter within substance of lung
	5. Hypertranslucency: increased radiolucency of lung lobe or segment
	6. Evidence of bronchial obstruction: collapse, consolidation, or pneumonitis in lung, lobe, or segment
Intrathoracic extrapulmonary structures	1. Mediastinal mass or widening: local or diffuse enlargement of normal mediastinal shadow
	2. Chest wall: erosion or interruption in normal contours of chest wall structures or vertebrae
	3. Pleural effusion
	4. Elevation of hemidiaphragm

Reproduced by permission from Byrd RB, Carr DT, Miller WE, et al: Radiographic abnormalities in carcinoma of the lung as related to histological cell type. Thorax 24:573–575, 1969.

Abnormal roentgenologic patterns of lung cancer can be related to tumor cell type (Table 10-2). Many factors are related to survival, but if lung cancer is diagnosed when it is still operable, cell type becomes a significant factor in anticipated survival (see Chapter 14). A peripheral mass most frequently occurs with adenocarcinoma (72 percent) and large cell carcinoma (63 percent). A peripheral mass is less common in squamous cell carcinoma (31 percent) and small cell carcinoma (32 percent) (Table 10-2). Because squamous and adenocarcinoma cell types are more common, a peripheral carcinoma that is demonstrated roentgenologically is most likely to be one of these two tumor types.

Data on alveolar cell or bronchiolar cell carcinoma are not included in Table 10-2, but this type of lesion has a bronchioalveolar lining growth pattern that is similar to the pattern of an adenocarcinoma.[14] The incidence of this form of lung cancer depends on how many of the adenocarcinomas are judged to have this growth pattern. Usually less than 5 percent of all primary lung carcinomas are classified as this cell type.

There are two types: localized and diffuse. In localized disease a solitary nodule (large or small) or an alveolar filling disease involving part or all of a lobe may be seen (without loss of volume) with air bronchograms and "alveolargrams." In diffuse disease both lungs usually are involved with an extensive alveolar pattern. The acinar shadow of peripheral airway filling with tumor may be scattered or may have a few or numerous areas of confluence or consolidation. Cavitations, pleural effusion, and adenopathy are uncommon.[13]

Pulmonary nodules (lesions 6 cm or less in diameter), when detected on chest roentgenograms (if no films are available for comparison), should be evaluated further by use of low-voltage (68-kV range) tomography. Tomograms will accurately localize the lesion, define the margins, and determine the presence of calcification within the lesion. If the margins are smooth and the nodule is less than 2 cm in diameter, the nodule is most likely a benign granuloma. However, even though neoplasms usually have ill-defined margins, carcinomas can be smoothly marginated. If the nodule

Table 10-2

Abnormal Radiographic Patterns in 600 Cases of Carcinoma of the Lung as Related to Histologic Cell Type

Radiographic Findings	Squamous Cell Carcinoma (263 Cases)			Adenocarcinoma (126 Cases)			Large Cell Carcinoma (97 Cases)			Small Cell Carcinoma (114 Cases)		
	S*	M*	%	S*	M*	%	S*	M*	%	S*	M*	%
Hilar or perihilar mass or prominence	34	70	40	6	16	17	10	21	32	23	66	78
Parenchymal pulmonary lesion												
Small mass (≤4.0 cm)	22	2	9	49	8	45	12	5	18	8	16	21
Large mass (>4.0 cm)	40	9	19	22	11	26	27	13	41	5	4	8
Apical mass	7	1	3	1	0	1	1	3	4	2	1	3
Multiple masses	1	0	0.5	3	0	2	1	1	2	1	0	1
Obstructive pneumonitis, collapse, or consolidation	59	80	53	7	25	25	2	30	33	5	38	38
Intrathoracic extrapulmonary involvement												
Mediastinal mass or widening	1	1	1	2	1	2	4	6	10	0	15	13
Chest wall lesion	0	0	0	0	0	0	0	0	0	0	0	0
Pleural effusion	1	8	3	1	5	5	0	2	2	0	6	5
Elevation of hemidiaphragm	1	2	1	0	5	4	0	1	1	0	4	4

*S, single abnormality; M, multiple abnormalities.

Reproduced by permission from Byrd RB, Carr DT, Miller WE, et al: Radiographic abnormalities in carcinoma of the lung as related to histological cell type. Thorax 24:573–575, 1969.

contains calcium, which is frequently seen on low-voltage tomograms but not on chest roentgenograms, the lesion almost certainly represents benign disease. If there is a centrally calcified nidus or a laminated calcium deposit, these findings are virtually pathognomonic for granuloma. The finding of "popcorn" calcification is reliable evidence of a hamartoma.[15]

If the patient is more than 40 years old and is a male smoker, thoracotomy should be considered. Tomograms can detect cavitation more reliably, unless an air–fluid level is present. Usually cavitation is best seen on the upright chest roentgenogram and is not well seen on the tomogram, which is taken with the patient prone or supine. Air in the cavity is seen because the cavity communicates with an airway. If there is no communication, only a solid mass is seen. If the cavity has a thick irregular inner wall, or if a "mural nodule" is present, the lesion is likely to be a neoplasm, although a lung abscess may have the same appearance. The cavitation can be in a lung abscess that has developed secondary to obstructive pneumonitis, but this is rare compared with cavitation in the lesion itself.[17] About 2 to 10 percent of bronchogenic carcinomas initially present with cavitation, which occurs most frequently in squamous cell carcinoma and almost never in small cell cancers.[13] When Pancoast's carcinoma or apical carcinoma is suspected clinically, tomography can be helpful in the detection of subtle apical soft tissue masses, especially in the detection of associated destruction of the posterior vertebral ends of the first or second ribs and adjacent vertebrae.

Occasionally, bronchogenic carcinoma can present as or can mimic a mediastinal mass; this can happen when small cell or large cell undifferentiated lesions are present. Prognosis in these cases is extremely poor. In these patients the pleural effusion is not the reason for the inoperability; obstructive pneumonitis is present, and the fluid is more likely to be due to this cause than to pleural involvement with tumor cells.

Obstructive emphysema from check valve obstruction probably would be a frequent finding of bronchogenic carcinoma if routine chest roentgenography included inspiratory and expiratory views.[18] Obstructive emphysema, if present, is so subtle that it is rarely detected on routine inspiratory chest roentgenograms, and expiratory chest roentgenography is seldom done.

ADVANCED LUNG CANCER

Intrathoracic findings of inoperability. In cases where curative resection seems possible before operation, but where tumor extension encountered at surgery makes curative resection impossible, the tumor extension is surprisingly roentgenologically occult. The most frequent cause for nonresectability at surgery is the presence of mediastinal nodal metastasis, but this is not detectable on chest roentgenograms, even in retrospect. Invasion of major blood vessels and pericardium is frequently not suspected before operation. A tumor may be considered unresectable roentgenographically (when direct extension is suspected) if the lesion is located immediately adjacent to pericardium, great vessels, or mediastinal nodes. Direct extension involving the chest wall is not evidence for nonresectability, and depending on the location of the lesion, operative cure is still feasible.

Pleural effusions can be caused by pleural involvement with tumor or can be secondary to obstruction of lymphatic vessels by metastasis to mediastinal lymph nodes. However, if obstructive pneumonitis is seen roentgenologically, the inflammatory nodes may cause lymphatic vessel obstruction with effusion.[13]

Lymphatic spread, in addition to involving adjacent hilar and mediastinal nodes, can occur to nodes in the opposite hemithorax. Lymphatic spread, causing right hilar adenopathy that is visible on the chest roentgenogram, occurs especially from cancer in the left lower lobe. Lymphogenous spread of bronchogenic carcinoma to diffusely involve bilateral pulmonary lymphatic vessels occurs, but it is uncommon.

Multiplicity of tumor origin is probably the cause when there is extensive alveolar cell carcinoma bilaterally.

Hematogenous spread frequently results in extrathoracic metastasis, but such spread also can be the mechanism for multiple intrapulmonary lesions.

Extrathoracic findings due to metastasis from bronchogenic carcinoma. The most commonly involved extrathoracic sites for metastasis that are seen roentgenologically are the brain, bones, liver, kidneys, and adrenals.[19] Occasionally, metastasis to the brain may be the first sign of disease, and the intracranial lesions can antedate the diagnosis of lung cancer. Neuroradiologic procedures, such as the brain scan, computerized axial tomography,[20] and cerebral angiography, may be necessary to diagnose the intracranial mass. On more than one occasion we have first detected bronchogenic carcinoma on a chest roentgenogram prior to craniotomy. Also, meta-static lesions to bones, liver, kidneys, or adrenals can cause symptoms and can be detected by radiologic studies (bone films, films of the abdomen, and excretory urograms, respectively) before the primary site is known, but this is rather rare, compared with the frequent involvement of these sites by metastasis in advanced lung cancer.

REFERENCES

1. Rigler LG: The roentgen signs of carcinoma of the lung. Am J Roentgenol Radium Ther Nucl Med 74:415–428, 1955

2. Boucot K, Cooper DA, Weiss W, et al: Appearance of first roentgenographic abnormalities due to lung cancer. JAMA 190:1103–1106, 1964

3. Weiss W, Boucot KR: The Philadelphia Pulmonary Neoplasm Research Project: Early roentgenographic appearance of bronchogenic carcinoma. Arch Intern Med 134:306–311, 1974

4. Fontana RS, Sanderson DR, Woolner LB, et al: The Mayo Lung Project for early detection and localization of bronchogenic carcinoma: A status report. Chest 67:511–522, 1975

5. Baker RR, Marsh BR, Frost JK, et al: The detection and treatment of early lung cancer. Ann Surg 179:813–818, 1974

6. Ikeda S: Atlas of Flexible Bronchofiberscopy. Baltimore, University Park Press, 1974

7. Molnar W, Riebel FA: Bronchography: An aid to diagnosis of peripheral pulmonary carcinoma. Radiol Clin North Am 1:303–314, 1963

8. Rinker CT, Garrotto LJ, Lee KR, et al: Bronchography: Diagnostic signs and accuracy in pulmonary carcinoma. Am J Roentgenol Radium Ther Nucl Med 104:802–807, 1968

9. Boucot KR, Weiss W: Is curable lung cancer detected by semiannual screening? JAMA 224:1361–1365, 1973

10. Fontana RS: The Philadelphia Pulmonary Neoplasm Research Project (editorial). JAMA 225:1372–1373, 1973

11. Brett GZ: Earlier diagnosis and survival in lung cancer. Br Med J 4:260–262, 1969

12. Nash FA, Morgan JM, Tomkins JG: South London lung cancer study. Br Med J 2:715–721, 1968

13. Fraser RG, Paré JA: Diagnosis of Diseases of the Chest: An Integrated Study Based on the Abnormal Roentgenogram, vol 2. Philadelphia, WB Saunders, 1970, pp 736–803

14. Belgrad R, Good CA, Woolner LB: Alveolar-cell carcinoma (terminal bronchiolar carcinoma): A study of surgically excised tumors with special emphasis on localized lesions. Radiology 79:789–798, 1962

15. Good CA: Roentgenologic appraisal of solitary pulmonary nodules. Minn Med 45:157–160, 1962

16. Liebow AA: Pathology of carcinoma of the lung as related to the roentgen shadow. Am J Roentgenol Radium Ther Nucl Med 74:383–401, 1955

17. Good CA, Holman CB: Cavitary carcinoma of the lung: Roentgenologic features in 19 cases. Dis Chest 37:289–293, 1960

18. Fleishner FG: Personal communication

19. Shields W, Gates O: Lung cancer and metastasis. Arch Pathol 78:467–473, 1964

20. Baker HL Jr, Campbell JK, Houser OW, et al: Computer assisted tomography of the head: An early evaluation. Mayo Clin Proc 49:17–27, 1974

Franco M. Muggia
Heine H. Hansen
Lakshman R. Chervu

11
Diagnosis in Metastatic Sites

The dictum of the late Dr. Karnofsky that "from the patient's point of view, in most instances, it is desirable to maintain an aggressive therapeutic approach"[1] also logically encompasses the initial diagnostic workup. The appropriate treatment decision can best be made after a thorough determination of the type and extent of disease at the time of diagnosis. Unfortunately, in many instances patients are categorized as having inoperable lung cancer, and treatment is instituted on the basis of data that may indicate only whether or not the primary lesion is resectable. This philosophy is unsatisfactory not only from the standpoint of investigation of new therapeutic approaches with intent to cure or to improve results but also from the standpoint of selection of the optimal palliative treatment. For example, a protracted course of radiotherapy to a primary lesion may be undesirable if accompanied by progressive liver involvement or by the appearance of brain metastases. Since systemic manifestations are already present in almost 50 percent of patients at the outset,[2] the importance of excluding metastatic disease in each and every patient with lung cancer cannot be overemphasized.

An initial diagnosis of lung cancer must be complemented by a systematic search for possible dissemination in preferred sites and a determination of prognosis and potentially lethal complications. The purpose of this chapter is to review diagnostic procedures that have been found useful or that may be promising in (1) detecting metastatic involvement once the diagnosis of lung cancer has been established and (2) initially diagnosing the disease when it presents in metastatic sites. With each of the diagnostic procedures the circumstances that render its application most desirable will be analyzed. A rigid schema of diagnostic procedures cannot be established, since the investigations used in any one case should in part be dictated by "Sutton's law" (i.e., "go where the money is"). Nevertheless, familiarity with the procedure and its yield will help the clinician to develop diagnostic approaches appropriate to a given setting. The methods to be employed in looking for metastases within the thoracic cavity and regional lymph nodes will not be reviewed, since they are covered elsewhere. However, metastases to the contralateral lung should usually be regarded as having similar therapeutic implications as extrathoracic dissemination of carcinoma.

The application of diagnostic procedures for the above purposes will certainly differ according to the patient's clinical presentation, the intrinsic yield of the procedure relative to its morbidity and expense, the availability of techniques and skills, and the therapeutic implications that one attaches to the staging. Histology is a major factor influencing therapy and prognosis, since the

137

Table 11-1
Preferred Sites of Distant Metastases at Autopsy: Incidence Percentage in Relation to Histology

Cell Type	Liver*	Adrenal*	Bone*	Brain†	Other*
Epidermoid	30.5	27.4	24.4	13.7	
Small cell	61.9	39.2	37.5	30.5	Abdominal lymph nodes 56.6%
Adenocarcinoma	44.8	42.9	39.9	25.4	
Large cell	39.6	36.4	28.9	29.4	Abdominal lymph nodes 36.0%

*Data from Hansen.[27]
†Data from 247 patients of the NCI-VA Medical Oncology Service including all clinical and autopsy incidence.[61]

various cell types differ in their growth rates and metastatic potential.[3] This is reflected in autopsy studies of metastatic patterns, as shown in Table 11-1. Metastases in general are most prevalent in small cell carcinoma and least prevalent in epidermoid carcinoma, with adenocarcinoma and large cell undifferentiated carcinoma showing an intermediate tendency to disseminate. However, these autopsy studies do not necessarily relate directly to our ability to detect disease at time of diagnosis.

More likely to reflect conditions at clinical presentation are studies showing the extent of involvement in patients dying shortly (1 month) after lung resection for cancer[4,5] (Table 11-2). Of 202 such patients in one study, 73 (35 percent) had persistent disease at autopsy. For epidermoid cancer, persistent disease was found in 33 percent of such patients (distant metastases and local dis-

ease only occurring in equal numbers); in small cell carcinoma and in adenocarcinoma, persistent disease was found more often (70 and 43 percent, respectively) and was only exceptionally localized to regional sites. The fact that these patients represented a special group selected for lung resection renders these figures even more impressive. Clearly, if all patients with lung cancer at the time of diagnosis are included and studied with sensitive diagnostic procedures, distant metastases should be detectable in at least 1 additional patient out of 3 patients now considered to have regional or localized disease.

Information on disease distribution at onset can be obtained by analyzing series of patients with inoperable disease. The NCI-VA Medical Oncology series included 200 consecutive patients with lung cancer deemed inoperable at time of diagnosis (1970–1972). For the 105

Table 11-2
Distribution of Lung Cancer at Autopsy in Patients Dying within 1 Month of "Curative" Resection

Cell Type	No. of Patients	No. with Persistent Disease		No. with Distant Metastases		Pattern of Distant Metastases
Epidermoid	131	44	33%	22	17%	Nonregional lymph nodes (LN) 6; adrenal 5; liver 5; contralateral lung and kidney 3
Small cell	19	13	70%	12	63%	Liver 7; LN 6; adrenal 4; brain and kidney 2
Adenocarcinoma	30	13	43%	12	40%	Adrenal 7; brain 5; LN 4; vertebrae 3
Large cell	22	3	17%	3	14%	Kidney 3; adrenal, liver, and contralateral lung 2
Total	202	73	35%	49	24%	Adrenal 18; LN 17; liver 16; kidney and contralateral lung 6

*Data from Matthews et al.[5]

Table 11-3
Site of Distant Metastases in Relation to Histology prior to Treatment*

Cell Type	No. with Distant Metastases	Percentage with Metastases to:					
		Liver	*Bone†*	*Brain*	*Thorax‡*	*LN§*	*Skin*
Epidermoid	25	8	16	20	36	24	8
Small cell	25	40	72	8	20	8	8
Adenocarcinoma	24	12.5	46	21	29	20	12.5
Large cell	31	6	26	13	38	35	13
Total	105	16%	40%	15%	30%	22%	10%

*Data from Hansen.[27]
†Excludes direct extension.
‡Refers to contralateral lung and mediatinum and pericardium.
§Refers to nonregional peripheral lymph nodes.

patients with extensive (nonregional) lung cancer, the localization of disease in relation to histology prior to treatment can be seen in Table 11-3. The distribution of metastases represents in part the staging measures used,[6] including routine bone marrow aspiration and needle biopsy and evaluation of the liver by peritoneoscopy. Not reflecting this bias would be an analysis of patients in whom the initial diagnosis was actually arrived at by biopsy of metastatic sites (Table 11-4). Bone was the major site of metastases in these patients.

Adenocarcinomas were diagnosed in metastatic sites at greater frequency than other cell types (Table 11-5). Overall, the diagnosis of metastatic lung cancer was made in 31 of 200 consecutive patients (15.5 percent) prior to any

staging. Any systematic search for metastases should easily exceed this minimum figure. The methods used will be reviewed by organ systems.

DETECTION OF BONE METASTASES

The skeletal system represents one of the four major sites of involvement by lung cancer at autopsy (Table 11-1). Sampling techniques used at autopsy probably underestimate its incidence; this becomes evident when one compares it with the incidence of skeletal involvement in the clinical study cited (Table 11-3). Clinically, the bones can be evaluated by bone marrow aspiration and

Table 11-4
Initial Diagnosis Established by Biopsy of Metastatic Sites in 31 of 200 Consecutive Nonsurgical Patients*

Diagnostic Procedure	No. of Patients
Chest wall and/or rib biopsy	10
Iliac bone marrow biopsy (needle)	6
Other bone biopsies	2†
Craniotomy	6
Liver biopsy	3
Soft tissue and nonregional lymph node	2
Pericardial biopsy	1
Laparotomy and adrenal biopsy	1
Total	31
Percentage of all patients: 31/200 = 15.5%	

*Data from Hansen.[27]
†One obtained at time of laminectomy.

Table 11-5
Initial Diagnosis Established by Biopsy of Metastatic Sites: Relationship to Histology*

| | No. of Patients | | | |
Cell Type	Metastatic Site Diagnosis	Total Studied	Percentage	Procedure and/or Site of Biopsy (No.)
Epidermoid	4	78	5.1	Chest wall/rib 3
				Distant soft tissue 1
Small cell	6	35	17.2	Chest wall/rib 1
				Bone marrow 3
				Craniotomy 1
				Liver 1
Adenocarcinoma	11	40	27.5	Chest wall/rib 4
				Bone marrow 1
				Open bone 1
				Craniotomy 2
				Liver 1
				Distant lymph node 1
				Adrenal 1
Large cell	10	47	21.3	Chest wall/rib 2
				Bone marrow 2
				Open bone 1
				Craniotomy 3
				Liver 1
				Pericardium 1
Total	31	200	15.5	

*Data from Hansen.[27]

biopsy, scans, and x-rays; they are generally more accessible to sampling than are visceral organs.

Bone Marrow Study

The technique of McFarland and Dameshek[7] for posterior iliac crest needle biopsy has been extensively evaluated in patients with lung cancer.[8-11] The initial report by Hansen and Muggia stressed the frequent occurrence of unsuspected metastases to bone in patients with small cell carcinoma of the lung.[10] Subsequent studies have confirmed a high rate of detection of unsuspected bone marrow metastases in these patients.[8-11] Bone pain, abnormal hematologic findings, or elevated serum calcium and alkaline phosphatase were usually absent in patients with marrow biopsies positive for tumor. Of 200 consecutive patients studied at the NCI-VA Medical Oncology Service, 15 of 35 (43 percent) with small cell carcinoma, 7 of 40 (17.5 percent) with adenocarci-

noma, 8 of 47 (17 percent) with large cell carcinoma, and 2 of 78 (2.6 percent) with epidermoid carcinoma had bone marrow metastases demonstrable at time of diagnosis. Patients in this series, having usually been referred because of unresectability, should be considered to be at a relatively more advanced stage than patients from a totally unselected series. Even so, in 141 consecutive patients with small cell carcinoma the incidence of marrow involvement was 19.9 percent. With the exception of thrombocytopenia (platelets less than 135,000/mm^3), no chemical or hematologic abnormalities were predictive of marrow involvement (unpublished observations of H. H. Hansen, 1975).

Bone marrow examination in some instances was useful in establishing the initial diagnosis (Table 11-4). Aspirates may be useful in prompt identification of bone marrow involvement; however, needle biopsies in addition to the aspirates are preferable in terms of yield, reliability, and information regarding cell type. The Jamzhidi needle and the Radner needle have proved to be suitable alternatives to the modified Silverman biopsy needle.

Bone Scanning

Osseous metastases commonly locate in spongy (trabecular) bone and are not demonstrable by radiologic examination until they are approximately 1–1.5 cm in diameter and until bone decalcification occurs at least to the extent of 50–75 percent to make decreased bone density detectable.[12,13] The use of radioactive compounds as diagnostic aids in the clinical study of bone and skeletal structures has now been widely accepted.[14,15] These agents offer greater sensitivity than x-rays in the early detection of primary and metastatic bone tumors. Although a number of radionuclides are bone-seekers, only a few are suitable for application in nuclear medicine from the viewpoint of their physical and biologic characteristics.

The radionuclides ^{85}Sr, ^{87m}Sr, and ^{18}F were introduced into clinical use for bone scanning.[16] ^{85}Sr has a long half-life (65 days) and results in high exposure levels (6 rads/200 μCi), thus precluding its use other than in patients with documented malignancy. ^{87m}Sr and ^{18}F have been used effectively,[17–20] but they have the drawbacks of too short a half-life and unavailability, respectively. The radionuclide ^{99m}Tc has ideal physical characteristics for imaging applications in nuclear medicine and is readily available from a generator system. Tumors in bones have been visualized directly with ^{99m}Tc-pertechnetate, but in this chemical state it is not a true bone-seeker. The development of ^{99m}Tc-Sn-polyphosphate and -diphosphonate complexes[21,22] is a major breakthrough in regard to the application of this radionuclide for skeletal imaging. The most effective imaging modality presently available for determining the presence and extent of skeletal metastases is offered through scanning with these newly developed agents.[16,23–25] The administration of a ^{99m}Tc complex results in minimal radiation dose (0.5 rads/10 mCi) to the skeleton when compared to ^{85}Sr. With these technical advances, one may anticipate more widespread use of this procedure for screening purposes in patients with lung cancer.

The NCI-VA experience of bone scanning with ^{85}Sr or ^{87m}Sr in 82 patients with lung cancer has been reported.[6] Scans were most helpful in detecting patients with diffuse bone marrow involvement secondary to small cell carcinoma. Scans were positive in 69.2 percent of patients with biopsy-proven bone marrow involvement. An additional 15.8 percent of the scans were positive in the absence of tumor identification on bone marrow biopsy, thus suggesting that the procedures are complementary. A high yield by the combined use of these procedures would also be expected in adenocarcinoma (Tables 11-1 and 11-3).

Skeletal X-Rays

For reasons cited in the preceding sections, the skeletal surveys requested almost as a routine investigation in cancer patients constitute an overrated procedure. The skeletal survey was positive in only 3.5 percent of patients with skeletal involvement proved by bone marrow biopsy. Nevertheless, radiologic investigations of areas positive on scan might be desirable when impending fracture is suspected or if serial measurements are intended. In addition, further comparative experience of x-rays and scans indicates instances of radiologically obvious lesions not apparent on the scan.[26] In 47 patients with lung cancer and radiographically demonstrable metastases exclusive of adjacent rib destruction, only 5 lesions of a total of 61 would not have been visualized by x-rays including the pelvis, abdomen, and thorax.[27] Three additional lesions would have been visualized on skull x-rays. This experience suggests that films confined to the pelvis and chest and a single lateral skull film should suffice as a baseline determination.

A relationship of histology to the type of bone lesion encountered has also recently become apparent.[28] An interesting observation was the propensity of small cell carcinoma to produce osteoblastic metastases.[29] This phenomenon, previously unnoticed, may have been uncovered as a result of prolongation in survival achieved by chemotherapy. Whether these blastic changes are related to ectopic calcitonin production by the tumor[30] must be investigated further. Adenocarcinomas can also be associated with osteoblastic lesions.[28] On the other hand, epidermoid cancer is predominantly osteolytic.[28]

The correlation of hypercalcemia and skeletal involvement in 200 patients with lung cancer has been analyzed by Bender and Hansen.[31] Noteworthy was the absence of hypercalcemia in 35 consecutive patients with small cell carcinoma and its occurrence in only 1 of 40 patients with adenocarcinoma. Six of 47 patients with large cell undifferentiated carcinoma and 18 of 78 patients with epidermoid carcinoma had hypercalcemia documented during their clinical course. Osseous metastases were documented in only 6 (one-third) of these patients with epidermoid carcinoma and in 4 (two-thirds) with the large cell type. Therefore hypercalcemia cannot be considered an indicator of bone metastases in the majority of patients with lung cancer. Presumably it is a result of ectopic elaboration of a hypercalcemic humoral substance. Such ectopic production could also account for the development of destructive bone lesions in epidermoid carcinoma by facilitating local bone resorption.

DETECTION OF LIVER METASTASES

Metastatic involvement of the liver can easily be recognized by serial observations in a few patients with small cell carcinoma who manifest a rapidly enlarging liver. In most patients with lung cancer, however, liver metastases are not commonly detected in the early stages.

In spite of their documented frequency at autopsy (Table 11-1), few studies have addressed themselves specifically to detection of liver metastases by standard or investigational diagnostic methods in lung cancer. There are pitfalls in extrapolating the validity of chemical determinations or scans in diagnosing lung cancer metastatic to the liver from series that have also included patients with gastrointestinal cancer.[32,33] Although hepatic dysfunction without actual involvement of the liver by tumor (as has been reported in patients with hypernephroma and Hodgkin's disease[34] has not been described in lung cancer, several other possible sources of error exist. For example, cirrhosis may be a more common source of false positives in the predominantly male population with lung cancer.[6] In addition, the frequent presence of bone metastases and the contribution of ectopic "placental" isoenzyme of alkaline phophatase[35] may invalidate the use of the serum alkaline phosphatase alone as an indicator of liver metastases. Further correlations

of chemical determinations with the various procedures outlined below are therefore needed in lung cancer.

Liver Scanning

Among the noninvasive diagnostic procedures for verifying metastatic spread to liver, the radionuclide scan has a very important role.[36,37] In fact, statistical comparison of liver scanning and a number of liver function tests has shown that the diagnostic value of liver scanning in metastatic disease is superior to that of any of the liver function tests studied.[38] Combined use of the laboratory test for serum alkaline phosphatase and liver scanning has been reported as a reliable indicator for detecting focal lesions, especially metastases in the liver.[39,40] Inability to visualize small metastatic deposits (less than 2–3 cm) on the radionuclide scan is a very common cause of false negative diagnosis, while unrelated conditions could contribute to false positive diagnosis.[41]

The radiopharmaceuticals developed for static liver scanning are the colloids labeled with a variety of radionuclides, including ^{99m}Tc-sulfur colloid, radiogold (^{198}Au), indium colloid (^{113}In), and small aggregates of human serum albumin labeled with ^{131}I or ^{99m}Tc. The ^{198}Au colloid results in a very large radiation dose to the liver (8 rads/150 μCi) and offers no distinct advantage compared to the ^{99m}Tc-sulfur colloid.[42] Newer techniques, to be described in a subsequent section, using radionuclides preferentially taken up by tumors may be combined advantageously with current liver scanning to aid in the differential diagnosis of hepatic lesions.[43]

Routine use of liver scanning with ^{99m}Tc-sulfur colloid in 64 patients with lung cancer in whom liver metastases were not suspected resulted in only three definitely positive and five suspicious scans.[37] Confirmation was eventually obtained in three of the latter cases, but the methods by which diagnoses were verified were not described. When there was clinical suspicion of liver metastases (basis for suspicion not stated), the scan was positive in 13 of 19 patients. The overall incidence of positive scans in the patient population was 16 of 83 patients.[37] A similar frequency (17 percent) of abnormal scans was obtained in our studies evaluating the use of peritoneoscopy for detection of liver metastases.[6]

The role of the scan in determining the application of additional tests will be discussed in the subsequent section.

Liver Biopsy and Peritoneoscopy

Because chemical tests and scans do not accurately distinguish metastatic disease in the liver from other intrahepatic processes such as abscess, cirrhosis, granuloma, etc., it is often imperative to obtain histologic proof of metastases. Percutaneous liver biopsy with the Menghini technique is a well-established procedure with little morbidity in experienced hands.[44] No study of the yield of this procedure confined to patients with lung cancer has been reported, as had been reported for Hodgkin's disease.[34]

An elegant study by Conn and Yesner in postmortem specimens demonstrated the limitations of diagnosing liver metastases by percutaneous liver biopsy.[45] The yield of liver biopsy was 45 percent if 25 or more nodules were scattered throughout the liver, and substantially less with lesser degrees of involvement. In view of this obvious limitation, peritoneoscopy with liver biopsy under direct vision was introduced as a staging procedure in patients with Hodgkin's disease and other lymphomas by DeVita and associates.[46,47] In Hodgkin's disease the yield by this procedure appears to be similar to that obtained by laparotomy.[46,47] In patients with suspected hepatic metastases from various origins, blind percutaneous biopsy followed by peritoneoscopy with a second biopsy under guidance have similarly been compared. The yield was 39.5 and 69 percent, respectively.[48]

The NCI-VA Medical Oncology Service utilized peritoneoscopy to establish the presence of liver metastases in 111 patients with unresectable lung cancer exclusive of the rare patient diagnosed by liver biopsy. Of 98 patients who underwent biopsy under visual guidance, 10 patients were documented to have liver metastases. The procedure was positive in 8 of 19 patients with small cell carcinoma, as opposed to only 1 of 41 and 1 of 24, respectively, with epidermoid carcinoma and adenocarcinoma. Of 70 patients considered to have disease limited to the involved hemithorax, 4 had their classifications changed on the basis of peritoneoscopy findings; 3 of them had small cell carcinoma. The yield of the procedure

was disappointing in patients with other cell types. However, the procedure was extremely valuable in defining causes for inaccuracies in ^{99m}Tc-sulfur colloid scans and chemistries.[49] Of note was the high frequency of positive and suspicious scans among the 94 patients studied (16 and 24, respectively). Six of the 16 patients with positive scans had subsequent documentation of liver metastases, whereas only two positive biopsies occurred in the suspicious group and two in the 54 patients with negative scans. Similarly, abnormalities in alkaline phosphatase, SGOT, or bilirubin were extremely common in the entire group who underwent peritoneoscopy. Seven of the 10 positive biopsies were recorded in the 18 patients where two of three tests were abnormal. Thus even when two chemical tests were combined, the true positive rate was only 38.9 percent, with a large percentage of false positives. Some causes for false positive scans and chemistries were Laennec's cirrhosis, miliary granuloma of tuberculous origin, hepatocellular necrosis, and fatty metamorphosis. The high incidence of false positives in this study therefore casts doubt on the validity of accepting the 18.6 percent positive scans obtained in lung cancer patients in previously cited studies[37] as representing liver metastases. On the other hand, our experience with peritoneoscopy does suggest that abnormal scans may be used to select those patients in whom use of additional procedures designed to obtain histologic documentation is desirable. If only patients with positive scans and patients with small cell carcinoma (regardless of their scans) had been selected for peritoneoscopy, liver metastases would have been established in 10 of 31 patients (32.3 percent).

Peritoneoscopy was more extensively evaluated in 130 patients with small cell carcinoma (unpublished observations of H. H. Hansen, 1975). The procedure was successful in 122 patients. Biopsy confirmation of liver metastases was obtained in 25 (20.4 percent); an additional 11 (9 percent) were considered to have metastatic disease, but biopsy either was not done or was unsuccessful. This study indicates that peritoneoscopy can exceed the potential of bone marrow biopsy in uncovering metastatic disease in this cell type of bronchogenic carcinoma. In fact, although 11.1 percent of patients had both bone marrow and liver involvement, 7 percent had marrow involvement only, as opposed to 10.3

percent who had liver involvement only. Obviously, if therapeutic planning depends on the presence or absence of extrathoracic spread, peritoneoscopy assumes an essential role in the staging of this disease.

Laparotomy

Two series have been reported dealing with prethoracotomy exploration of the abdomen in patients suspected of having lung cancer, one by the transdiaphragmatic route[50] and the other by standard laparotomy.[51] The incidence of liver metastases was 14.9 percent (of 127 patients) in the first series and 13.6 percent (of 88 patients) in the second series. The latter study documented an additional 5.7 percent of intraabdominal metastases located in the adrenal and retroperitoneal lymph nodes and ribs. The conclusion was that this approach was desirable in sparing sizable numbers of patients unwarranted reductive surgery.

Comparison with our peritoneoscopy series in evaluating liver metastases is not strictly valid. The patient selection and preexploration staging studies were not stated in the surgical series, and differences in histologic cell type would further render the comparison invalid. Thus the somewhat lower yield obtained at peritoneoscopy cannot presently be interpreted as a deficiency in the procedure. Although no mortality was associated with laparotomy in the study reported,[51] it should be noted that peritoneoscopy had distinct advantages over laparotomy in patients who could be expected to be at high risk of developing infectious complications following general anesthesia.[47] On the other hand, laparotomy does permit palpation of subcapsular nodules and examination of retroperitoneal structures.

In conclusion, histologic documentation of liver metastases would appear desirable in many lung cancer patients. The inaccuracies of diagnosing metastatic disease on the basis of scans and chemistries alone require reemphasis. Peritoneoscopy in patients with small cell carcinoma (regardless of their scans) and in patients with other cell types in the presence of abnormal scans would be expected to establish metastatic liver disease in one-third of patients. Although laparotomy might improve on the yield in unselected patients, the desirability of such a major proce-

dure strictly for staging purposes in patients who are often poor surgical risks is questionable.

DETECTION OF CENTRAL NERVOUS SYSTEM METASTASES

Brain metastases occur in 20–40 percent of patients with lung cancer at autopsy (Table 11-1). Forty percent of all cerebral metastases were found at the time of initial staging, 40 percent developed subsequently, and 20 percent were found at autopsy.[61] Occasionally, neurologic signs and symptoms are the first manifestations of the disease, and the diagnosis of lung cancer is first made at craniotomy even before the primary site has been identified (Table 11-4). The diagnosis of lung cancer must be considered in any adult patient presenting with sudden or gradual onset of neurologic deficits, particularly in the absence of preexisting cardiovascular disease. In neurosurgical series the lung is the most frequent primary site of origin of brain metastases;[52,53] in radiotherapy series, brain metastases from lung cancer and breast cancer predominate.[54,55] The metastases are most often multiple, but are occasionally single and rarely also solitary (i.e., no other metastases present).[56]

Early detection of spread to the central nervous system is crucial if its disastrous consequences are to be avoided. Examination for signs and symptoms of neurologic disease, brain scanning, electroencephalograph, computer tomography, spinal fluid examination, and arteriography are the major diagnostic procedures employed. The brain scan occupies the central role as a screening procedure because of its simplicity and high yield of positive findings. Computerized tomography, as it becomes more readily available, will undoubtedly supplement or replace scan information.[26,57–60]

Symptoms such as headache, dizziness, disorientation, unexplained vomiting, and newly appearing ulcer diathesis are prominent indicators of brain metastases in the absence of focal findings. Focal seizures and findings on neurologic examination assume diagnostic significance even in the absence of confirmatory tests. The incidences of specific neurologic signs and symptoms in a large series of patients treated for brain metastases have been analyzed by Nisce et al.[55] Although motor deficits predominated (75 percent), personality changes, lethargy, and coma occurred in 41 percent, often without focal findings. Other causes for neurologic dysfunction such as vascular accidents, emboli from marantic endocarditis, infection, or metabolic derangements including hypercalcemia must be excluded. In addition, cerebellar degeneration, dementia, and rarely optic atrophy have been noted as distant effects of the tumor, without actual central nervous system invasion.

Histology influences the incidence of brain metastases. Small cell and large cell carcinomas spread to the brain more often than do other cell types (Table 11-1).[3,56,61] However, other cell types also metastasize in excess of 20 percent to the brain (Table 11-1) and may present clinically with brain metastases as the only metastatic lesion (Table 11-3). The risk of developing brain metastases in small cell carcinoma has been shown to increase during the course of the disease.[56] For this reason, elective irradiation of the brain has been advocated in these patients,[56] and treatment protocols evaluating the effects of such prophylactic therapy have been initiated by the Acute Leukemia Group B and the Working Party for Therapy of Lung Cancer. We have noted an increased risk of brain metastases in patients presenting with superior vena caval obstruction; retrograde embolization of tumor is a possible explanation for this phenomenon. In general, however, spread to the brain has been considered to occur via arterial routes.[63,64] Meningeal carcinomatosis is another complication associated with lung cancer, and it must be suspected in patients with cranial nerve deficits.

Cord compressions are also frequently reported in association with lung cancer but rarely are the presenting manifestation (Table 11-4). This occurs often as a result of direct extension of the tumor to vertebrae and the epidural space. Patients with Pancoast tumors and with superior vena caval obstruction are prone to develop this complication. Radiation-induced myelopathy must be considered in the differential diagnosis of previously irradiated patients developing cord signs.

Brain Scanning

Brain scanning techniques have proved to be efficient methods of demonstrating metastatic deposits, with a high degree of positive correlation with documented metastatic spread of a variety of primary malignancies.[66,67] The scanning procedure has been applied as part of the initial workup of the lung cancer patient to detect metastatic disease.[36,37] The size of the lesion and the concentration of the nuclide radioactivity in the lesion in relation to background radioactivity somewhat limit the sensitivity of the method. Only 3 percent of lesions greater than 2.7 cm in diameter are missed on scanning, with only 1.3 percent false positives.[68]

The use of ^{99m}Tc-pertechnetate for brain scanning for initial screening has been most extensive, owing to its favorable physical characteristics and its ready availability from the generator system, even though the tumor-to-background ratio is not very high and the pertechnetate accumulates in salivary glands, choroid plexus, and thyroid. Total body radiation dose for the procedure is very low, 0.15 rads/10 mCi. Metastatic brain lesions are usually multiple and peripheral and are noticed as small round areas of increased uptake with a somewhat low differential. Improved delineation of the lesion is noticed on the brain scan 3–4 hr after injection.[66,67] The delayed scan is also useful in disclosing multiple metastatic lesions in cases in which the initial scan reveals only a single lesion. The use of multiple radiopharmaceuticals may improve the accuracy of brain scanning, particularly when the ^{99m}Tc-pertechnetate scans are equivocal (^{67}Ga brain scan, see below).

Brain scanning may establish the presence of metastases from lung cancer prior to any neurologic manifestations.[69] When used as a routine procedure, the yield is low in those patients not suspected of having metastatic disease; three positive (3.7 percent) and four equivocal scans were obtained among 80 such patients studied.[37] One of the patients with equivocal scans was subsequently proved to have brain metastases. When metastases were suspected, the yield rose to 12 of 26 patients (46 percent).[37] Scans that might have been positive can revert to negative as a result of diminution of the edema surrounding the tumor if the patient has received corticosteroids. Raskind et al. have commented on the need for surgical exploration of patients with cancer suspected of having solitary lesions.[52] In their series, a number of nonmetastatic lesions of the brain were documented at craniotomy in these patients. However, the interval between diagnosis of the cancer and the appearance of suspicious brain lesions exceeded 2 years in all these patients, and none had lung cancer.

Other CNS Studies; Computerized Tomography

In one series[54] both the electroencephalogram and the spinal fluid examination for protein were abnormal in 50 percent of patients with brain metastases; these procedures, however, lack specificity and are likely to be impractical for screening purposes. Detection of abnormal cells on cytologic examination of the cerebrospinal fluid by Millipore techniques or by use of the cytocentrifuge occasionally indicates the diagnosis.

Computerized axial tomography or computed tomography is a new type of body-layer visualization in which projections of the radiations detected at multiple angles are used to reconstruct the anatomic layer with the aid of a computer. The procedure permits one to appreciate differences in absorption in various tissues so small as to produce no perceptible differences in film blackening in conventional radiography. The success of this technique in neuroradiology is impressive, and data from large patient series indicate that familiar procedures such as angiography, pneumography, and radionuclide brain scanning may be relegated to less prominent positions for the detection of metastatic neoplasms in the brain.[26,57−60]

DETECTION OF OTHER SITES; NEW PROCEDURES

The retroperitoneal lymph nodes and other organs such as the adrenals and kidneys are major sites of involvement by lung cancer that cannot readily be assessed by currently used procedures. The diagnostic procedures that have been introduced, some of which may assume practical importance, will be reviewed below. Subcutaneous or peripheral lymph node metastases are readily diagnosed by excision, but fine needle aspiration can be used advantageously with no morbidity. Because of their scanty stroma, cells are easily aspirated and identified in metastases from small cell carcinoma.[70] Cytologic examination has also been shown to increase the yield of

tumor identification at the time of percutaneous needle biopsy of the liver.[71,72] Metastases to the eye usually localize in the choroid and can be identified further by the use of fluorescein angiography. Carcinoma of the lung appears to be the tumor most frequently metastatic to the eye.[73]

Adrenal Metastases

In males lung cancer is the most common neoplasm metastasizing to the adrenal glands, and in most instances there are few recognizable clinical manifestations from these metastases. Studies have demonstrated the value of adrenal venography and its superiority to arteriography for their detection.[74] However, the procedure is not suitable for screening purposes. The technique of adrenal photoscanning for diagnosis of adrenal tumors was developed following the introduction of radiopharmaceuticals such as ^{131}I-19-iodocholesterol.[75,76] The avid uptake and retention of this agent by the adrenals and cortical tumors is the basis of its application. Optimum adrenal scanning is accomplished 5 to 14 days after dose administration. The estimated absorbed dose in humans is 30.0 rads/mCi, 2.88 rads/mCi, and 2.01 rads/mCi to the adrenals, ovaries, and testes, respectively.[77] Experience is lacking in the use of this procedure for detection of metastases to the adrenal or for adrenal hyperplasia.

Miscellaneous Techniques

Ultrasound has been advocated as an adjunct to liver biopsy in guiding the needle to an area of suspected involvement.[78] Echography also has a role in the evaluation of brain metastases. A recently introduced combined x-ray and brain scanner developed by EMI, Ltd. in Britain has become a valuable tool in the diagnosis of brain disorders.[56] The technique has been extended toward development of fractional computer-assisted tomography for organs in various parts of the body other than the head. In fact, identification of pancreatic masses appears promising by this noninvasive technique.

Bipedal lymphangiography is probably too cumbersome to be used in routine evaluation of retroperitoneal involvement by lung cancer; such a study does not appear justified, with the possible exception of use in selected patients with small cell carcinoma. ^{198}Au colloid scanning by the endolymphatic route has been used to detect retroperitoneal involvement, but this procedure probably lacks the specificity of newer scanning procedures that utilize tumor-seeking radiopharmaceuticals or radiolabeled antibodies.[79]

Scanning with Tumor-Seeking Markers

Several radiopharmaceuticals that have tumor affinity, although not tumor specificity, have been proposed for use in recent years; these include ^{67}Ga-citrate, ^{75}Se-selenite, ^{197}HgCl$_2$, ^{111}In-chloride, ^{131}I-fibrinogen, and ^{169}Yb-citrate. ^{67}Ga-citrate has been evaluated clinically in a number of patient series in the scintigraphy of brain tumors.[43,80-86] The increased uptake of gallium by certain tumors lends itself to better delineation because of the more favorable target-to-nontarget ratio, since the time from injection to scan is 2–3 days (^{67}Ga half-life, 78 hr) and gallium is rapidly cleared from the bloodstream. The usual intravenous dose is 1–3 mCi of ^{67}Ga-citrate, and the total body radiation dose has been estimated to be 0.26 rads/mCi.[86] The ^{67}Ga scan is of value as an adjunctive scanning procedure and has been shown to be useful in the diagnosis of metastatic brain tumors.[82] Similarly, combined use of the ^{67}Ga scan and ^{99m}Tc-sulfur colloid has been valuable in diagnosing space-occupying lesions of the liver.[43] Lung cancer is one of the tumors that most actively picks up gallium.[80,85] Inflammatory conditions and sarcoidosis[87] have been reported to give false positives.

The radiopharmaceuticals that have specific affinity for malignant tumors are still in developmental stages. The labeling of the chemotherapeutic agent Bleomycin (which is known to concentrate actively in certain types of neoplastic tissue) with ^{111}In, ^{57}Co, ^{67}Ga, ^{59}Fe, and ^{99m}Tc has been reported with somewhat varied clinical experience and findings.[88-91] Scanning with radiolabeled antitumor platinum compound has also been reported.[92] Large classes of these organometallic complexes that have antitumor activity, when labeled with radionuclide, might prove to exhibit the desired specificity in tumor delineation not achieved thus far. Similarly, labeled tumor-specific antibodies have also been investigated as tumor-scanning agents,[93,95] and clinical application of these is awaited.

CONCLUSION

Detection of metastatic disease at the time of diagnosis is likely to have great influence on our therapeutic approach and our ability to prevent critical complications. In addition, accurate staging can provide valuable information on patterns of disease and can establish the standards of comparability required for evaluation of new therapeutic modalities. For these reasons the application of a schema in the search for metastatic involvement and in the search for knowledge of useful procedures is likely to play a major role in optimizing the treatment of patients with lung cancer. In the development of such a diagnostic evaluation the intimate relationship of possible yield with histologic cell type of bronchogenic carcinoma has been emphasized. In a great percentage of patients with small cell carcinoma, for example, a search for metastases to bone, liver, brain, and retroperitoneal areas is likely to be productive. Sequential examination of these areas prior to treatment with local measures is almost mandatory. Patients showing minimal metastatic burden at the time of diagnosis are likely to benefit from intensive therapeutic programs, including chemotherapy.

In other histologic cell types, clinical circumstances dictate the selection of diagnostic procedures to be applied. Unfortunately for many patients who manifest widespread disease at the time of diagnosis, treatment is at present ineffective. Even so, proper application of diagnostic procedures may spare the patient the morbidity associated with unwarranted tests or misguided treatment.

REFERENCES

1. Karnofsky DA: Chemotherapy of lung cancer, in Mayer E, Maier HC (eds): Pulmonary Carcinoma. Philadelphia, Lippincott, 1956, pp 384–397

2. Cutler SJ: End Results in Cancer. Report No. 3 prepared for NIH-NCI, GPO, Washington, D.C. No. 30, 1968, pp 81–85

3. Selawry OS, Hansen HH: Lung cancer, in Holland JF, Frei E III (eds): Cancer Medicine. Philadelphia, Lea & Febiger, 1973, pp 1473–1518

4. Winstanley DP: Fruitless resection. Thorax 23:327, 1968 (abstract)

5. Matthews MJ, Kanhouwa S, Pickren J, et al: Fre-

quency of residual and metastatic tumors in patients undergoing curative surgical resection for lung cancer. Cancer Chemother Rep (Part 3) 4:63–67, 1973

6. Hansen HH, Muggia FM: Staging of inoperable patients with bronchogenic carcinoma with special reference to bone marrow examination and peritoneoscopy. Cancer 30:1395–1401, 1972

7. McFarland W, Dameshek W: Biopsy of bone marrow with the Vim-Silverman needle. JAMA 166:1464–1468, 1958

8. Hansen HH, Muggia FM, Selawry OS: Bone marrow examination in 100 consecutive patients with bronchogenic carcinoma. Lancet 2:433–445, 1971

9. Hansen HH, Muggia FM, Andrews R, et al: Intensive combined chemotherapy and radiotherapy in patients with nonresectable bronchogenic carcinoma. Cancer 30:315–324, 1972

10. Hansen HH, Muggia FM: Early detection of bone-marrow invasion in oat-cell carcinoma of the lung. N Engl J Med 284:962–963, 1971

11. Maurer LH, Tullon M, Eagan RT, et al: Combination chemotherapy and radiation therapy for small cell carcinoma of the lung. Cancer Chemother Rep (Part 3) 4:171–176, 1973

12. Bachman AL, Sproul EE: Correlation of radiographic and autopsy findings in suspected metastases in the spine. Bull NY Acad Med 31:146–148, 1955

13. Edelstyn GA, Gillespie PJ, Grebbell FS: The radiological demonstration of osseous metastases: Experimental observations. Clin Radiol 18:158–162, 1967

14. DeNardo GL, Jacobson SJ, Raventos A: ^{85}Sr bone scan in neoplastic disease. Semin Nucl Med 2:18–30, 1972

15. Merrick MV: Bone scans or skeletal surveys? Lancet 2:382–383, 1972

16. Bell EG: Nuclear medicine and skeletal disease. Hosp Practice 7:49–60, 1972

17. Briggs RC: Detection of osseous metastasis. Evaluation of bone scanning with ^{85}Sr. Cancer 20:392–395, 1967

18. Milner TH, Maynard CD, Cowan RJ: Evaluation of strontium-85 bone scans and roentgenograms in 100 patients. Arch Surg 103:371–372, 1971

19. Sharma SM, Quinn JL: Sensitivity of ^{18}F bone scans in the search for metastases. Surg Gynecol Obstet 135:536–540, 1972

20. Shirazi PH, Stern AJ, Sidell MS, et al: Bone scanning in the staging and management of bronchogenic carcinoma: Review of 206 cases. J Nucl Med 14:451, 1973 (abstract)

21. Subramanian G, McAfee JG, Bell EG, et al: Tc-99m labeled polyphosphate as a skeletal imaging agent. Radiology 102:701–704, 1972

22. Yano Y, McRae J, Van Dyke DC, et al: Tc-99m labeled stannous ethane-1-hydroxy-1-diphosphon-

ate: A new bone scanning agent. J Nucl Med 14:73–78, 1973

23. Pendergrass HP, Potsaid MS, Castronovo FP: The clinical use of ^{99m}Tc-diphosphonate (HEDSPA). Radiology 107:557–562, 1973

24. Eckelman WC, Reba RC, Kubota H, et al: ^{99m}Tc-pyrophosphate for bone imaging. J Nucl Med 15:279–283, 1974

25. Subramanian G, McAfee JA, Blair RJ, et al: ^{99m}Tc-methylene diphosphonate—A superior agent for skeletal imaging: Comparison with other technetium complexes. J Nucl Med 16:744–755, 1975

26. Galasko CSB: The value of scintigraphy in malignant disease. Cancer Treatment Reviews 2:225–272, 1975

27. Hansen HH: Bone Metastases in Lung Cancer—A Clinical Study in 200 Consecutive Patients with Bronchogenic Carcinoma, and Its Therapeutic Implications for Small Cell Carcinoma. Copenhagen, Denmark, Christian Christensen & Co, 1974

28. Napoli L, Hansen HH, Muggia FM, et al: The incidence of osseous involvement in lung cancer with special reference to the development of osteoblastic changes. Radiology 108:17–21, 1973

29. Muggia FM, Hansen HH: Osteoblastic metastases in small cell (oat cell) carcinoma of the lung. Cancer 30:801–805, 1972

30. Hansen HH, Muggia FM: Ectopic production of calcitonin. Lancet 2:915, 1973

31. Bender RA, Hansen HH: Hypercalcemia in bronchogenic carcinoma—A prospective study of 200 patients. Ann Intern Med 80:205–208, 1974

32. Yesner R, Conn HO: Liver function tests and needle biopsy in the diagnosis of metastatic cancer of the liver. Ann Intern Med 59:62–73, 1963

33. Hitzelberger AL, Parker GW, Durden WD, et al: Peritoneoscopy and radioisotope scintiscanning of the liver in the detection of hepatic metastases. Gastrointest Endosc 13:12–17, 1967

34. Bagley CM, Roth JA, Thomas LB, et al: Liver biopsy in Hodgkin's disease. Clinicopathologic correlations in 127 patients. Ann Intern Med 76:219–225, 1972

35. Stolbach LL, Krant MJ, Fishman WH: Ectopic production of an alkaline phosphatase isoenzyme in patients with cancer. N Engl J Med 281:757–762, 1969

36. McCormack KR, Greenlaw RH, Hopkins C: Scanning of liver and brain in evaluation of patients with bronchogenic carcinoma. J Nucl Med 9:222–224, 1968

37. Hayes TP, Davis LW, Raventos A: Brain and liver scans in the evaluation of lung cancer patients. Cancer 27:362–363, 1971

38. Liewendahl K, Schauman KO: Statistical evaluation of liver scanning in combination with liver function tests. Acta Med Scand 192:395–400, 1972

39. Castagna J, Benfield JR, Yamada H, et al: The

reliability of liver scans and function tests in detecting metastases. Surg Gynecol Obstet 134:463–466, 1972

40. Wilson FE, Preston DF, Overholt EL: Detection of hepatic neoplasm. JAMA 209:676–679, 1969

41. Covington EE: The accuracy of liver photoscan. Am J Roentgenol Radium Ther Nucl Med 109:742–744, 1970

42. Cantor RE, Cohn EM, Park CH, et al: Comparative liver scanning. Technetium sulfide Tc-99m vs. Gold Au-198. JAMA 211:1677–1680, 1970

43. Lomas F, Dibos PE, Wagner HN Jr: Increased specificity of liver scanning with the use of ⁶⁷Ga citrate. N Engl J Med 286:1323–1329, 1972

44. Menghini G: One-second biopsy of the liver— Problems of its clinical application. N Engl J Med 283:582–585, 1970

45. Conn HO, Yesner R: A re-evaluation of needle biopsy in the diagnosis of metastatic cancer of the liver. Ann Intern Med 59:53–61, 1963

46. DeVita VJ Jr, Bagley CM, Goodell E, et al: Peritoneoscopy in the staging of Hodgkin's disease. Cancer Res 31:1746–1750, 1971

47. Bagley CM, Thomas LB, Johnson KE, et al: Diagnosis of liver involvement by lymphoma: Results in 96 consecutive peritoneoscopies. Cancer 31:840–847, 1973

48. Jori GP, Peschle C: Combined peritoneoscopy and liver biopsy in diagnosis of hepatic neoplasm. Gastroenterology 63:1016–1019, 1972

49. Margolis R, Hansen HH, Muggia FM, et al: Diagnosis of liver metastases in bronchogenic carcinoma—A comparative study of liver scans, function tests and peritoneoscopy with liver biopsy in 111 patients. Cancer 34:1825–1829, 1974

50. Yashar J: Transdiaphragmatic exploration of the upper abdomen during surgery for bronchogenic carcinoma. J Thorac Cardiovasc Surg 52:599–603, 1966

51. Bell JW: Abdominal exploration in 100 lung cancer suspects prior to thoracotomy. Ann Surg 167:199–203, 1968

52. Raskind R, Weiss SR, Manning JJ, et al: Survival after surgical excision of single metastatic brain tumors. Am J Roentgenol Radium Ther Nucl Med 111:323–328, 1971

53. McGee EE: Surgical treatment of cerebral metastases from lung cancer plus the effect on quality and duration of survival. J Neurosurg 35:416–420, 1971

54. Order SE, Hellman S, Von Essen CF, et al: Improvement in quality of survival following whole-brain irradiation for brain metastasis. Radiology 91:149–153, 1968

55. Nisce LZ, Hilaris BS, Chu FCH: A review of experience with irradiation of brain metastasis. Am J Roentgenol Radium Ther Nucl Med 111:329–333, 1971

56. Hansen HH: Should initial treatment of small cell carcinoma include systemic chemotherapy and brain irradiation? Cancer Chemother Rep (Part 3) 4:239–241, 1973

57. Editor: Computer assisted tomography. JAMA 232:941–942, 1975

58. New PF, Scott RR, Schnur JA, et al: Computerized axial tomography with the EMI scanner. Radiology 110:109–123, 1974

59. Baker HL, Campbell JK, Hauser OW, et al: Early experience in the EMI scanner for study of the brain. Radiology 116:327–333, 1975

60. Du Boulay GH, Marshal J: Comparison of EMI and radioisotope imaging in neurological disease. Lancet 2:1294–1297, 1975

61. Newman SJ, Hansen HH: Frequency, diagnosis, and treatment of brain metastases in 247 consecutive patients with bronchogenic carcinoma. Cancer 33:492–496, 1974

62. Deeley TJ, Rice Edwards JM: Radiotherapy in the management of cerebral secondaries from bronchial carcinoma. Lancet 1:1209–1212, 1968

63. Chason H, Walker FB, Landers IW: Metastatic carcinoma in the central nervous system and dorsal root ganglia: A prospective autopsy study. Cancer 16:781–787, 1963

64. Kindt CW: The pattern of location of cerebral metastatic tumors. J Neurosurg 21:54–57, 1969

65. Rubin P, Hicks GL: Biassociation of superior vena caval obstruction and spinal cord compression. NY State J Med 73:2176–2182, 1973

66. Gates GF, Done EK, Taplin GV: Interval brain scanning with sodium pertechnetate Tc-99m for tumor detectability. JAMA 215:85–88, 1971

67. Ramsey RG, Quinn JL III: Comparison of accuracy between initial and delayed ⁹⁹ᵐTc-pertechnetate brain scans. J Nucl Med 13:131–134, 1972

68. Boller F, Pattern DH, Howes D: Correlation of brain scan results with neuropathological findings. Lancet 1:1143–1146, 1973

69. Cohen Y, Robinson E: Radionuclide examination for detection of metastases to brain from cancer of the lung. Harefuah 79:295–297, 1970

70. Muggia FM, DeVita VJ Jr: In vivo tumor cell kinetic studies: Use of local thymidine injection followed by fine-needle aspiration. J Lab Clin Med 80:297–301, 1972

71. Sherlock P, Kim YS, Koss LG: Cytologic diagnosis of cancer from aspirated material obtained with liver biopsies. Am J Dig Dis 12:396–402, 1967

72. Grossman E, Goldstein MJ, Koss LG, et al: Cutological examination as adjuvant to liver biopsy in diagnosis of hepatic metastases. Gastroenterology 62:56–60, 1972

73. Kurimoto S, Ito E: A case of metastatic tumor of the choroid. Folia Ophthalmol Jpn 21:308–315, 1970

74. Reuter SR: Demonstration of adrenal metastases

by adrenal venography. N Engl J Med 278:1423–1425, 1968

75. Lieberman LM, Beierwaltes WH, Conn JW, et al: Diagnosis of adrenal disease by visualization of human adrenal glands with [131]I-19-iodo-cholesterol. N Engl J Med 285:1387–1397, 1971

76. Conn JW, Morita R, Cohen EL, et al: Primary aldosteronism, photoscanning of tumors after administration of [131]I-19-iodocholesterol. Arch Intern Med 129:417–425, 1972

77. Kirschner AS, Ice RD, Beierwaltes WH: Radiation dosimetry of [131]I-19-iodocholesterol. J Nucl Med 16:248–249, 1975

78. Rasmussen SN, Hom HH, Kristensen JK, et al: Ultrasonically guided liver biopsy. Br Med J 2:500–502, 1972

79. Order SE, Bloomer WD, Jones AG, et al: Radionuclide immunoglobulin lymphangiography. Cancer 35:1487–1492, 1975

80. Okuyama S, Ito Y, Awanto T, et al: Prospects of ^{67}Ga scanning in bone neoplasms. Radiology 107:123–128, 1973

81. Langhammer H, Glaubitt G, Grebe SF, et al: [67]Ga for tumor scanning. J Nucl Med 13:25–30, 1972

82. Henskin RE, Quinn JL, Weinberg PE: Adjunctive brain scanning with ^{67}Ga in metastases. Radiology 106:595–599, 1973

83. Higasi T, Nakayama Y, Murato A, et al: Clinical evaluation of ^{67}Ga citrate scanning. J Nucl Med 13:196–201, 1972

84. Jones AE, Koslow M, Johnston GS, et al: [67]Ga citrate scintigraphy of brain tumors. Radiology 105:693–697, 1972

85. Edwards CL, Hayes RL: Scanning malignant neoplasms with gallium-67. JAMA 212:1182–1190, 1970

86. MIRD dose estimate report No. 2—Summary of current radiation dose estimates to humans from [66]Ga, ^{67}Ga, ^{68}Ga, and [72]Ga citrate. J Nucl Med 14:755–756, 1973

87. McKusick KA, Singh Soin J, Chiladi A, et al: Gallium 67 accumulation in pulmonary sarcoidosis. JAMA 223:688, 1973

88. Mori T, Hammato K, Torizuka K: Studies on the usefulness of ^{99m}Tc-labeled Bleomycin for tumor imaging. J Nucl Med 14:431, 1973 (abstract)

89. Goodwin DA, Lin MS, Diamanti CI, et al: ^{111}In-labeled Bleomycin for tumor localization by scintiscanning. J Nucl Med 14:401, 1973 (abstract)

90. Grove RB, Eckelman WC, Reba RC: Preparation, distribution, and tumor imaging properties of ^{111}In, [57]Co, ^{67}Ga, and ^{59}Fe-labeled Bleomycin. J Nucl Med 14:627, 1973 (abstract)

91. Grove RB, Reba RC, Eckelman WC, et al: Clinical evaluation of radiolabeled Bleomycin for tumor detection. J Nucl Med 15:386–390, 1974

92. Monod O, Rymer M: Chemotherapeutic drugs marked with radioactive isotopes. Cancer Chemother Rep (Part 3) 4:245–249, 1973

93. Lange RC, Spencer RP, Harder HC: The antitumor agent CIS-Pt (NH$_3$) 2 Cl$_2$: Distribution studies and dose calculations for [193m]Pt and [195m]Pt. J Nucl Med 14:191–195, 1973

94. Spar IL, Bales HF, Goodland RL, et al: Preparation of purified ^{131}I-labeled antibody which reacts with human fibrin. Preliminary tracer studies on tumor patients. Cancer Res 24:286–293, 1964

95. Hoffer PB, Lathrop K, Bekerman C, et al: Use of ^{131}I-CEA antibody as a tumor scanning agent. J Nucl Med 15:323–327, 1974

David T. Carr
Clifton F. Mountain

12

Staging Lung Cancer

In addition to the characteristics of the organ in which a cancer originates, there are many other factors that influence the choice of treatment for a specific patient with cancer, as well as the patient's chance of long-term survival following that treatment. As pointed out elsewhere in this book (see Chapter 4), the histologic cell type and the grade of malignancy are important determinants of both proper treatment and prognosis. Other important influences are the presence of symptoms due to the tumor, the nature of the symptoms, the duration of the symptoms, the age and sex of the patient, the presence of concomitant disease, the growth rate of the tumor, and stage of the tumor. The stage of the tumor means the anatomic extent of the tumor. Of all these variables, the histologic cell type and the stage are probably the most important factors in determining treatment and estimating prognosis.

The anatomic extent of the tumor could be described in a narrative statement giving details of the extent of the primary lesion, the presence or absence of spread to the regional lymph nodes, and the presence or absence of metastases to distant lymph nodes and various other parts of the patient's body. But in order to avoid the infinite variety of such descriptive statements, classification systems have been developed using a type of shorthand for the designation of the various categories of extent of the primary tumor,

the involvement of regional nodes, and the presence of distant metastases. In the most commonly used system, the capital letters T, N, and M are used to designate Tumor, Nodes, and Metastasis, and various modifiers are used to indicate the category of that component of the patient's cancer.

The American Joint Committee for Cancer Staging and End Results Reporting (AJC) has enunciated[1] general guidelines for the use of T, N, and M and their modifiers, as shown in Table 12-1. TNM assignments may be grouped into a small number of *stages* related to appropriate treatment and probable survival rates. According to the AJC,[1] the purposes of staging each patient with cancer are:

1. To aid in more precise communication about patients with cancer.
2. To aid in selection of the most effective treatment.
3. To assist in determining prognosis.
4. To make possible meaningful comparisons of end-results reporting from different sources.
5. To help evaluate cancer control measures.

Obviously the description of the anatomic extent or the stage will depend on the thoroughness of the patient's diagnostic and evaluative

Table 12-1
Guidelines for Use of T, N, and M and Their Modifiers

Tumor		
	T0	No evidence of primary tumor
	TIS	Carcinoma in situ
	T1, T2, T3, T4	Progressive increase in tumor size and involvement
	TX	Tumor cannot be assessed
Nodes		
	N0	Regional lymph nodes not demonstrably abnormal
	N1, N2, N3, etc.	Increasing degrees of demonstrable abnormality of regional lymph nodes
	NX	Regional lymph nodes cannot be assessed clinically
Metastasis		
	M0	No evidence of distant metastasis
	M1, M2, M3	Ascending degrees of distant metastasis, including metastasis to distant lymph nodes

studies. In addition, as cancer is a dynamic disease process, the description of its anatomic extent will depend on the time during its life history that the stage is determined and recorded.

Consider first the effect of the thoroughness of examination on the staging of a cancer. It is obvious that different types of evaluative evidence may be used to stage cancers at each step in the diagnostic study of a patient or during the initial phase of treatment for some patients. Each patient can be assigned a *clinical classification* based on the pretreatment study of that patient using generally available techniques of physical examination, laboratory tests, and minor surgical diagnostic procedures.

For cancers at sites inaccessible to adequate clinical evaluation, such as cancer of the ovary, stomach, colon, and kidney, it is generally agreed that such a clinical classification is usually inadequate; and the information obtained by a major surgical exploration, including appropriate biopsies, may be used to establish a more valid staging, which is called a *surgical-evaluative classification*.

When a cancer is therapeutically resected, the information obtained by a thorough examination of the resected specimen should be combined with previously available data to determine the *postsurgical treatment classification*. In this way the precise stage and the examinations used to determine that stage can be recorded for clear and concise communication from one physician to another and for proper grouping of cases in reports in the medical literature.

Once the extent of disease or the stage has been determined according to any or all of the above classifications, that classification should not be changed. The subsequent course of the cancer or the results of reexaminations of the patient must not be used to alter the original description of the extent of the tumor or its stage, whether it is a clinical classification, a surgical-evaluative classification, or a postsurgical treatment classification. This rule should be observed whether follow-up examinations detect no evidence of residual cancer or whether such examinations reveal local recurrence or development of regional or distant metastases.

Consider next the problem of describing the extent of disease in a previously treated patient with a local recurrence or a newly diagnosed metastasis. Prior to further anticancer treatment, such a patient may be assigned a *retreatment classification* based on the anatomic extent of the cancer known to be present at the time the retreatment is initiated. Such cases cannot be grouped with original treatment cases for analysis of the efficacy of treatment. These retreatment cases should be grouped together and reported as a separate, special group. However, they must not be deleted from the original primary treatment series to which they were assigned prior to initial therapy.

STAGING SYSTEM

Although many staging systems for lung cancer have been proposed over a period of years,[2-12] none has been accepted generally by the medical profession or widely and uniformly used. For this reason a Task Force on Carcinoma of the Lung was created by the AJC, and a staging system for lung cancer based on TNM principles was developed and published.[1,13] This staging system was based on a thorough study of more than 2000 cases of proven carcinoma of the lung that included 111 items of information about each patient. Physicians in six medical centers participated in the study. The data included size and location of each primary tumor, the presence of extrapulmonary extension, and complications such as obstructive pneumonitis, atelectasis, and pleural effusion. The presence of metastases to lymph nodes in the hilar region and in the mediastinum and the presence of more distant metastases were recorded. Although histologic proof of the diagnosis may have been obtained by exploratory thoracotomy, only the information obtained by prethoracotomy diagnostic examination was used to measure the anatomic extent of the disease. A patient was admitted to the study only if the cancer had been diagnosed 4 years or more prior to the start of the study and if follow-up information was available, either to the time of death or to survival for at least 4 years.

Because there is convincing evidence that the four major cell types of lung cancer differ significantly, data for patients with each cell type were analyzed separately. More than 300 survival curves for these patients were plotted for various characteristics of the primary tumor and for metastases to the regional lymph nodes and more distant metastases in various combinations.

All the survival curves for patients with undifferentiated small cell (oat cell) carcinoma indicate that these patients have very poor prognoses regardless of the demonstrable anatomic extent of their cancers (Fig. 12-1). However, for purposes of communication and for future research studies of the retrospective type, it seems worthwhile to record the anatomic extent of the cancer for each patient with small cell (oat cell) carcinoma.

Analysis of the other survival curves shows that for patients with squamous cell carcinoma, adenocarcinoma, and undifferentiated large cell carcinoma the prognosis is related to the size of the tumor, its location, and its extension, as well as complications such as atelectasis, obstructive pneumonitis or pleural effusion, metastasis to regional lymph nodes, and the presence of more distant metastasis. Consequently the primary tumor, designated by the letter T, is classified by its size, location, extension, and complications; involvement of the regional lymph nodes is indi-

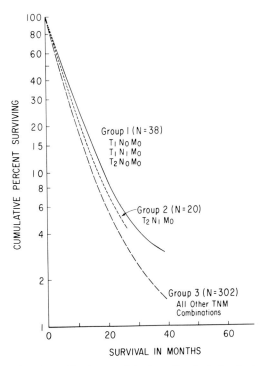

Fig. 12-1. Carcinoma of the lung. Survival of patients with undifferentiated small cell carcinoma (oat cell) by classification group.

cated by an appropriate category of N; the presence or absence of distant metastasis is indicated by an appropriate category of M. The definitions for each category of T, N, and M currently recommended by the Task Force on Carcinoma of the Lung of the AJC are as shown in Table 12-2. Survival curves for each of these stages of squamous cell carcinoma, large cell undifferentiated carcinoma, and adenocarcinoma are shown in Figs. 12-7, 12-8, and 12-9.

It is evident that there is a marked and statistically significant difference in the prognostic implications for each stage and that these implications vary according to cell type. The prognosis in squamous cell carcinoma is consistently better in each stage of disease than that in undifferentiated large cell carcinoma and adenocarcinoma. If the primary tumor is large, metastasis to the hilar lymph nodes has a more deleterious effect in adenocarcinoma and large cell carcinoma. A grave prognosis is associated with mediastinal node metastasis, pleural effusion, or distant metastasis.

Patients with other malignancies of the lung, such as bronchial carcinoids, mucoepidermoids, and lymphomas, were not included in this study;

T1

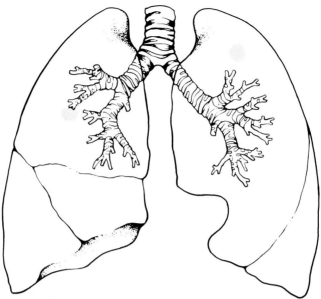

Fig. 12-2. T1: Solitary tumor 3.0 cm or less in greatest diameter, surrounded by lung or visceral pleura and without evidence of invasion proximal to a lobar bronchus at bronchoscopy. Two examples of T1 lesions are shown. (Reproduced by permission of the American Joint Committee for Cancer Staging and End Results Reporting.)

T2

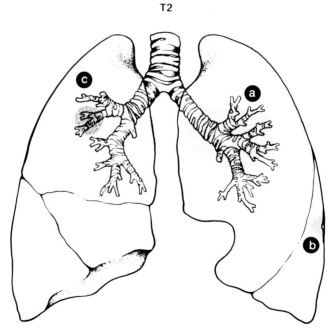

Fig. 12-3. T2: The primary tumor is more than 3.0 cm in greatest diameter, as depicted in (a), or a tumor of any size that invades visceral pleura (b) or that, with its associated atelactasis or obstructive pneumonitis, extends to the hilar region (c). At bronchoscopy the proximal extent of demonstrable tumor must be within a lobar bronchus or at least 2 cm distal to the carina. Any associated atelectasis or obstructive pneumonitis must involve less than an entire lung, and there must be no pleural effusion. (Reproduced by permission of the American Joint Committee for Cancer Staging and End Results Reporting.)

T3

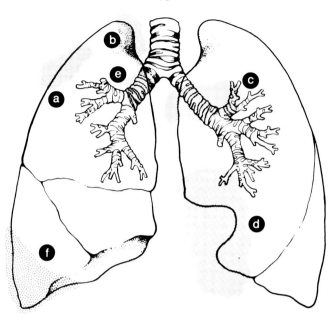

Fig. 12-4. T3: A primary tumor of any size with direct extension into an adjacent structure such as chest wall (a) or mediastinum and its contents (b), with direct invasion of the aorta, main pulmonary artery or veins, or recurrent or phrenic nerves (c), or with invasion of the pericardium or diaphragm (d). T3 lesions include tumors demonstrable bronchoscopically to involve a main bronchus less than 2.0 cm distal to the carina (e) and any tumor associated with a pleural effusion (f) or with atelectasis or obstructive pneumonitis of an entire lung. (Reproduced by permission of the American Joint Committee for Cancer Staging and End Results Reporting.)

this staging system is not thought to be applicable to them.

The clinical classification of patients with carcinoma of the lung should be based on the anatomic extent of the disease, which can be detected by examination prior to any treatment. Such an examination may include a medical history, physical examination, routine and special roentgenograms, bronchoscopy, esophagoscopy, mediastinoscopy, mediastinotomy, thoracocentesis, thoracoscopy, and other special examinations including those used to demonstrate the presence of extrathoracic metastasis. Information obtained by an exploratory or therapeutic thoracotomy should not be used for the clinical classification.

The surgical-evaluative classification should be based on all the data obtained for the clinical classification and on information obtained at the time of exploratory thoracotomy, including biopsy information but not including that information obtained by complete examination of a therapeutically resected specimen. That information and all other previously available data should be used to assign a postsurgical treatment classification to those patients having such a resection.

All patients should have a clinical classification. Those patients having a thoracotomy should have, in addition, a surgical-evaluative classification and/or a postsurgical treatment classification.

When appropriate, a retreatment classification may be assigned to a patient prior to treatment of a recurrence based on the anatomic extent of the cancer known to be present at the time the retreatment is initiated. Obviously it is possible for a patient to have a second or even additional retreatment classifications if he has two or more distinct recurrences.

All the survival data in this chapter are based on the clinical classification. Application of this staging system for the assignment of a surgical-evaluative classification, a postsurgical treatment classification, or a retreatment classification seems reasonable but has not been tested.

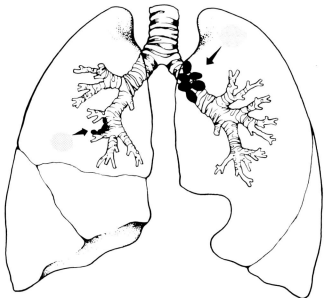

Fig. 12-5. N1: Spread to lymph nodes in peribronchial and/or ipsilateral hilar regions (including direct extension). (Reproduced by permission of the American Joint Committee for Cancer Staging and End Results Reporting.)

N2

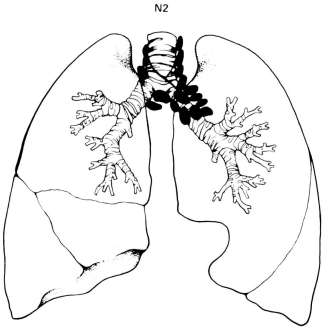

Fig. 12-6. N2: Spread to mediastinal lymph nodes.

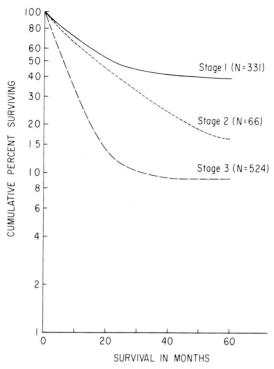

Fig. 12-7. Carcinoma of the lung. Survival of patients with squamous cell carcinoma by stage. (Reproduced by permission of the American Joint Committee for Cancer Staging and End Results Reporting.)

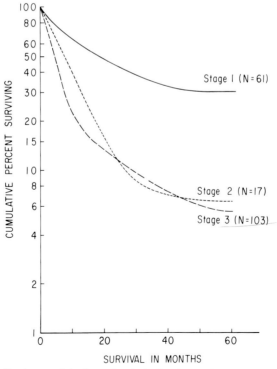

Fig. 12-8. Carcinoma of the lung. Survival of patients with undifferentiated large cell carcinoma by stage. (Reproduced by permission of the American Joint Committee for Cancer Staging and End Results Reporting.)

157

Table 12-2
AJC Definitions of TNM Categories

Primary tumors

T   Primary tumor

T0 No evidence or primary tumor

TX Tumor proven by presence of malignant cells in bronchopulmonary secretions but not visualized roentgenographically or bronchoscopically

TIS Carcinoma in situ

T1 Tumor that is 3.0 cm or less in greatest diameter, surrounded by lung or visceral pleura and without evidence of invasion proximal to a lobar bronchus at bronchoscopy (Fig. 12-2)

T2 Tumor more than 3.0 cm in greatest diameter, or tumor of any size that invades the visceral pleura or with its associated atelectasis or obstructive pneumonitis and extends to the hilar region. At bronchoscopy the proximal extent of demonstrable tumor must be within a lobar bronchus or at least 2.0 cm distal to the carina. Any associated atelectasis or obstructive pneumonitis must involve less than an entire lung, and there must be no pleural effusion (Fig. 12-3).

T3 Tumor of any size with direct extension into an adjacent structure such as chest wall, diaphragm, or mediastinum and its contents, or tumor demonstrated bronchoscopically to involve a main bronchus less than 2.0 cm distal to the carina; any tumor associated with atelectasis or obstructive pneumonitis of an entire lung or pleural effusion (Fig. 12-4)

Regional lymph nodes

N   Regional lymph nodes

N0 No demonstrable metastasis to regional lymph nodes

N1 Metastasis to lymph nodes in peribronchial and/or ipsilateral hilar region (including direct extension) (Fig. 12-5)

N2 Metastasis to lymph nodes in the mediastinum (Fig. 12-6)

Distant metastasis

M   Distant metastasis

M0 No distant metastasis

M1 Distant metastasis such as in scalene, cervical, or contralateral hilar lymph nodes, brain, bones, lung, liver, etc.

These categories of T, N, and M may be combined into the following groups or stages:

Occult carcinoma

TX N0 M0   Occult carcinoma with bronchopulmonary secretions containing malignant cells but without other evidence of the primary tumor or evidence of metastasis to the regional lymph nodes or distant metastasis

Table 12-2
AJC Definitions of TNM Categories (continued)

Stage I

TIS N0 M0	Carcinoma in situ
T1 N0 M0	Tumor that can be classified T1 without any metas-
T1 N1 M0	tasis or with metastasis to the lymph nodes in the
T2 N0 M0	ipsilateral hilar region only, or a tumor that can
	be classified T2 without any metastasis to nodes
	or distant metastasis

Note: TX N1 M0 and T0 N1 M0 are also theoretically possible, but such a clinical diagnosis would b ' difficult if not impossible to make. If such a diagnosis is made, it should be included in stage I.

Stage II

T2 N1 M0	Tumor classified as T2 with metastasis to the lymph
	nodes in the ipsilateral hilar region only

Stage III

T3 with any N or M	Any tumor more extensive than T2, or any tumor
N2 with any T or M	with metastasis to the lymph nodes in the
M1 with any T or N	mediastinum, or with distant metastasis

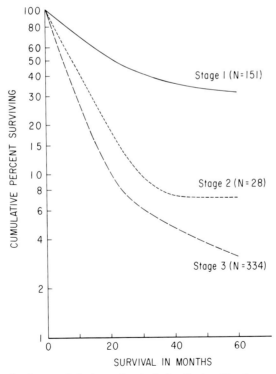

Fig. 12-9. Carcinoma of the lung. Survival of patients with adenocarcinoma by stage. (Reproduced by permission of the American Joint Committee for Cancer Staging and End Results Reporting.)

A worksheet to facilitate the use of this staging system has been developed and is reproduced in Fig. 12-10. This may be copied or modified freely by the reader. It may be used as a worksheet and discarded after the data have been entered into the patient's medical record, or the worksheet itself may be incorporated into the patient's medical record.

This relatively simple TNM system of classification and staging should meet the needs of most investigators and cancer registries. Certain groups of workers and institutions may require a more complex system to separate the subsets within each TNM category. The basic system is responsive to such a need by use of the decimal-point system of expanded notation. For example, the exact size of a primary tumor classified as T1 could be indicated by using T1.1 for lesions 1 cm in diameter, T1.2 for those 2 cm in diameter, and T1.3 for those 3 cm in diameter. In a similar manner the characteristics of the tumor that make it a T2 lesion could be specified by the use of the designations T2.1, T2.2, etc. Likewise, the designations N1.1, N1.2, N2.1, and N2.2 may be used to specify certain subgroups of lymph nodes within the broader categories designated by N1 and N2. The same sort of subdivisions of M1 may be used to satisfy the needs of any investigator or group of investigators. The extent of such an expansion is limited only by the imagination. For example, multiple digits to the right of the decimal point might be used to indicate the presence or the absence of metastases to specific organs and whether the diagnosis was clinical or histologic; e.g., the first digit to the right of the decimal point might be assigned to the ipsilateral scalene or supraclavicular lymph nodes, the second digit to the contralateral scalene or supraclavicular nodes, the third digit to other cervical nodes, the fourth digit to the brain, the fifth digit to the liver,

WORK SHEET FOR STAGING LUNG CANCER

No. _____ Name _____ Date _____

Directions: Encircle the T, N, and M rating following the description that is most accurate for the patient's cancer. Encircle the value for each rating and add to obtain the total value. Consult the table at the bottom of the form to determine the stage.

This form may be used for 4 staging classifications: (1) CLINICAL (2) SURGICAL (3) POST–SURGICAL (post-resection) (4) RETREATMENT (upon failure of initial treatment, patient is restaged prior to retreatment).

Check appropriate classification: Clinical ___ Surgical ___ Post-Surgical ___ Retreatment ___

	CLASSIFICATION:	Value
PRIMARY TUMOR – T		
No evidence of primary tumor	T0	0
Tumor proven by the presence of malignant cells in broncho-pulmonary secretions but not visualized roentgenographically or bronchoscopically	TX	0
Carcinoma in situ	T1S	1
A tumor that is 3.0 cm or less in greatest diameter, surrounded by lung or visceral pleura and without evidence of invasion proximal to a lobar bronchus at bronchoscopy	T1	1
A tumor more than 3.0 cm in greatest diameter, or a tumor of any size, which invades the visceral pleura or with its associated atelectasis or obstructive pneumonitis extends to the hilar region. At bronchoscopy the proximal extent of demonstrable tumor must be within a lobar bronchus or at least 2.0 cm distal to the carina. Any associated atelectasis or obstructive pneumonitis must involve less than an entire lung, and there must be no pleural effusion	T2	2
A tumor of any size with direct extension into an adjacent structure such as the chest wall, the diaphragm, or the mediastinum and its contents; or demonstrable bronchoscopically to involve a main bronchus less than 2.0 cm distal to the carina; any tumor associated with atelectasis or obstructive pneumonitis of an entire lung or pleural effusion	T3	4
REGIONAL LYMPH NODES – N		
No demonstrable metastasis to regional lymph nodes	N0	0
Metastasis to lymph nodes in peribronchial and/or the ipsilateral hilar region (including direct extension)	N1	1
Metastasis to lymph nodes in the mediastinum	N2	4
DISTANT METASTASIS – M		
No distant metastasis	M0	0
Distant metastasis such as in scalene, cervical, or contralateral hilar lymph nodes, brain, bones, lung, liver, etc.	M1	4

Cell type:

Squamous ☐   Small ☐   Adenocarcinoma ☐   Large ☐

Other (specify) _____

TOTAL VALUE   STAGE
0 . . . . Occult Carcinoma
1 or 2 I
3 II
4 or more III

SUMMARY
OF
STAGING

T _____
N _____
M _____
Stage _____

If patient had a resection, indicate whether post-surgical treatment classification was based on pathological evaluation of:

primary tumor mass   ☐ yes   ☐ no   ☐ unknown
regional lymph nodes   ☐ yes   ☐ no   ☐ unknown

Fig. 12-10. Suggested worksheet for staging lung cancer. (Permission is hereby granted to reproduce the worksheet as desired to expedite the use of this staging system in the classification of patients with lung cancer.)

the sixth digit to osseous metastases, and the seventh digit to other sites. A 0 would be used to indicate no evidence of metastasis to the designated site, 1 to indicate clinical evidence of such metastasis, and 2 for microscopic proof of such metastasis. Accordingly, biopsy-proven metastasis to the ipsilateral supraclavicular nodes plus clinical evidence of metastasis to the brain without any evidence of other metastasis would be designated M1.2001000.

It is essential, however, that the basic rules and definitions for assigning TNM values and stages be followed in creating such subsets. Only by doing so can various series of cases be compared by combining the subsets to create comparable groups.

It is recognized that changes in any staging system may become necessary as time passes and new knowledge is acquired. For that reason any publication in which cases of cancer are staged should carefully specify which staging system was used in the classification of the cases analyzed in the report. Furthermore, all lung cancer research workers should search for ways to improve the staging system. All suggestions should be sent to the Task Force on Lung Cancer, American Joint Committee for Cancer Staging and End Results Reporting, 55 East Erie Street, Chicago, Illinois 60611.

REFERENCES

1. American Joint Committee for Cancer Staging and End Results Reporting: Clinical Staging System for Carcinoma of the Lung. Chicago, Ill, Sept, 1973

2. Slazer G: Vorscheag einer Einteilung des Brorchuskarzinoms nach pathologisch-anatomischklinischen Gesichtspunkten. Wein Med Wochenschr 101:102–103, 1951

3. Nohl HC: A three-year follow-up of classified cases of bronchogenic carcinoma after resection. Thorax 15:11–16, 1960

4. Cliffton EE: Criteria for operability and resectability, in Watson WL (ed): Lung Cancer. A Study of Five Thousand Memorial Hospital Cases. St Louis, Mosby, 1968, pp 258–262

5. TNM Classification of Malignant Tumors. Geneva, International Union Against Cancer, 1968

6. Feinstein AR: A new staging system for cancer and reappraisal of "early" treatment and "cure" by radical surgery. N Engl J Med 279:747–753, 1968

7. Rakov AI, Kabishev EN, Lakshtanova IP: Evaluation of the TNM clinical classification for the lung cancer. Neoplasma 16:325–333, 1969

8. Dold U, Schneider V, Krause F: Applicability of the TNM system on lung carcinoma, field trial. Proposal of advanced TNM classification including a category for diagnostic certainty degree. Z Krebsforsch 78:317–325, 1972

9. Larsson S: Pretreatment classification and staging of bronchogenic carcinoma. Scand J Thorac Cardiovasc Surg [Suppl] 10:1–147, 1973

10. Cliffton EE, Martini N, Beattie EJ Jr: A classification of lung cancer: Value for prognosis and comparison of series and methods of treatment. Proc Natl Cancer Conf 7:729–737, 1973

11. Guinn GA, Tomm KE, North L, et al: Clinical staging of primary lung cancer. Chest 64:51–54, 1973

12. Ishikawa S: Staging system on TNM classification for lung cancer. Jpn J Clin Oncol 6:19–30, 1973

13. Mountain CF, Carr DT, Anderson WAD: A system for the clinical staging of lung cancer. AM J Roentgenol Radium Ther Nucl Med 120:130–138, 1974

Robert E. Lee

13
Radiotherapy for Lung Cancer

In the United States lung cancer is the number one cancer killer,[1,2] and radiotherapy is administered to the majority of these patients. Nevertheless, the role of radiotherapy for the patient with bronchogenic carcinoma is frequently misunderstood. Radiotherapy is a regional treatment, and frequently with lung cancer that is apparently confined to one hemithorax there are distant subclinical metastases. Sufficient knowledge regarding radiotherapy for bronchogenic carcinoma is available to increase the survival in some patients and to improve the quality of life in many patients. Successful radiotherapy controls local disease but does not affect distant subclinical metastases. Recent studies suggest that combinations of radiotherapy and other modalities of treatment can improve the survival rates and the quality of life for patients with lung cancer. Because no single treatment is uniformly effective against bronchogenic carcinoma there must be a spirit of cooperation among surgical, medical, and radiation oncologists.

The role of the radiotherapist in lung cancer is to cure some patients and to palliate many. We should attempt to make the remaining life of these patients as comfortable, physically and emotionally, as is possible. Thus our efforts may be directed toward relieving symptoms caused by the primary tumor or by mediastinal metastasis or distant metastasis. The length of the course of radiotherapy may represent a significant portion of the patient's remaining life; so if the same benefit can be achieved without undue complications, we prefer a short and thereby economic course of radiotherapy. Moreover, because hospitalization is expensive, outpatient radiotherapy usually lessens the financial burden considerably. The overall cost-effectiveness of radiotherapy for patients with lung cancer is difficult to ascertain.

Not the least of the radiotherapist's responsibilities is his obligation to communicate with the patient as a person in need of support. We think it is important to keep the patient informed about all tests he needs and why he needs them. We explain treatment planning and dosimetry. We review the complications of radiotherapy before starting treatment and again at the end of each course. We encourage the family to ask questions. We see the patient briefly at the time of each treatment in order to deal promptly with any new problems and to offer whatever reassurance we can. We hope each patient will realize that he can rely on his radiotherapist for information and counsel.

Furthermore, although we are involved in scientific evaluation of the results of our treatments, we must never forget that we are dealing with *people,* not subjects for research.

The author gratefully acknowledges the helpful editorial counsel provided by Drs. Richard A. Kirkpatrick and Charles G. Roland during the preparation of this manuscript.

163

PRINCIPLES OF MANAGEMENT

Cell Type and Stage

Management of lung cancer depends on the cell type and the stage of disease (see Chapter 12). Surgery is usually recommended for patients with stage I and stage II malignancy, and the chances of 5-year survival are 30–40 percent and 10–15 percent, respectively.[3] If surgery is not possible because of medical problems or other considerations, radiotherapy is the treatment of choice. Stage III disease is any disease more extensive than stage II, and it may include pleural effusion or atelectasis of an entire lung. From the radiotherapeutic viewpoint, stage III disease can be subdivided into the limited and extensive categories. Limited stage III disease is confined to one hemithorax and may be encompassed by a single portal for radiotherapy. Extensive stage III disease includes disease spread beyond the hemithorax. Treatment usually involves radiotherapy or chemotherapy or both, and five-year survival is less than 10 percent. According to statistics of the American Joint Committee,[3] about 29 percent of lung cancer patients have stage I disease. Stage II accounts for 7 percent, and the remaining 64 percent have stage III disease. About 48 percent of lung cancer is squamous cell epithelioma, 25 percent is adenocarcinoma, 9 percent is large cell carcinoma, and 18 percent is small cell carcinoma.[3]

According to Galofre et al.,[4] squamous cell epitheliomas (SCE) involve major bronchi in 72 percent of cases. In their series 54 percent of resected specimens were found to have metastases to lymph nodes on routine pathologic examination. Mountain[5] reported that 50 percent of patients with SCE undergoing resection had hilar or mediastinal nodal metastasis. In a study of autopsies, Deeley and Line[6] reported metastasis outside the chest in 61 percent of patients with SCE. This tendency of SCE to spread via regional lymphatic channels rather than by hematogenous dissemination is greater than in the other cell types. Frequently, in situ SCE involves the bronchial mucosa adjacent to the gross tumor; this is of significance because if it cannot be recognized clinically, in situ tumor may be left in the bronchial stump inadvertently. If tumor involves the lines of resection, postoperative radiotherapy should be considered to try to prevent recurrence in the bronchial stump. In addition, Matthews et al.[7] have reported a retrospective study of autopsy findings from 202 patients who had had curative lobectomies or pneumonectomies for lung cancer and who died within 1 month of surgery. Of 131 patients who had SCE, 44 (33 percent) had persistent tumor identified at autopsy. Half of these patients had disease limited to the bronchial stump or to the hilar or mediastinal nodes. This residual disease could be encompassed by ports suitable for radical or curative radiotherapy. (The remaining 22 of these patients had distant metastases.) Deeley[8] reported a 3-year survival of 12 percent in a group of 30 such patients receiving postoperative radiotherapy.

Small cell carcinomas (SMC) are central in location in 97 percent of patients. Lymph node involvement by tumor occurred in 91 percent of the specimens in routine pathologic examination in one series,[7] and vascular invasion was almost always demonstrable by microscopic examination. Mountain[5] reported that 76 percent of patients with SMC undergoing resection had hilar or mediastinal nodal metastases. Deeley and Line[6] reported metastases outside the chest in 94 percent of patients with SMC at autopsy. Thus SMC is probably widely disseminated before the primary tumor can be identified and resected.

In about 80 percent of patients with adenocarcinoma (AC) the primary tumor is located in the peripheral portions of the lung. Although lymph node involvement was found in 44 percent of resected specimens in routine pathologic examination in one series,[8] blood-borne metastasis is the more important mode of spread. Mountain[5] reported that 68 percent of patients with AC undergoing resection had hilar or mediastinal nodal metastases. Deeley and Line[6] reported metastases outside the chest in 84 percent of patients with AC at autopsy.

Large cell carcinoma (LC) also tends to occur (i.e., 60 percent) in the peripheral portion of the lung. About 50 percent of resected specimens show lymphatic involvement on routine pathologic examination.[8] Of patients with LC undergoing resection, Mountain[5] reported that 57 percent had hilar or mediastinal nodal metastases. These tumors most often spread by hematogenous dissemination. Deeley and Line[6] reported metastases outside the chest in 82 percent of patients with anaplastic (large cell) carcinoma at autopsy.

In view of these statistics of the four cell types of bronchogenic carcinoma, it may be said that radiotherapy should usually encompass the regional lymph nodes. Adjuvant chemotherapy should be considered in all cases of small cell carcinoma treated with radiotherapy. As more effective chemotherapeutic agents are found for the other cell types of bronchogenic carcinoma, chemotherapy should be strongly considered as an adjuvant to radiotherapy for patients with all cell types.

Routes of Lymphatic Metastases

A knowledge of the lymphatic system is essential for planning treatment and establishing proper ports for radiotherapy. In general, lymphatics of the periphery of the lung drain subpleurally and lymphatics of the deep portions of the lung drain toward the hilus (Fig. 13-1).

The subpleural lymphatics of the superior portion of the upper lobes drain to mediastinal lymph nodes (on the right, to the nodes near the junction of the azygos vein and superior vena cava; on the left, to a node near the ligamentum arteriosum between the aortic arch and the left pulmonary artery). Involvement of this node in carcinoma of the lung may, by affecting the left recurrent laryngeal nerve, cause vocal cord paralysis (Fig. 13-1).

The subpleural lymphatics of the inferior portions of the lungs drain to the nodes of the right or left anterior pulmonary ligament. These nodes are in communication with the subcarinal nodes, according to Rouviere,[9] and with the nodes near the cisterna chyli, according to Weinberg.[10] This latter drainage allows direct spread of carcinoma of the lung to nodes in the upper retroperitoneal area and may explain the poorer prognosis of carcinoma of the lower lobes reported by Deeley.[8]

The deep lymphatics and the subpleural lymphatics of the rest of the peripheral lung drain to hilar lymph nodes. The lymph from paratracheobronchial nodes of the right lung drains into the right lymphatic duct, and that from nodes of the left lung flows into the thoracic duct. The crossover flow of lymph occurs from the lingula of the left upper lobe and the superior portion of the left lower lobe via subcarinal nodes to the right lymphatic duct.

Once the parietal pleura is involved with lung cancer there are direct routes of spread to axillary nodes and subdiaphragmatic organs such as the liver, kidney, and adrenal glands.

There is crossover drainage between right and left paratracheal nodes; from these nodes, lung cancer may spread to paraesophageal and anterior mediastinal lymph nodes. Metastasis to contralateral paratracheal nodes is generally con-

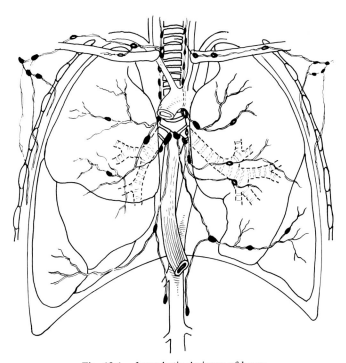

Fig. 13-1. Lymphatic drainage of lungs.

sidered a contraindication to surgical resection of bronchogenic carcinoma.

According to Weinberg,[10] supraclavicular nodal metastases are more frequently seen in lung carcinoma at the stage of disease when it is first diagnosed than in any other form of carcinoma. In bronchogenic carcinoma, tumor emboli reach the supraclavicular nodes via the mediastinal lymphatic trunks, and they may lodge in nodes on either side of the neck. There is lively disagreement as to the pathway of metastasis from the lungs. Rouviere studied this question in newborn fetuses and concluded that most of the left lower lobe drained through the subcarinal nodes to the right supraclavicular region, along with the lymph from the entire right lung. Only the left upper lung drains to the left side of the neck. Warren and Drinker reached this same conclusion in their study of the flow of lymph from the lungs in dogs. But Correll and Langston, who also studied the question in dogs, concluded that the pattern of lymph drainage from the lungs is ipsilateral.

Surgery

Surgical considerations are discussed in detail in Chapter 14. However, a few facts[5] may be of particular interest. In operable patients with bronchogenic carcinoma, complete resection is possible in fewer than half the cases (48 percent of SCE, 40 percent of LC, 30 percent of AC, and 12 percent of SMC).[5] The surgical mortality rate varies between 5 and 10 percent, and this exceeds the surgical survival rate for SMC.

Radiotherapy for Stage I and II Disease

When stage I or stage II cancer cannot be treated by surgery, radiotherapy offers a chance for cure. Smart selected 40 patients and referred them to Hilton for radiotherapy for cure.[11,12] They were in good general condition; they had localized primary lesions, so that surgery could have been undertaken; and they had no clinical evidence of lymph node metastases. Histologic proof of diagnosis was established by bronchoscopic biopsy or sputum cytology. Of the 40, 27 had squamous cell carcinoma, 8 had undifferentiated carcinoma, and 5 had malignant cells of an unidentified cell type. Kilovoltage equipment (4000–5500 rads in 6 to 7 weeks) was used. Nine patients (23 percent) survived 5 years, and 3 patients (8 percent) survived 10 years. Although

these survival rates were somewhat lower than surgical survival rates, they were substantial. Moreover, this series may have included patients with lesions thought to be operable but that would have proved unresectable at thoracotomy (a common occurrence).

Morrison et al.[13] also conducted a clinical trial with 58 patients to compare surgery and supervoltage radiotherapy in the treatment of operable bronchogenic carcinoma. These included 37 patients with squamous cell carcinoma and 19 with oat cell and anaplastic carcinomas. The type of therapy was decided by random selection. Those in the radiotherapy group received 4500 rads in 4 weeks using 8 million volt roentgen rays. For squamous cell carcinoma, surgical resection proved to be the better treatment (4-year survival of 30 percent compared to 6 percent for radiotherapy). For anaplastic carcinomas, however, the 4-year survival was 10 percent in patients who underwent operation versus 11 percent in those treated with radiotherapy. These latter groups were too small for meaningful comparison.

The Medical Research Council of Great Britain conducted a comparative clinical trial[14,15] of surgical resection and radical radiotherapy in the treatment of operable small cell or oat cell carcinoma of the bronchus. Diagnosis in all cases was made by bronchoscopic biopsy. Of the 144 patients in the trial, 71 were randomly allocated to the surgical group and 73 to the radical radiotherapy group. The only 5-year survivors (5 percent of the total series) were patients treated with radiotherapy. Moreover, the surgical patients had a mean survival of only 199 days—significantly less than the mean survival (284 days) of radiotherapy patients ($p = 0.05$). The conclusion drawn was that radical radiotherapy is generally preferable to operation for patients with resectable small cell or oat cell bronchogenic carcinoma.

Radiotherapy for Limited Stage III Disease

Radical radiotherapy, or radiotherapy aimed at cure, may be attempted for unresectable squamous cell carcinomas, adenocarcinomas, and large cell carcinomas under certain conditions. In such patients with stage III disease, invasion must be limited to the hemithorax, including the mediastinum and ipsilateral supraclavicular nodes. Curative radiotherapy may also be tried for *all* small cell carcinomas limited to the hemithorax and for those patients with potentially

Table 13-1
Survival in Bronchogenic Carcinoma at Various Institutions

	No. of Patients	1-Year Survival	5-Year Survival
Duke University[17]	347	40%	6%
Stanford University[18]	284	30%	6%
Hammersmith Hospital[19]	513	36%	6%
Columbia University[20] (unresectable at thoracotomy)	103	59%	9%
Columbia University[21] (clinically inoperable)	150	40%	3%
Ellis Fischel Hospital[22]	277	30%	6%
Mayo Clinic*[23]	188	37%	3%

*Of these 188 patients, 56 percent were clinically inoperable, 25 percent had thoracotomy without resection, 3 percent had thoracotomy with partial resection, and 16 percent did not have thoracotomy for medical reasons or because of the patient's refusal.

Reproduced by permission from Lee RE: Radiotherapy of bronchogenic carcinoma. Semin Oncol 1:245–252, 1974.

resectable tumors whose general condition, pulmonary function, or refusal of surgery precludes operation.

Roswit et al.[16] randomized radiotherapy versus placebo and found 18 percent and 14 percent 1-year survivals—which were significantly different. The results of others disclose higher 1-year survival rates than 18 percent for patients with limited stage III disease treated by radiotherapy (Table 13-1).

Survival rates after radical radiotherapy for patients with inoperable or unresectable carcinoma remain poor (Table 13-1). However, several studies have shown that even in those who are not cured the area encompassed by treatment is often free of residual tumor. When surgical specimens were analyzed histologically after radical radiotherapy, localized lung cancer was found to be destroyed in almost half of the cases (29 of 66) reported by Bromley and Szur.[24] The average radiation dose had been 4700 rads over a period averaging 6 weeks using orthovoltage radiation. In a similar series of 82 patients, Bloedorn[25] reported a sterilization rate of 35 percent for the primary tumor and 77 percent for the regional lymph nodes. The dose was 5500 rads in 6 weeks using Co[60] teletherapy. An autopsy series of 67 patients with inoperable bronchogenic carcinoma treated by curative megavoltage radiotherapy was reported by Rissanen et al.[26] No carcinoma

was found at autopsy at the site of the primary lesion in 18 of 60 patients; all patients whose carcinoma had disappeared completely had received a total dose of 4800 to 6250 rads. Of these 18 patients with no residual carcinoma, 14 had been treated by a split-course technique. Although this series was not randomized, it is interesting to note that the primary lesion was sterilized in 37 percent of patients treated by split-course radiotherapy but in only 14 percent of patients treated by continuous radiotherapy. Abadir and Muggia[27] have also shown the tumoricidal effectiveness of radiotherapy. In an autopsy analysis of 48 cases, radical irradiation had achieved local control in 38 percent.

In patients with disseminated bronchogenic carcinoma, chemotherapy is often the treatment of choice, with radiotherapy being kept in reserve as a palliative measure. Consequently, if a patient receiving chemotherapy develops particularly distressing metastatic problems, such as cerebral metastases, superior mediastinal obstruction, painful osseous metastases, or ulceration of a subcutaneous mass, then adjunctive radiotherapy may give him relief.

Selection of Patients

The complications and costs of radiotherapy can be substantial. Therefore attempts have been made to determine the characteristics of patients who "do well."* This factor is being taken into account in current protocols.

A suitable patient should have a hemoglobin concentration above 10 g/dl. He should be able to climb one flight of steps without severe dyspnea and should not be hypercapniac at rest; he should have a 1-sec forced expiratory volume of 700 ml or more and a maximum breathing capacity of at least half of the predicted normal.[28] If he is to receive 5000 rads in 5 weeks to one lung, he must be able to survive a functional pneumonectomy; thus unless the opposite lung is physiologically adequate, radiotherapy will probably result in a respiratory cripple.

If the patient with lung cancer also has pneumonitis or tuberculosis, the appropriate antibiotics should be given; radiotherapy can then be started.[8,29]

In summary, curative radiotherapy should be attempted for patients with carcinoma confined to one hemithorax, including the mediastinum and ipsilateral supraclavicular nodal region. The ports for radiotherapy should encompass all known disease. Curative radiotherapy should not be attempted when the patient's general condition is poor or when distant dissemination of the disease has occurred.

TECHNIQUES OF RADIOTHERAPY

Dose of Radiotherapy

As of February 1976 the most effective and efficient doses of radiotherapy for the four cell types of bronchogenic carcinoma were not known. It is hoped that the randomized prospective clinical trials now in progress will provide this needed data.

Normally ventilated lung transmits more ionizing radiation than does a comparable volume of fat, muscle, or bone. Emphysematous lung transmits still more radiation, and atelectatic lung less. A solid tumor separated from the skin portal by normal lung would naturally receive a higher dose of radiation than would a similar tumor embedded in an equal volume of muscle. The magnitude of this difference depends on the thickness of intervening normal lungs, ribs, and vertebrae, on

*See Chapter 20 in which Lagakos discusses prognosis, including initial performance status as a significant prognostic factor.

pleural effusion, and on the quality of the beam. Normal lung immediately beyond the mass may alter backscatter to the mass slightly. The complexity of this problem increases still further as one encounters different thicknesses of these tissues for each of several directed beams. For beams passing through the mediastinum the dose to the tumor may be truly represented by standard depth dose tables, whereas for beams passing through large thicknesses of aerated lung, sizable correction factors should be added, according to Moss et al.[30]

The quality of radiation alters the magnitude of the correction factor. Megavoltage beams will, in general, require smaller correction factors than medium-voltage beams. The correction may vary from 0 to 40 percent more than the standard depth dose tables would suggest.

We have three possible alternative methods for considering the dose distribution of radiation within the chest.[8] First, we may assume unit tissue density, knowing that there is an obvious error that may vary throughout the course of treatment. Second, we may calculate a correction factor from measurements taken from radiographs, which is an approximation only because the absorption of radiation varies during the course of treatment. Third, we can calculate the absorption factor before each treatment by giving a test dose of radiation, measuring the exit dose, and then calculating the incident dose to be given as an equal treatment. This method, although obviously impractical with the numbers of patients involved, would be the ideal method. The variation of dose distribution within the lungs makes it extremely difficult to state exactly what dose a particular tumor has received. According to Deeley,[8] over the years most radiotherapists have attempted to give higher and higher doses of irradiation, but when a given dose of 6000 may actually be 8000 rads, it is obviously excessive. So, if in the past we have been administering excessive doses of radiation, then some of our failures may be due to the effects of radiation on normal tissues. Deeley[8] therefore recommends a reduced tumor dose.

Split-Course Radiotherapy

In the past most patients have received continuous radiotherapy totaling 3000 rads in 2 weeks as a minimum and 6500 rads in 7 weeks as a maximum. Recently we and others have turned to split-course schedules.

Split-course radiotherapy was first advocated by Scanlon[31] in 1959. Although the exact radiobiologic mechanism remains unknown, theoretically, reduction in tumor size by the first course may result in improved vascularization of the tumor, and reoxygenation of hypoxic tumor cells renders them more susceptible to destruction by the second course of radiotherapy.[32] Increased tumor oxygen tension after completion of radiotherapy has been documented.

Scanlon[33] has suggested that mitotic suppression, with later rebounding and recovery, if sufficient time elapses, allows the second course to occur at an especially radiovulnerable time in the cell cycle. Sambrook[34] believes that studies of cell population kinetics endorse split-course radiotherapy rather than continuous radiotherapy because ionizing radiation stimulates reparative proliferation more slowly in tumor cells than in normal cells; split-course schedules allow normal tissue to recover before the second course, but tumor tissue is attacked before it has recovered. Theoretical arguments, however, are not as important as clinical trials.

Holsti[35] found no significant difference in survival rates between continuous and split-course radiotherapy for bronchogenic carcinoma. Levitt et al.[36] found no difference in symptomatic relief or survival between the two groups. Hazra et al.[37] had a 1-year survival rate of 96 percent and a 2-year survival of 43 percent using split-course radiotherapy (3000 rads in 10 days, then 2 weeks of rest, then 1500 rads in 5 days). It will be interesting to see the 5-year results with this method.

Abramson and Cavanaugh[38] reported a better survival rate for patients with bronchogenic carcinoma treated with split-course radiotherapy than for those treated with continuous radiotherapy. Their study was not a randomized clinical trial. The split-course radiotherapy consisted of 2000 rads in 5 days, followed by a 3-week rest period, and then a second course of 2000 rads in 5 days. The continuous radiotherapy consisted of 6000 rads over 6 weeks. The 1-year survival rates were 43 percent for the split-course radiotherapy and 15 percent for the continuous radiotherapy. These authors have extended their study of the short split-course technique and have reported on a series of 347 patients.[17] The survival rates were 40 percent at 1 year (347 at risk) and 6 percent at 5 years (85 at risk). Partial or complete relief of symptoms was attained in 78 percent of the patients, whereas there was minimal or no improvement in 22 percent. Cough, dyspnea, hemoptysis, and pain were the most common symptoms.

Subjective side effects and complications of radiation are often difficult to assess, but in this series such symptoms as nausea and esophagitis occurred frequently without interfering with therapy or the ultimate status of the patient. Clinical radiation pneumonitis was uncommon. The major complication in this large group of 347 patients was chronic progressive radiation myelitis (4 patients). These cases occurred 8 to 24 months after therapy and produced the typical Brown-Séquard neurologic picture with decrease in pain and temperature sensation on one side and decrease in motor function on the other. The specific etiology for these cases of myelitis is not clear, but some theoretical technical reasons can be suggested: first, too small a gap between the supraclavicular and mediastinal portals; second, failure to compensate for the slope of the chest; third, failure to block the midline of the supraclavicular portal down to the sternal notch; fourth, poor positioning of the patient; fifth, failure to use a lung factor in severely emphysematous patients. The most obvious possible reason is that the dose rate may exceed the tolerance of the spinal cord.

In each of these 4 patients the midline supraclavicular block used to protect laryngeal structures did not extend to the sternal notch, thereby possibly allowing an increased dose at the thoracic inlet due to the small gap between mediastinal and supraclavicular portals. In the last 225 patients a midline block extending to the sternal notch was used routinely, and no further cases of radiation myelitis occurred.

After this report, Abramson modified the technique to reduce spinal cord dosage by adding a spinal cord block in the posterior port during the second course. For Co^{60} therapy this block measured 1 cm by 5 cm by the length of the port. For 6-MV linear-accelerator therapy the block measured 1 cm by 7 cm by the length of the port. No difference in survival was noted with this modification.

The Working Party for Therapy of Lung Cancer has a randomized clinical trial in progress to compare short-course radiotherapy with long-course radiotherapy for regional (confined to one hemithorax) SCE of the lung. The short course is 2000 rads in 5 days, a 3-week rest period, then 2000 rads in 5 days. The long course is 3000 rads in 3 weeks, then a 2-week rest period, and then

2000 rads in 2 weeks. By March 1975 case accrual had reached 167 patients, and there was no significant difference in survival rates or complication rates between these two courses of radiotherapy.

Continuous versus Split-Course Radiotherapy

We conducted a clinical trial[23,39] to compare continuous radiotherapy with split-course radiotherapy for the treatment of 188 patients with unresectable bronchogenic carcinoma confined to one hemithorax. The patients were stratified by cell type, TNM staging, and prior surgery; thereafter they were randomized to receive continuous radiotherapy (5000 R in 5 weeks) or split-course radiotherapy (2500 R in 2.5 weeks, followed by a 4-week interval, then 2500 R in 2.5 weeks). There was no difference in objective improvement between the two groups. The 5-year results were

similar for continuous radiotherapy and split-course radiotherapy (Fig. 13-2), although the survival rate in the small number of patients with large cell carcinoma was better after split-course radiotherapy. Objective response, judged by chest roentgenograms, was 74 percent with SMC (median survival time 32 weeks), 47 percent with AC (median survival time 52 weeks), 41 percent with LC (median survival time 39 weeks), and 40 percent with SCE (median survival time 43 weeks). Only in SCE was objective response accompanied by improvement in survival.

We concluded that split-course radiotherapy is superior to continuous radiotherapy for several reasons. First, it is better tolerated by the patient. Second, reexamination of the patient prior to the second half of split-course therapy permits detection of metastatic disease that is manifested during the rest period, and thus the patient is spared futile additional radiotherapy to the primary site. Third, if the general condition of a patient is

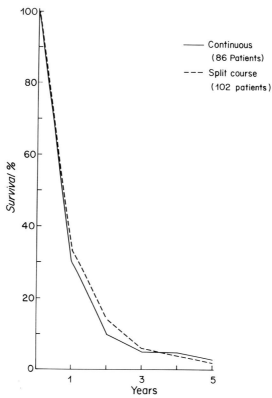

Fig. 13-2. Percentage survival by year for patients with each of the four cell types of bronchogenic carcinoma treated with split-course radiotherapy (102 patients) or continuous radiotherapy (86 patients).

borderline at the time he starts radiotherapy, he may be significantly improved by the end of the rest period, and then the second course can be given. Fourth, it is often difficult to delineate the border between the lung cancer and atelectasis or obstructive pneumonitis seen on chest roentgenograms. Frequently, shrinkage of the lesion with correction of atelectasis or obstructive pneumonitis following the first course of split-course radiotherapy permits the second course to be given through smaller ports. Fifth, if there is a question of distant metastasis (for example, abnormal liver function tests and suspicious liver scan but negative peritoneoscopy and liver biopsy) we give the patient the benefit of the doubt and proceed with the first course of radiotherapy. Three weeks later the patient is reevaluated. If his general condition is the same or better and the tests for metastasis to liver and other sites are negative, the second course of radiotherapy is given to complete the planned tumor dose, and no time has been lost.

Current Mayo Clinic Technique

In the past year almost all Mayo Clinic patients with potentially curable lung cancer have received split-course radiotherapy using the following technique. They receive supervoltage radiotherapy with a 4- or 10-MV linear accelerator with a minimum target-skin distance of 100 cm. Anterior and corresponding posterior ports include the primary tumor, the mediastinal lymph nodes, and usually the ipsilateral supraclavicular region. Both ports are treated daily. The mediastinal target volume extends superiorly from the suprasternal notch to not less than 5 cm below the carina inferiorly, then across the midline to include 1 cm of contralateral lung; it is continuous with the primary target volume, which includes the involved portion of the lung plus a suitable margin of at least 2 cm. The midplane central axis dose in the thoracic region is 2000 rads in five fractions over 5 to 7 days, then 3 weeks of rest, followed by a second course of 2000 rads in five fractions over 5 to 7 days. This dose is for unit-density material. An anterior and posterior cervical lead block over the larynx and spinal cord extends down to the level of the suprasternal notch. A posterior thoracic spinal cord lead block is used to decrease the dosage to the spinal cord to a maximum of 3600 rads, as indicated by the isodose plots (Figs. 13-3 and 13-4). Transverse and sagittal isodose plots are made for each patient.

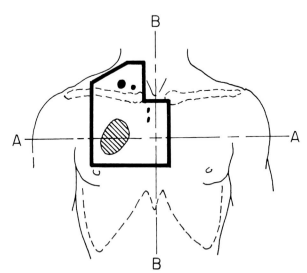

Fig. 13-3. Portal drawing. Primary lung tumor, mediastinal nodes, and supraclavicular nodes are included in two parallel, opposed fields. The risk of overdose to spinal cord (because of junction of separate supraclavicular and thoracic fields) is thus avoided. Lines AA and BB indicate planes of isodose plots: AA, cross section through central axis; BB, sagittal section through midline.

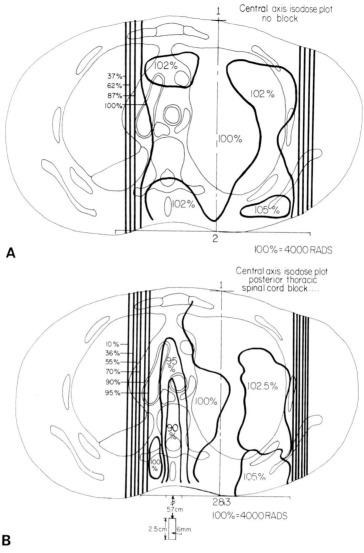

Fig. 13-4. Isodose plots for treatment with 4-MV linear accelerators, opposing 15- by 20-cm fields. (A) Cross section through central axis without spinal cord block. (B) Cross section through central axis with posterior lead block over the thoracic spinal cord region. (C) Sagittal section through midline without spinal cord blocks. (D) Sagittal section through midline with lead blocks over spinal cord in the posterior thoracic area and anterior and posterior cervical areas.

RADIOTHERAPY WITH OTHER MODES OF TREATMENT

Radiotherapy and Surgery

The aims of preoperative radiotherapy are to increase the resectability of a tumor, control lymph node metastases that are unresectable, decrease local and distant dissemination of viable tumor cells, and control subclinical extension of tumor outside the margins of resection.

A cooperative clinical trial was conducted under the aegis of the Committee for Radiation Therapy Studies[40] to evaluate preoperative radiotherapy for cancer of the lung. There were 568 patients classified as initially operable, and approximately half received preoperative radiotherapy. Of 425 patients classified as potentially

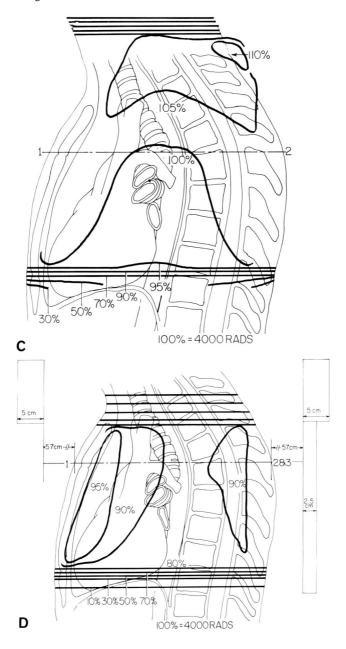

C

100% = 4000 RADS

D

100% = 4000 RADS

operable there were 152 patients considered resectable following radiotherapy, and about half underwent surgery. A dose of 4000 rads in 4 weeks was followed in 4 to 6 weeks by surgery. There were no significant differences in the survival rates, but survival was somewhat less in patients who had resections following radiotherapy.

Preoperative radiotherapy was evaluated in a cooperative clinical trial conducted by the VA Lung Study Group.[41] Of 339 patients with operable carcinoma of the lung, half of the patients received preoperative radiotherapy with 3000–6000 rads, followed in 6 weeks by surgery. There was decreased survival in the patients who had curative resection following irradiation. It was suggested that radiation injury to the lungs, heart, and mediastinum is too large a burden for the patient who is undergoing major pulmonary resection. Based on these two clinical trials, the routine use of preoperative radiotherapy is contraindicated.

Preoperative radiotherapy has been shown to improve survival in selected patients with operable oat cell carcinoma[42] and superior sulcus tumor,[43,44] as well as in patients with SCE tumors of trachea, carina, or mainstem bronchus when the patients are suitable for sleeve resection but cannot tolerate pneumonectomy.[45] These studies were not controlled clinical trials.

The aim of postoperative radiotherapy is to control subclinical and known residual tumor. Paterson and Russell conducted a clinical trial[46] of postoperative radiotherapy in 202 patients with lung cancer. Half of the patients had pneumonectomy alone, and the other half had postoperative radiotherapy after an interval of 6 weeks. A dose of 4500 rads in 3 weeks was given to the region of the hilum and adjuvant mediastinum. The 3-year survival rates were 36 percent for pneumonectomy only and 33 percent for pneumonectomy plus radiotherapy. This difference was not statistically significant. In a reassessment of this trial by Sherrah-Davies[47] it was pointed out that the portal size (5 × 10 cm) was probably too small to cover the potentially involved volume of mediastinum. If roentgenographic studies (including tomograms) demonstrate mediastinal metastases, the prognosis is poor with radiotherapy. Of 70 patients with demonstrable nodal metastases only 3 patients (4 percent) were 5-year survivors. In contrast, of 17 patients without demonstrable mediastinal nodal metastases, 7 patients (41 percent) were 5-year survivors. Uncontrolled observations in selected patients with metastases in mediastinal lymph nodes (particularly patients with SCE[48] and to a lesser degree those with other cell types) indicate that postoperative radiotherapy improves survival.[49]

These failures with routine use of both preoperative radiotherapy and postoperative radiotherapy to improve survival rates are largely due to the high incidence of subclinical distant metastases in these patients.

Superior Pulmonary Sulcus Tumors

Superior pulmonary sulcus tumors are peripheral bronchogenic carcinomas in the upper lobe that invade the superior sulcus of the chest.

These tumors are usually low-grade squamous cell carcinomas that grow slowly and metastasize late.

Paulson[50] has emphasized the importance of defining and staging (T3 N0 M0) superior pulmonary sulcus tumors. According to the guidelines of Pancoast, such tumors at the thoracic inlet may involve ribs, vertebrae, the brachial plexus, and the sympathetic chain, but not scalene, hilar, or mediastinal lymph nodes. Paulson recommends preoperative radiotherapy with 3000 rads in 10 fractions over 2 weeks to the involved region; surgery is performed approximately 4 weeks after radiotherapy.

Combined preoperative radiotherapy and an extended resection (to include the chest wall, involved nerve roots, lower trunk, and sympathetic chain) were completed in 52 patients in Paulson's report.[50] Fifteen of 44 patients with such treatment have survived 5 years, and 8 of 26 have lived 10 years. Only 12 of 44 had lymph node metastases. There were no survivors among 11 patients with hilar or mediastinal node metastases.

Radiotherapy and Chemotherapy

Radiotherapy has been compared to chemotherapy in 68 patients with small cell carcinoma of the bronchus by Laing et al.[51] Overall survival was poor, but radiotherapy (3000–3500 rads in 25 days plus a booster dose of 1000 rads if disease remained) resulted in significantly longer survival, better amelioration of symptoms, and fewer side effects. Those receiving chemotherapy (six 14-day courses of nitrogen mustard, vinblastine, procarbazine, and prednisolone) relapsed in the lungs, whereas those receiving radiotherapy developed disease elsewhere.

Chemotherapeutic agents may be used in combination with radiation in a variety of ways, according to Bleehen.[52] The most common use, as adjuvant therapy, is when the drugs and radiation kill tumor and normal cells in an additive manner. This is obviously of little significance if the same effect can be obtained more simply by an increase in the radiation dose. However, systemic therapy has the theoretically possible advantage of attaining simultaneous control of distant metastases. Secondly, drugs may also be used to potentiate the radiation effect. This situation occurs when the effects of both treatment modalities given together are greater than the sum of the effects of the individual treatments given separately. Radiosensitizers are included in this class of drugs; theoretically they should have little or no effect on cell viability on their own, but they produce a marked increase in the cell killing caused by radiation. 5-Bromodeoxyuridine (5-BUdR) is one such sensitizer. Other agents such as 5-fluorouracil (5-FU) and actinomycin D may act partially as sensitizers of the radiation effect, but they probably have their main value as adjuvant therapy. A potentiation of the radiation effect with increased cell killing may be associated with one or both of two radiobiologic phenomena. There may be a decrease in the capacity of the cells to recover from what otherwise would have been sublethal radiation damage, with a reduction in the values of quasi threshold (D_q) and extrapolation number (N); thus at the lower radiation doses more often used in clinical practice there would be proportionally greater cell killing than in the unsensitized state. Alternatively, there may be a change in the slope of the exponential part of the survival curve (D_0), as seen with 5-BUdR sensitization.

Some potentiation effects may be due to partial age synchronization of cells within the mitotic cycle, so that the subsequent radiation, if administered at the more sensitive part of the cycle, will be more effective. This has been attempted, particularly with methotrexate and hydroxyurea, but without much clinical success.[52] Another role for the adjunctive drugs could be to produce some tumor shrinkage, with consequent reduction in the total number of hypoxic cells requiring subsequent irradiation.[52] As yet this has not been tested adequately by clinical trial.

A newly discovered class of radiosensitizers includes electronaffinic compounds such as metronidazole (Flagyl)[53-55] and related compounds. These drugs sensitize hypoxic cells with no effect on well-oxygenated normal tissue. Animal studies suggest that these drugs are effective radiosensitizers, and studies in man are under way.

Combined radiotherapy and chemotherapy were superior to radiotherapy alone in 3 of 23 prospective studies,[56] but had *lessened* survival in some studies.[2] Toxicity may be additive or even potentiated. Polychemotherapy appears to be better than single-agent therapy, and small cell carcinoma is the type most susceptible to chemotherapy. The combinations of curative radiotherapy and adjunctive chemotherapy should also be considered for stage III disease associated with mediastinal compression syndrome when no distant metastases are present. Patients with small cell carcinoma confined to one hemithorax and with metastasis involving only the ipsilateral supraclavicular nodes should receive curative radiotherapy and probably adjunctive chemotherapy.[57] Chemotherapy is usually the treatment of choice for patients with distant metastases to any of the following sites: liver, brain, bones, kidneys, adrenal glands, and lymph nodes beyond the ipsilateral scalene and supraclavicular region. Adjunctive radiotherapy should then be considered for relief of specific symptoms.

Radiotherapy and Immunotherapy

The effects of radiotherapy on the immune system may actually lessen survival by interfering with body defenses. However, in a more positive manner, effects on the immune system may be helpful. In the study of Dellon et al.[58] serial determination of T-cell (thymus-dependent lymphocyte) levels commencing with radiotherapy or shortly after the start of radiotherapy was used to assess prognosis. In all patients the T-cell levels fell precipitously during radiotherapy, probably because of damage of the thymus or lymphocytes circulating in the heart and great vessels encompassed by the portals. However, in 15 of 16 responders T-cell levels were abruptly increased after completion of radiotherapy, and in 12 of 14 nonresponders the decline in T-cell levels during radiation therapy persisted in the interval after therapy. (The responders had somewhat less extensive disease, however.) Correlations with T-cell levels and clinical course showed that successive falls in T-cell levels coincided with or heralded later recurrence or metastasis. Thus monitoring T-cell levels offers a means of predicting the course of the individual patient and affords an opportunity to institute adjuvant chemotherapy or immunotherapy. In addition, relatively short survival intervals were seen in patients with T-cell levels less than 400 cells/mm³ prior to or during radiotherapy. These values may serve as criteria for cessation of radiotherapy or for the addition of agents that stimulate the immune response.

We are now conducting a study to determine whether MER (a nonviable methanol extraction residue of Calmette-Guerin bacillus) immunotherapy will prevent the immunosuppressive effects of radiotherapy in patients with inoperable and unresectable SCE. The Radiation Therapy Oncology Group, the Working Party for Therapy of Lung Cancer, and other groups also have studies in progress to evaluate combined radiotherapy and immunotherapy.

Theoretically, radiotherapy may help prepare patients for immunotherapy by lessening the tumor bulk to levels that can be held in check by immunotherapy, and immunotherapy may help radiotherapy by offsetting the immunodepression associated with radiotherapy.

PALLIATIVE RADIOTHERAPY

Unfortunately, as Table 13-1 shows, radiotherapy rarely cures lung cancer. However, radiotherapy can usually improve the quality of remaining life by relieving symptoms of the primary tumor or metastases. Doses smaller than those used for cure are often employed—from 2000 rads in 1 week to 3500 rads in 3.5 weeks. No serious complications are warranted if palliation is the aim of radiotherapy.

Hemoptysis, a common symptom with bronchogenic carcinoma, and one dreaded by most patients, can be improved in 95 percent of patients, according to Line and Deeley, and cough can be helped in 58 percent.[59] Pain due to involvement of the lung, chest wall, or mediastinum can be relieved in 72 percent.[59] Tumor extension causing pain in Pancoast's syndrome can be relieved in 70 percent;[60] and the fields should include the involved intervertebral foramina. Dyspnea can be relieved in 60 percent of patients,[60] but it is more likely to be relieved in those with lesions obstructing the bronchus rather than permeating the lung. Symptoms due to pleural effusion can be controlled in 50 to 80 percent.[61] Dysphagia due to esophageal obstruction by mediastinal metastasis can frequently be relieved by radiotherapy.[62] (However if the lesion extends into the lumen of the esophagus, radiotherapy may create a fistula; so this is a contraindication to radiotherapy.) Mediastinal compression with obstruction of the trachea or superior vena cava can be relieved in 75 percent of patients.[62]

Cerebral metastases are common with bronchogenic carcinoma, and symptoms can be relieved in up to 83 percent of patients.[63,64] Cardiac metastases, although uncommon, are related to the type of primary tumor, and among solid tumors, lung tissue is one of the most frequently implicated.[65] External radiotherapy resulted in improvement for 1 month and 9 months in 2 of 7 patients treated by Cham et al.[65]

The general feeling of well-being improves dramatically after radiotherapy in about 70 percent of patients.[59] In 75 percent of patients radiotherapy can relieve bone pain from metastasis; it also may help prevent pathologic fractures.

Conditions rarely if ever palliated by radiotherapy include paralysis of the phrenic nerve or the recurrent laryngeal nerve and bronchoesophageal or tracheoesophageal fistulas.

COMPLICATIONS

Unfortunately, radiation therapy has side effects and toxicity. It harms both the normal and the abnormal tissue in its beam. Patients commonly experience weakness and malaise after radiotherapy, but nausea and vomiting are uncommon with radiotherapy of the lung; if they occur they usually respond to prochlorperazine (Compazine). Because only about 20 percent of the active bone marrow in adults is present in the hemithorax,[66] radiotherapy rarely causes a significant fall in the white blood cell count unless the marrow is already depleted.

Radiation esophagitis, dermatitis, and subcutaneous fibrosis occur, but the three most life-threatening consequences are radiation myelitis, myocarditis or pericarditis, and pneumonitis.

Myelitis

Radiation myelitis is a calculated risk of radical radiotherapy. However, it usually requires a year or more to become clinically apparent.[67] Rubin and Casarett[68] have estimated that it will develop in 1–5 percent of patients within 5 years after a spinal cord dose of 5000 rads in 25 fractions over 5 weeks. Because a few large fractions in a short course appear to increase the risk of myelitis, many radiotherapists have lengthened the treatment course and reduced the dose.

Myocarditis and Pericarditis

Fajardo et al.[69] have recently reviewed radiation-induced heart disease. Connective tissue proliferation in the heart occurred in their patients after 3000 to 9800 rads of gradually administered radiotherapy. The most frequent alteration was organizing pericarditis with extensive fibrosis, which was clinically apparent as diffuse myocardial constriction or tamponade. Diffuse interstitial myocardial fibrosis also occurred; and the endocardium was affected least. Focal fibrous thickening was the major finding, but vessels showed no consistent change even though endothelial proliferation was observed in half the cases. Lawson et al.[70] also have reviewed the subject. They found a 4 percent incidence of radiation pericarditis after mediastinal irradiation following pulmonary resection for bronchogenic carcinoma. It appeared to develop at about 1 year after treatment (4500 to 5000 rads over 4 to 5 weeks through anterior and posterior oblique fields using a 4-MV linear accelerator in which at least half of the heart volume was exposed to full dose). Others have said that radiation pericarditis occurs in a low percentage of patients in whom the left lower lobe of the lung (and consequently the heart) is irradiated. The low overall incidence probably reflects the fact that it takes 6 months to 8 years to develop, and at 1 year only a fraction of patients with inoperable and unresectable bronchogenic carcinoma treated by radiotherapy are still alive (Table 13-1).

Pneumonitis

Radiation pneumonitis, or radiation fibrosis, has been recognized for many years. Roentgenographically it appears as a hazy infiltration in the acute stage, followed by varying degrees of resolution and transition to fibrosis, with loss of lung volume in the chronic stage. Usually the first signs are roentgenographically apparent within 2 to 6 months after radiation therapy, and fibrosis is seen on roentgenograms of most patients by 12 months.[71] Pleuritis with or without effusion is sometimes an additional complication. The pathologic changes have been studied carefully.[72-74] The acute radiation pneumonitis reaction usually reaches its peak within 45 days after therapy, but the earliest changes (hyperemia and edema) have been described as soon as 4 hr after irradiation. The reaction peak is characterized by degenerative and inflammatory changes consisting of hyaline membrane formation, thickening of alveolar septum, hyalinization of alveolar and arteriolar walls, edema of alveoli and the interstitium, desquamation of alveolar cells, endothelial swelling and thrombosis of capillaries, and fibrosis in all tissues. Resolution is accompanied by further fibrosis, vascular obliteration, slight bronchial proliferation, and connective tissue sclerosis. Cilia loss, areas of atelectasis, congestion and edema, secondary infection, fibrosis, and in some cases bronchiectasis may occur also.

The mechanisms for radiation pneumonitis are poorly understood. Total dose, total volume of irradiation, and length of therapy are certainly significant, but their effects are highly variable. Reactions vary greatly from patient to patient, and most are asymptomatic. Based on a study of 109 patients whose postirradiation roentgenograms were available for review, Hellman et al.[75] reported that fibrosis eventually becomes demonstrable in 100 percent of patients treated with radiation for lung cancer. Yet only 5 of their 109 patients developed *clinically significant* pulmonary fibrosis, and of their 9 patients who survived 2 years, pulmonary fibrosis was clinically significant in only 1 patient. When radiation pneumonitis produces severe shortness of breath, corticosteroid therapy may give prompt relief. However, it is not uniformly effective, and progressive roentgenographic changes usually occur.

When an infection occurs, culture of a sputum specimen may be helpful (no one single pathogen predominates), and the appropriate antibiotic should be given if the patient has fever or other evidence of pneumonia.

Minor Complications of Radiotherapy

When the esophagus is included in treatment ports that encompass mediastinal nodes, exposure to 5000 rads in 5 weeks produces transient esophagitis with dysphagia in about 50 percent of patients. This dysphagia usually starts after 2 weeks of therapy, lasts from 1 to 2 weeks, and then subsides spontaneously.

Skin reactions are usually mild; they include alopecia, desquamation, and tanning (increased pigmentation). Subcutaneous fibrosis is variable, but it usually occurs with higher doses and large treatment volumes. It may result in limitation of motion of the shoulder. Damage to connective tissue is increased with higher doses per fraction. Radiation-induced brachial plexopathy is not commonly seen in patients with lung cancer.[76,77]

Finally, in dealing with complications, a concept of absolute tolerance must be replaced by a flexible concept that takes into consideration the control of the tumor versus the incidence and severity of complications.[78]

Radiotherapy and Chemotherapy

When radiation and chemotherapy are given concurrently, toxicity is enhanced in some instances. Because some drugs seem to sensitize cells to radiotoxicity (increased cell killing per rad), it is necessary to look into this question further.

Phillips et al.[79] have summarized reports of increased tissue or cell damage in vivo and in tissue cultures. Actinomycin D reduces the tolerated radiation dose in the lung by at least 20 percent.[80] The pulmonary toxicity of bleomycin may increase the chances of radiation pneumonitis.[79] The studies of Phillips et al.[79] showed that in mice actinomycin D increased radiation damage but BCNU did not. Rosen et al.[81] found that radiation therapy coupled with high doses of methotrexate and citrovorum factor rescue caused pulmonary fibrosis and pneumonitis 3 months after administration of 1400 to 1600 rads to the lung. Wara et al.[82] studied radiation pneumonitis complicating combined radiotherapy and actinomycin D therapy; they suggested that a safe treatment for avoiding radiation pneumonitis with whole lung radiation is 1500 rads in 10 fractions with actinomycin D and 2500 rads in 20 fractions without actinomycin D. Baeza et al.[83] found that radiation pneumonitis developed in 21 percent of irradiated patients (a slightly higher percentage with doses greater than 1500 rads); that rose to 25 percent if actinomycin D was added.

In another study, cyclophosphamide increased injury only in the lung, and vincristine and hydroxyurea caused minimal damage or none.[79] Only prednisone provided any significant radioprotection.[79]

Corder and Flannery[84] have reported that radiation pericarditis may be precipitated by actinomycin D. In the intestine, radiation damage has been greater with doxorubicin hydrochloride (Adriamycin) than with any other agent.[79] Adriamycin cardiomyopathy has been reported[85,86] to develop at lower cumulative doses of Adriamycin in patients who have had prior radiotherapy to any portion of the heart. Bleomycin has increased damage in the esophagus but not in the lung or intestine.[79]

Specifics in Minimizing Complications

Several procedures minimize toxicity. First, we rarely begin radiotherapy immediately after surgery, because healing might be delayed. If pneumonectomy has been performed we usually wait 4 weeks before beginning radiotherapy. If lobectomy has been performed there is residual lung covering the bronchial stump; so we usually start about 1 to 2 weeks after surgery if the patient's general condition is satisfactory. Second, a computer program (Programmed Console 12 Radiotherapy Planning System, PC-12RS) for calculating and plotting dose distribution helps with individualized treatment planning to assure adequate dose to the tumor and to minimize the dose to adjacent normal tissues. Third, meticulous care is taken to exclude the noncancerous lung from the beams of irradiation.

FUTURE DEVELOPMENTS

Changes in dose schedules, applications of cell kinetics, and combinations of different modalities that will benefit the patient with lung cancer are hoped for in the near future.

Cellular Kinetics and Fractionation

A knowledge of the cellular kinetics of a given tumor would be helpful. In both normal and neoplastic tissues there is a cell renewal system with a spectrum of responses. Some cells undergo mitosis frequently, some occasionally, some after unusual stress, and some never. The response of a tissue to irradiation is related to the proportion of cells ordinarily destined to undergo early and frequent mitosis, as well as to the proportion that is destined to remain in a mature, nonmitotic state. The current fractionation scheme of 175 to 200 rads per day for 5 to 6 weeks may be optimal for some lung cancers, but it is certainly not ideal for all. Knowledge of tumor kinetics before irradiation might provide more efficient tumor cell killing; however, it has been shown that the doubling times of metastases and the primary tumor may differ and that the doubling time within a given metastasis may increase or decrease as it enlarges. Ultimately, kinetics may be used for determining the treatment strategy for each patient (see Chapter 2).

Tumor dose, fractionation, size of treatment ports, and overall period of treatment are interrelated. Ellis[87] has suggested a formula based on clinical results of radiotherapy that relates total dose, number of fractions, and overall treatment time to a quantity termed nominal standard dose (NSD). The NSD formula of Ellis is based on the isoeffect curve for skin (vasculoconnective tissue); total dose = $NSD \cdot N^{0.24} \cdot T^{0.11}$, where total dose is in rads, N is the number of fractions, T is elapsed time in days, and NSD is the nominal standard dose in rets (rads equivalent therapy).

The effect of total elapsed days is due to the proliferation of critical stem cells and to a lesser extent to the changes in radiosensitivity of cells. The effect of the number and size of fractions is related to cell killing and intracellular repair, the "Elkind recovery." Changes of circulation, oxygenation, and nutrition and selection of resistant cell types modify predicted outcome. A spectrum of sensitivities changes unpredictably during fractionated radiotherapy. (Fowler[88] has discussed the various factors.) Ellis,[89] in summarizing the effects of the number of fractions and the number of days, said that in vitro studies have failed to show consistent differences between normal and malignant cells in regard to radiation-induced damage, intracellular recovery, and proliferation rates. For both normal and malignant cells damage and recovery depend on the size and number of doses. The exponents of N and T for normal tissue injury and recovery do not apply to malignant cells because there is no homeostatic control of malignant cells. This should not be confused with the response of some tumors to hormonal regulation.

Thus the Ellis formula is based on the radiation tolerance of normal cells. With greater experience the NSD formula probably will be revised, although it may prove accurate because it applies to vasculoconnective tissue, which is the key to healing in many anatomic sites. In addition, it may apply, at least in general, to tumor cells. High extrapolation numbers seem to be characteristic of radioresistant tumors,[90] but there is no way to determine cell characteristics for individual human neoplasms. Finally, with high extrapolation numbers the sterilizing effect (for the same NSD values) of a small number of large fractions is greater than that of a large number of small fractions (the conventional schedule). Recently

Fletcher et al.,[78] Fischer and Moulder,[91] Wara et al.,[82] and others[92] have criticized the Ellis NSD formula.

Cohen and Scott[93] have suggested a cell population kinetic model for use with a computer program to predict the outcome of fractionated radiotherapy and to generate tumor lethal doses and normal tissue tolerance doses.

Brown and associates[94] have proposed a model based on proliferation kinetics with which the effects of both fractionated high dose rate and low dose rate can be simulated. This allows prediction of the responses to new time-dose schedules, such as giving several fractions daily, 4 hr or more apart.

Hyperfractionated Radiotherapy

Repair of sublethal radiation damage in aerobic mammalian cells is essentially completed within 2 to 4 hr.[95] Accordingly, when a rapidly proliferating tumor cell population is growing in normal tissue (the cells of which are proliferating slowly or not at all), an advantage accrues to the tumor cells if the intertreatment interval lasts more than 4 hr. In addition, at least theoretically, tumor tissue, with its disorganized vascular supply and often lazy cell cycling, may recover less rapidly. So, placing 24 hr between fractions may allow the tumor to gain ground. In such situations greater therapeutic efficacy would be expected by employing two or three treatment sessions per day with a standard dose per fraction and less than 4 hr between fractions. Even in situations where there is no difference in proliferative activity a treatment schedule using several fractions per day would be attractive for certain tumor-versus-normal-tissue situations where low to moderate dose levels are planned for palliation. The significant reduction in total time of treatment also would mean greater convenience for patients who are hospitalized or who come for daily outpatient visits. Rapid radiation treatment utilizing two to three treatment sessions per day has been performed in patients with extensive soft tissue sarcoma,[95] Burkitt's lymphoma,[96] and glioblastoma multiforme of the brain.[97] These treatments were well tolerated, and the normal tissue reaction was approximately the same as in a conventional schedule of one treatment per day. The total dose employed in these instances was reduced at least 10 percent.

According to Suit[98] and Brown et al.,[94] the effects of the number of fractions and the time interval between fractions depend on the kinetics of at least eight biologic processes in the irradiated tissues: (1) repair of radiation damage by the individual cell, (2) cell proliferation, (3) progression of cells through the cell replication cycle and hence changes in age (cell radiosensitivity) distributions, (4) cell differentiation, (5) changes in oxygen tension distributions, (6) immunologic rejection response by host against tumor, (7) changes in normal tissues of tumor bed that affect tumor cell viability in unspecified ways, and (8) possible migration of nonirradiated normal tissue cells into the irradiated area. Apparently the target for cell reproductive death at low doses is nuclear DNA. Modification of the repair of radiation-damaged DNA to differentially affect the tumor and normal tissue would be of great clinical value.

Although most radiotherapy courses for lung cancer deliver the tumor dose by identical daily fractions over a period of 3 to 11 weeks, Hill and Bush[99] recently concluded that frequent fractionation may have advantages. Jakobsson and Littbrand[100] and Backstrom et al.[101] obtained good clinical results by giving three sessions of radiotherapy per day. Svoboda[102] showed that normal tissue tolerances were similar with one or three daily fractions.

Recently Choi and Suit[95] have also evaluated rapid radiation treatment schedules (two regular-size doses per day with total course dose reduced by 10 percent to 3440 rads) in regard to skin reaction, local control of tumor, and relief of pain. Tumor regression and pain relief were achieved faster in the rapid fractionation schedules, and skin reactions were nearly the same.

In contrast to hyperfractionation, Ellis[90] has stated that "resistant neoplasms" might be better treated by small numbers of large doses than by conventional large numbers of small doses. Schumacher[103] has successfully employed a smaller number of larger fractions in bronchogenic carcinoma.

Clinical Trials

Interesting uncontrolled studies suggest the need for randomized clinical trials to provide answers to questions yet unanswered in the literature. Some are planned and others are under way to answer questions in the following areas.

RADIOTHERAPY AND CHEMOTHERAPY

We believe that most patients with stage III lung cancer limited to one hemithorax have occult distant metastases, even when careful pretreatment evaluation shows no evidence of widespread disease. Many oncologists are attempting to find the proper chemotherapeutic agent or agents for each cell type of lung cancer. Because single agents as adjunctive treatments to radiotherapy have not increased survival above that of radiotherapy alone, many protocols involve radiotherapy with adjunctive polychemotherapy.

RADIOTHERAPY AND IMMUNOTHERAPY

Clinical trials are under way to study the effects of combinations of radiotherapy and immunotherapy for patients with lung cancer. Also, investigations are currently being conducted to correlate the immune response with prognosis of patients with bronchogenic carcinoma. The possible enhancement of tumor growth by immunosuppressive effects of radiotherapy needs further study.

ELECTIVE RADIOTHERAPY OF SUBCLINICAL METASTASES

Although in patients with disseminated cancer radiotherapy is often held in reserve for use if and when specific palliation is needed, studies are now under way to determine the effectiveness of elective or so-called prophylactic radiotherapy to the brain for subclinical metastases as an adjunct to polychemotherapy for patients with small cell carcinoma (the most radiosensitive type). Elective irradiation of the upper abdomen as an adjunct to polychemotherapy is also being investigated. A third type of investigation centers around the use of polychemotherapy and radiotherapy administered to the entire brain, chest lesions, regional lymph nodes, and upper abdomen.

HIGH-LET RADIATION

Many patients have local recurrences of their bronchogenic carcinoma after conventional radical radiotherapy. The major reason for recurrence at the original site is thought to be relative anoxia and concomitant radioresistance of tumor cells as compared to normal cells. Therefore other forms of radiotherapy are being investigated.

These include accelerated particles (neutrons, pi-mesons, and stripped nuclei), which more effectively destroy anoxic cells than do conventional roentgen rays and gamma rays. Some high-linear-energy-transfer (high-LET) particles also offer dose distribution advantages over conventional irradiation. Preliminary results of a clinical trial at Hammersmith Hospital in London have confirmed the biologic and physical predictions of earlier investigations, and similar projects are under way in the United States. Eventually the use of high-LET accelerated particles may provide the means for local control in a substantial number of patients with bronchogenic carcinoma.

Based on past calculations of Suit,[98] it can be estimated that of the 81,000 persons who were expected to die of lung cancer in 1975 about 7350 would die because of failure to control the primary lesion. If the radiotherapeutic use of optimum-dose fractionation schedules or the use of accelerated particles could reduce these treatment failures by half, 3675 lives per year could be saved.

CONCLUSION

The most important consideration for the radiotherapist is whether he can encompass all the tumor-bearing tissues in the treatment ports and give a cancericidal radiation dose without unduly damaging vital tissues. Both surgery and curative radiotherapy are applicable to only a localized region.

Surgery is the treatment of choice for any stage I or stage II squamous cell carcinoma, adenocarcinoma, or large cell carcinoma. The percentage of patients in these categories surviving 5 years varies from 10 to 35 percent. For stage III carcinoma of these cell types limited to one hemithorax, radiotherapy is the treatment of choice. All small cell carcinomas limited to one hemithorax should be treated with radiotherapy and chemotherapy. In these patients curative radiotherapy is indicated if the general condition and pulmonary function are satisfactory. The 5-year survival rate for patients so treated ranges from 0 to 9 percent. For patients with distant metastases chemotherapy is the treatment of choice, but adjunctive radiotherapy often relieves symptomatic lesions. Palliative radiotherapy does not often extend life, but it does achieve the important goal of enhancing the quality of life.

It is hoped that current clinical trials of combinations of radiotherapy with surgery, chemotherapy, and immunotherapy will result in more cures of bronchogenic carcinoma. While seeking cures, let us not forget that for most of our patients with lung cancer radiotherapy is the most effective palliative treatment.

REFERENCES

1. Cancer statistics. CA 25:12, 1975
2. Carter S: cited in lung cancer studies supported by NCI-VA; outlined in reports to advisors. Cancer Letter May 9, 1975, pp 4–7
3. Mountain CF, Carr DT, Anderson WAD: A system for the clinical staging of lung cancer. Am J Roentgenol Radium Ther Nucl Med 120:130–138, 1974
4. Galofré M, Payne WS, Woolner LB, et al: Pathologic classification and surgical treatment of bronchogenic carcinoma. Surg Gynecol Obstet 119:51–61, 1964
5. Mountain CF: Surgical therapy in lung cancer: Biologic, physiologic, and technical determinants. Semin Oncol 1:253–258, 1974
6. Deeley TJ, Line DH: Solitary metastases in carcinoma of the bronchus. Br J Dis Chest 63:150–154, 1969
7. Matthews MJ, Kanhouwa S, Pickren J, et al: Frequency of residual and metastatic tumor in patients undergoing curative surgical resection for lung cancer. Cancer Chemother Rep 4:63–67, 1973
8. Deeley TJ: Radiotherapy for carcinoma of bronchus. Cancer Treat Rev 1:39–64, 1974
9. Rouvière H: cited by Weinberg JA: The intrathoracic lymphatics, in Haagensen CD, Feind CR, Herter FP, et al (eds): The Lymphatics in Cancer. Philadelphia, WB Saunders, 1972
10. Weinberg JA: The intrathoracic lymphatics, in Haagensen CD, Feind CR, Herter FP, et al (eds): The Lymphatics in Cancer. Philadelphia, WB Saunders, 1972, p 231
11. Smart J: Can lung cancer be cured by irradiation alone? JAMA 195:1034–1035, 1966
12. Smart J, Hilton G: Radiotherapy of cancer of the lung: Results in a selected group of cases. Lancet 1:880–881, 1956
13. Morrison R, Deeley TJ, Cleland WP: The treatment of carcinoma of the bronchus: A clinical

trial to compare surgery and supervoltage radiotherapy. Lancet 1:683–684, 1963

14. Scadding JG (chairman): Comparative trial of surgery and radiotherapy for the primary treatment of small-celled or oat-celled carcinoma of the bronchus. Lancet 2:979–986, 1966

15. Miller AB, Fox W, Tall R: Five-year follow-up of the Medical Research Council comparative trial of surgery and radiotherapy for the primary treatment of small-celled or oat-celled carcinoma of the bronchus. Lancet 2:501–505, 1969

16. Roswit B, Patno ME, Rapp R, et al: The survival of patients with inoperable lung cancer: A large-scale randomized study of radiation therapy versus placebo. Radiology 90:688–697, 1968

17. Abramson N, Cavanaugh PJ: Radiation therapy in carcinoma of the lung: The short-course method. Thirteenth International Congress of Radiology, Madrid, Spain, October 15–19, 1973

18. Caldwell WL, Bagshaw MA: Indications for and results of irradiation of carcinoma of the lung. Cancer 22:999–1004, 1968

19. Deeley TJ, Singh SP: Treatment of inoperable carcinoma of the bronchus by megavoltage x rays. Thorax 22:562–566, 1967

20. Guttmann R: Radical supervoltage therapy in inoperable carcinoma of the lung, in Deeley TJ (ed): Carcinoma of the Bronchus. New York, Appleton-Century-Crofts, 1972, p 181

21. Guttmann RJ: Results of radiation therapy in patients with inoperable carcinoma of the lung whose status was established at exploratory thoracotomy. Am J Roentgenol Radium Ther Nucl Med 93:99–103, 1965

22. Perez-Tamayo R, Soberon M: The place of radiotherapy in the treatment of bronchogenic carcinoma. Mo Med 66:876–880, 1969

23. Lee RE, Carr DT, Childs DS Jr: Comparison of split-course radiotherapy and continuous radiotherapy for unresectable bronchogenic carcinoma: 5-year results. Am J Roentgenol Radium Ther Nucl Med 126:116–123, 1976

24. Bromley LL, Szur L: Combined radiotherapy and resection for carcinoma of the bronchus: Experiences with 66 patients. Lancet 2:937–941, 1955

25. Bloedorn FG: Rationale and benefit of preoperative irradiation in lung cancer. JAMA 196:340–341, 1966

26. Rissanen PM, Tikka U, Holsti LR: Autopsy findings in lung cancer treated with megavoltage radiotherapy. Acta Radiol [Ther] (Stockh) 7:433–442, 1968

27. Abadir R, Muggia FM: Irradiated lung cancer: An autopsy analysis of spread pattern. Radiology 114:427–430, 1975

28. Lee RE: Radiotherapy of bronchogenic carcinoma. Semin Oncol 1:245–252, 1974

29. Fulkerson LL, Perlmutter GS, Zack MB, et al: Radiotherapy in chest malignant tumors associated with pulmonary tuberculosis. Radiology 106:645–648, 1973

30. Moss WT, Brand WN, Battifora H: Radiation Oncology: Rationale, Technique, Results (ed 4). St Louis, CV Mosby, 1973

31. Scanlon PW: The effect of mitotic suppression and recovery after irradiation on time-dose relationships and the application of this effect to clinical radiation therapy. Am J Roentgenol Radium Ther Nucl Med 81:433–455, 1959

32. Sambrook DK: Split-course radiation therapy in malignant tumors. Am J Roentgenol Radium Ther Nucl Med 91:37–45, 1964

33. Scanlon PW: Split-dose radiotherapy. Prog Clin Cancer 2:143–163, 1966

34. Sambrook DK: Fractionation technique, in Deeley TJ (ed): Carcinoma of the Bronchus. New York, Appleton-Century-Crofts, 1972, p 196

35. Holsti LR: Alternative approaches to radiotherapy alone and radiotherapy as a part of a combined therapeutic approach for lung cancer. Cancer Chemother Rep (Part 3) 4:165–169, 1973

36. Levitt SH, Bogardus CR, Ladd G: Split-dose intensive radiation therapy in the treatment of advanced lung cancer: A randomized study. Radiology 88:1159–1169, 1967

37. Hazra TA, Chandrasekaran MS, Colman M, et al: Survival in carcinoma of the lung after a split course of radiotherapy. Br J Radiol 47:464–466, 1974

38. Abramson N, Cavanaugh PJ: Short-course radiation therapy in carcinoma of the lung. Radiology 96:627–630, 1970

39. Carr DT, Childs DS Jr, Lee RE: Radiotherapy plus 5-FU compared to radiotherapy alone for inoperable and unresectable bronchogenic carcinoma. Cancer 29:375–380, 1972

40. Collaborative Study: Preoperative irradiation of cancer of the lung: Preliminary report of a therapeutic trial. Cancer 23:419–430, 1969

41. Roswit B, Higgins GA, Shields W, et al: Preoperative radiation therapy for carcinoma of the lung: Report of a national VA controlled study. Front Radiation Ther Oncol 5:163–176, 1970

42. Bates M, Hurt R, Levison V, et al: Treatment of oat-cell carcinoma of bronchus by preoperative radiotherapy and surgery. Lancet 1:1134–1135, 1974

43. Mallams JT, Paulson DL, Collier RE, et al: Presurgical irradiation in bronchogenic carcinoma, superior sulcus type. Radiology 82:1050–1054, 1964

44. Paulson DL: The survival rate in superior sulcus tumors treated by presurgical irradiation. JAMA 196:342, 1966

45. Saxena VS, Hendrickson FR, Jensik RJ, et al:

Conservative surgery following preoperative radiation therapy of lung cancer. Am J Roentgenol Radium Ther Nucl Med 114:93–98, 1972

46. Paterson R, Russell MH: Clinical trials in malignant disease. Part IV—Lung cancer: Value of postoperative radiotherapy. Clin Radiol 13:141–144, 1962

47. Sherrah-Davies E: Does postoperative irradiation improve survival in lung cancer? JAMA 196:345–347, 1966

48. Kirsh MM, Kahn DR, Gago O, et al: Treatment of bronchogenic carcinoma with mediastinal metastases. Ann Thorac Surg 12:44–48, 1971

49. Green N, Kurohara SS, George FW III, et al: Postresection irradiation for primary lung cancer. Radiology 116:405–407, 1975

50. Paulson DL: The importance of defining location and staging of superior pulmonary sulcus tumors (editorial). Ann Thorac Surg 15:549–551, 1973

51. Laing AH, Berry RJ, Newman CR, et al: Treatment of small-cell carcinoma of bronchus. Lancet 1:129–132, 1975

52. Bleehen NM: Combination therapy with drugs and radiation. Br Med Bull 29:54–58, 1973

53. Urtasun RC, Sturnwind J, Rabin H, et al: High-dose metronidazole: A preliminary pharmacological study prior to its investigational use in clinical radiotherapy trials (letter to the editor). Br J Radiol 47:297–299, 1974

54. Asquith JC, Foster JL, Willson RL: Metronidazole ("Flagyl") a radiosensitizer of hypoxic cells. Br J Radiol 47:479–481, 1974

55. Sutherland RM: Selective chemotherapy of noncycling cells in an in vitro tumor model. Cancer Res 34:3501–3503, 1974

56. Selawry OS: The role of chemotherapy in the treatment of lung cancer. Semin Oncol 1:259–272, 1974

57. Maurer LH, Tulloh M, Eagan RT, et al: Combination chemotherapy and radiation therapy for small cell carcinoma of the lung. Cancer Chemother Rep (Part 3) 4:171–176, 1973

58. Dellon AL, Potvin C, Chretien PB: Thymus-dependent lymphocyte levels during radiation therapy for bronchogenic and esophageal carcinoma: Correlations with clinical course in responders and nonresponders. Am J Roentgenol Radium Ther Nucl Med 123:500–511, 1975

59. Line D, Deeley TJ: Palliative therapy, in Deeley TJ (ed): Carcinoma of the Bronchus. New York, Appleton-Century-Crofts, 1972, p 298

60. Mantell BS: Superior sulcus (Pancoast) tumours: Results of radiotherapy. Br J Dis Chest 67:315–318, 1973

61. Strober SJ, Klotz E, Kuperman A, et al: Malignant pleural disease: A radiotherapeutic approach to the problem. JAMA 226:296–299, 1973

62. Schulz MD: Palliation by radiotherapy, in Rubin P (ed): Bronchogenic Carcinoma (Current Concepts in Cancer No. 9). New York, American Cancer Society, 1966, p 33

63. Deutsch M, Parsons JA, Mercado R Jr: Radiotherapy for intracranial metastases. Cancer 34:1607–1611, 1974

64. Chu FCH, Hilaris BB: Value of radiation therapy in the management of intracranial metastases. Cancer 14:577–581, 1961

65. Cham WC, Freiman AH, Carstens PHB, et al: Radiation therapy of cardiac and pericardial metastases. Radiology 114:701–704, 1975

66. Ellis RE: The distribution of active bone marrow in the adult. Phys Med Biol 5:255–258, 1961

67. Reagen TJ, Thomas JE, Colby MY Jr: Chronic progressive radiation myelopathy: Its clinical aspects and differential diagnosis. JAMA 203:106–110, 1968

68. Rubin P, Casarett GW: Clinical Radiation Pathology. Philadelphia, WB Saunders, 1968

69. Fajardo LF, Stewart JR, Cohn KE: Morphology of radiation-induced heart disease. Arch Pathol 86:512–519, 1968

70. Lawson RAM, Ross WM, Gold RG, et al: Postradiation pericarditis: Report on four more cases with special reference to bronchogenic carcinoma. J Thorac Cardiovasc Surg 63:841–847, 1972

71. Libshitz HI, Southard ME: Complications of radiation therapy: The thorax. Semin Roentgenol 9:41–49, 1974

72. Warren S, Spencer J: Radiation reaction in the lung. Am J Roentgenol Radium Ther 43:682–701, 1940

73. Boushy SF, Helgason AH, North LB: The effect of radiation on the lung and bronchial tree. Am J Roentgenol Radium Ther Nucl Med 108:284–292, 1970

74. Braun SR, doPico GA, Olson CE, et al: Low-dose radiation pneumonitis. Cancer 35:1322–1324, 1975

75. Hellman S, Kligerman MM, von Essen CF, et al: Sequelae of radical radiotherapy of carcinoma of the lung. Radiology 82:1055–1061, 1964

76. Match RM: Radiation-induced brachial plexus paralysis. Arch Surg 110:384–386, 1975

77. Thomas JE, Colby MY Jr: Radiation-induced or metastatic brachial plexopathy? A diagnostic dilemma. JAMA 222:1392–1395, 1972

78. Fletcher GH, Barkley HT Jr, Shukovsky LJ: Present status of the time factor in clinical radiotherapy. Part II. The nominal standard dose formula. J Radiol Electrol Med Nucl 55:745–751, 1974

79. Phillips TL, Wharam MD, Margolis LW: Modification of radiation injury to normal tissues by

chemotherapeutic agents. Cancer 35:1678–1684, 1975

80. Wharam MD, Phillips TL, Jacobs EM: Combination chemotherapy and whole lung irradiation for pulmonary metastases from sarcomas and germinal cell tumors of the testis. Cancer 34:136–142, 1974

81. Rosen G, Tefft M, Martinez A, et al: Combination chemotherapy and radiation therapy in the treatment of metastatic osteogenic sarcoma. Cancer 35:622–630, 1975

82. Wara WM, Phillips TL, Margolis LW, et al: Radiation pneumonitis: A new approach to the derivation of time-dose factors. Cancer 32:547–552, 1973

83. Baeza MR, Barkley HT Jr, Fernandez CH: Total-lung irradiation in the treatment of pulmonary metastases. Radiology 116:151–154, 1975

84. Corder MP, Flannery EP: Possible radiation pericarditis precipitated by actinomycin D. Oncology 30:81–84, 1974

85. Minow RA, Benjamin RS, Gottlieb JA: Adriamycin (NSC-123127) cardiomyopathy—An overview with determination of risk factors. Cancer Chemother Rep (Part 3) 6:195–201, 1975

86. Cortes EP, Lutman G, Wanka J, et al: Adriamycin (NSC-123127) cardiotoxicity: A clinicopathologic correlation. Cancer Chemother Rep (Part 3) 6:215–225, 1975

87. Ellis F: Dose, time and fractionation: A clinical hypothesis. Clin Radiol 20:1–7, 1969

88. Fowler JF: Experimental animal results relating to time–dose relationship in radiotherapy and the "RET" concept. Br J Radiol 44:81–90, 1971

89. Ellis F: Nominal standard dose and the RET. Br J Radiol 44:101–108, 1971

90. Ellis F: The NSD concept and radioresistant tumours (letter to the editor). Br J Radiol 47:909, 1974.

91. Fischer JJ, Moulder JE: Time-dose relationships for tumor control, in: Proceedings of the Time-Dose Conference, Madison, Wisc, Oct 4–5, 1974

92. Orton C (ed): Communications. Med Phys 2:85–92, 1975

93. Cohen L, Scott MJ: Fractionation procedures in radiation therapy: A computerized approach to evaluation. Br J Radiol 41:529–533, 1968

94. Brown BW, Thompson JR, Barkley T, et al: Theoretical considerations of dose rate factors influencing radiation strategy. Radiology 110:197–202, 1974

95. Choi CH, Suit HD: Evaluation of rapid radiation treatment schedules utilizing two treatment sessions per day. Radiology 116:703–707, 1975

96. Norin T, Clifford P, Einhorn J, et al: Conventional and superfractionated radiation therapy in Burkitt's lymphoma. Acta Radiol [Ther] (Stockh) 10:545–557, 1971

97. Simpson WJ: Studies at the clinical level, in Bond BP, Suit HD, Marcial V (eds): Proceedings of Conference on Time and Dose Relationships in Radiation Biology as Applied to Radiotherapy. Carmel, Calif, Sept 15–18, 1969. BNL 50203 (C-57). Upton, NY, Brookhaven National Laboratory, 1969, p 301

98. Suit HD: Introduction, in Bond BP, Suit HD, Marcial V (eds): Proceedings of Conference on Time and Dose Relationships in Radiation Biology as Applied to Radiotherapy. Carmel, Calif, Sept 15–18, 1969. BNL 50203 (C-57). Upton, NY, Brookhaven National Laboratory, 1969, p vii

99. Hill RP, Bush RS: The effect of continuous or fractionated irradiation on a murine sarcoma. Br J Radiol 46:167–174, 1973

100. Jakobsson PÅ, Littbrand B: Fractionation scheme with low individual tumour dose and high total dose. Acta Radiol [Ther] (Stockh) 12:337–346, 1973

101. Bäckström A, Jakobsson PÅ, Littbrand B, et al: Fractionation scheme with low individual doses in irradiation of carcinoma of the mouth. Acta Radiol [Ther] (Stockh) 12:401–406, 1973

102. Svoboda VHJ: Radiotherapy by several sessions a day. Br J Radiol 48:131–133, 1975

103. Schumacher T: cited by Ellis F: The NSD concept and radioresistant tumours (letter to the editor). Br J Radiol 47:909, 1974

Clifton F. Mountain

14

Biologic, Physiologic, and Technical Determinants in Surgical Therapy for Lung Cancer

Observation of the disease which is independent of and falls short of a knowledge of its cause has told us in unmistakable terms that whatever its origin, it is at first confined to the part of the body it attacks and has further shown us the precise methods and routes by which it spreads. And surgeons, by making use of this knowledge in devising the technique of their operations have proved that in situations where it is removable it is quite possible to cure it . . . depending on a knowledge of the behavior of the tumor.

Childe, *Cancer and the Public,* 1925

Given the state of our present knowledge, it is a regrettable truism that the only real promise for extending survival for primary lung cancer patients depends on our ability to successfully implement definitive surgical therapy. However, the technical development of thoracic surgery has reached the point where it becomes doubtful that further advances will have significant impact on the overall problem. Essentially, a state of equilibrium has been reached between the technique of the surgeon and the biology of the disease. In order to advance further in the development of new management strategies, a quantitative appreciation of the contributions of surgery, as well as its limitations, is essential. Capitalizing on such insights appears to be the optimum pathway to improved end results in the near term.

It must be appreciated that survival following definitive surgical therapy in lung cancer is dependent on a large number of complex interacting variables that may be expected to affect the delicate balance between tumor and host. These relate principally to the immunologic and physiologic status of the host, the biologic characteristics of the tumor, and the location and extent of the total tumor burden imposed. Available diagnostic and evaluative methods enable preoperative judgments to be made in regard to the individual and in regard to the collective influence of these variables on the force of mortality. In addition, independently predictive factors of extended cancer-free survival can be identified. The rational application of surgery in the individualization of therapy involves a weighted balance between these factors. The care and judgment exercised in this analysis profoundly affects prognosis in the surgically "curable" patient. With respect to the patient, it is important to distinguish between what is technically possible and what is functionally sound. With respect to the tumor, the surgeon should develop an appreciation for the distinction between what is technically resectable and what is biologically rational. An understanding of these biologic, physiologic, and technical

185

determinants is the basis for proper selection of the surgical patient, and it can provide reasonably reliable and valid estimates of prognosis.

BIOLOGIC DETERMINANTS RELATED TO SURVIVAL

Distinct morphologic groups exist within the spectrum of lung cancer, each exhibiting a unique pattern of biologic behavior. It is important to realize that this malignant process cannot be considered as a single disease entity. Four major histologic patterns of disease comprise more than 95 percent of all bronchogenic carcinomas. Epidemiologic studies in the United States indicate that epidermoid (squamous cell) carcinoma constitutes approximately 50 percent of all primary lung cancers, adenocarcinoma about 20 percent, undifferentiated small cell (oat cell) carcinoma about 20 percent, and undifferentiated large cell carcinoma the remaining 10 percent.

With rare exceptions this morphologic hierarchy is constant throughout the world, although the relative frequency of each type may vary between countries and ethnic groups. Oat cell carcinoma is reported in localized endemic areas where it constitutes up to 35 percent of lung cancer. It appears that in the past few years the pattern has been changing within the United States, with increasing frequencies of adenocarcinoma and oat cell carcinoma being reported. If this is true it will become important to our interpretation of end results. The observation probably relates to a more critical and more accurate pathologic classification. Studies that correlate the findings of electron microscopy with those of light microscopy have stimulated considerable progress in this important area. Our studies of surgically resected cases clearly demonstrate that the morphology of the tumor is a significant factor in survival, regardless of any other variable.[1] With respect to the histologic classification alone, three distinct survival patterns are evident. When all stages of disease are combined, epidermoid carcinoma has the best prognosis following surgical resection, with an overall accumulative 5-year survival rate of 37 percent. The survival dynamics for surgically treated adenocarcinoma and undifferentiated large cell carcinoma are almost identical, with a 5-year cumulative survival rate of 27 percent. In a highly selected group of patients with oat cell carcinoma undergoing surgi-

cal resection there were no survivors beyond 39 months, and the surgical mortality rate exceeded the cumulative survival rate at 18 months.

Regardless of the appearance of the primary lesion, oat cell carcinoma is known to be widely disseminated in an overwhelming preponderance of cases at the time of first diagnosis.[2] Regardless of which index of disease extent is examined, no significant relationship can be demonstrated between the clinical estimate of tumor burden and survival.[3] Although long-term survival is an elusive goal, some promising new leads are being developed through multimodality treatment with combined chemotherapy, radiotherapy, and immunotherapy regimes. Comparison of this information with the results of surgery leads to the conclusion that surgical resection, as the primary treatment modality, is not a rational policy. Oat cell carcinoma presenting as a peripheral lesion of unknown etiology continues to be resected, but this is regarded as diagnostic surgery. The role of adjunctive reductive surgery in oat cell carcinoma, where surgery is employed to reduce the total tumor burden in conjunction with planned adjunctive treatment, remains to be evaluated. Our survival experience in 835 resected patients with primary bronchogenic carcinoma, stratified by cell type, is shown in Table 14-1.

The relationships among various clinical variables and their contributions to the force of mortality in lung cancer have been carefully studied for each major morphologic pattern of disease.[4] The influence of factors such as size, location, proximal margination, distribution and extent of lymph node involvement, and presence or absence of more extensive disease varies within each histologic subset. It was observed that in epidermoid carcinoma approximately two-thirds of the lesions were centrally located, with a cumulative 5-year survival rate of 22 percent for those within the hilar region, as compared to 10 percent for those originating within the mainstem bronchus.

The remaining one-third were in the periphery of the lung or the apical region, with survival rates of 29 and 21 percent, respectively. In the group of patients with undifferentiated large cell carcinoma and adenocarcinoma, lesions were more evenly distributed between the hilar region and the periphery, with a very small number originating within a mainstem bronchus. The cumulative 5-year survival was 21 percent for peripheral lesions, as compared to 5 percent for

Table 14-1
Survival Pattern of Resected Cases of Lung Cancer by Morphology

Cell Type	Number of Cases	Cumulative Percentage Surviving		
		18 mo	*36 mo*	*60 mo*
Epidermoid carcinoma	528	55	41	37
Adenocarcinoma	183	47	32	27
Undifferentiated large cell carcinoma	83	44	31	27
Undifferentiated small cell carcinoma	41	9	3	0

more centrally placed tumors. The presence of any degree of atelectasis or obstructive pneumonitis had an unfavorable effect on prognosis in large cell carcinoma and adenocarcinoma. On the other hand, in epidermoid carcinoma these associated secondary manifestations of disease had little relationship to survival unless the entire lung was involved. Total atelectasis is brought about by obstruction of the mainstem bronchus. Accordingly, this effect for prognosis is a simple reflection of a central proximal tumor margination. The size of the primary tumor, as measured both by clinical criteria and by the pathologist, is highly correlated with survival. In surgically staged patients having tumors 3 cm or less in diameter, the 5-year survival for adenocarcinoma was 72 percent, and for epidermoid carcinoma 56 percent. Increasing tumor size had more serious implications in large cell carcinoma and adenocarcinoma than in epidermoid carcinoma, with respective survival rates of 31 percent, 28 percent, and 42 percent for that group of tumors greater than 3 cm in diameter. Size was a proportionately less effective predictor in undifferentiated large cell carcinoma.

Concomitant pleural effusion occurred more frequently in association with adenocarcinoma and oat cell carcinoma than with other cell types. The presence of fluid is a very serious prognostic sign, especially in adenocarcinoma and in oat cell carcinoma. In the presence of any effusion with demonstrated malignant cells or an exudate without malignant cells, survival rarely exceeds 1 year. Accordingly, except in the case of a cell-free transudate accompaning otherwise resectable epidermoid or large cell carcinoma, the clinical presence of any effusion is a contraindication to surgery; the rationale for resection is debatable, and the results are marginal.

Any degree of lymph node involvement pro-

duces a significant drop in the survival rate. The relative prognostic influence of regional lymphatic metastases is demonstrated in Fig. 14-1. Viewing this single disease parameter in patients with no clinical evidence of disseminated disease, but without consideration of other related variables affecting prognosis, the cumulative 5-year survival rate is 46 percent in the absence of demonstrated lymph node involvement. On extension to the

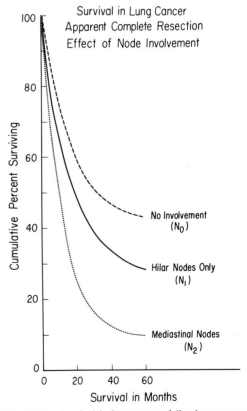

Fig. 14-1. Survival in lung cancer following apparent complete resection: Relationship of lymph node metastasis to prognosis (all cell types).

peribronchial or hilar lymph nodes, the equiva- lent survival drops to 33 percent, and in the pres- ence of mediastinal lymph node metastases it drops to 8 percent. Thus even limited lymphatic extension peripheral to the mediastinal pleural reflection at the hilum reduces estimated survival by 13 percent at 5-years. With further extension to the intrathoracic mediastinal lymph nodes, sur- vival drops 38 percentage points. With respect to the prognostic effect of lymph node involvement, survival estimates based on clinical criteria paral- lel these data based on surgical staging.

In the section on technical factors, the limit- ed circumstances under which definitive resec- tion appears justified in the presence of proven mediastinal lymph node involvement will be dis- cussed. The important principle that these data support is that any evidence of disease within the mediastinal lymph nodes forewarns of a very poor prognosis. Approximately 25 percent of resected cases of epidermoid carcinoma with hilar lymph node involvement will also have mediastinal lymph node metastases. The propor- tions in large cell carcinoma and adenocarcinoma are nearly twice as high. These observations strongly support the rationale for advising objec- tive assessment of the mediastinum by mediasti- noscopy or mediastinotomy prior to thora- cotomy.

The actual distribution and frequency of lymph node involvement in bronchogenic carci- noma are unknown. Reports in the literature vary widely and are conditioned by the stage distribu- tion of the cases being reported and by the magni- tude of the diagnostic and evaluative profile and the care with which it is obtained. Estimates based on a collected series of published reports[5-9] suggest that 50 percent of patients with epider- moid carcinoma will have positive hilar or mediastinal lymph node metastases at first diag- nosis. This compares to an estimated 68 percent with adenocarcinoma, 57 percent with undifferen- tiated large cell carcinoma, and 76 percent with undifferentiated small cell carcinoma. Further insight may be gained from our evaluation of 835 patients undergoing resection. It must be remem- bered that all of these patients were judged resectable on clinical grounds. An apparent com- plete resection was possible in almost 40 percent of the total group. This refers to those cases with the highest expectation for survival and, by defi- nition, embodies the following criteria: (1) the surgeon is morally certain that he has encom- passed all known disease; (2) the proximal mar- gins of the resected specimen are microscopically free of malignant disease; (3) within each major lymphatic drainage region (subcarinal, peritra- cheal, subaortic, periesophageal, etc.) the most peripheral node in the dissection is microscopi- cally free of tumor; (4) capsules of resected nodes are intact. Table 14-2 shows the proportion of patients in our lung cancer population who com- prised this select resected group, as well as the incidence of nodal involvement in each cell type. A number of patients in this series were operated on before our present policies evolved. This accounts for the presence of resected oat cell carcinoma cases and for the inclusion of adeno- carcinoma patients with positive mediastinal nodes.

The presence of metastases in the supraclav- icular and scalene lymph nodes carries an extra-

Table 14-2

Frequency of Apparent Complete Resection and Lymph Node Involvement by Cell Type

Cell Type	Apparent Complete Resections (%)	All Nodes Negative (%)	Hilar Nodes Only Positive (%)	Mediastinal Nodes Positive (%)
Epidermoid carcinoma	49	62	25	13
Adenocarcinoma and undifferentiated large cell carcinoma	34	45	31	24
Undifferentiated small cell (oat cell) carcinoma	9	50	44	6

heavy burden of mortality and precludes surgical intervention. In practiced hands such asssssment is highly correlated with the results of biopsy. In the presence of such extensive disease less than 0.5 percent of patients will survive 5 years. Any other manifestation of distant spread, beyond the confines of one hemithorax and its adjacent mediastinum, has similar prognostic implications. With the exception of a few cases that are highly selected by precise criteria, direct extension of the primary tumor into mediastinal structures portends a similar outcome.

The postsurgical treatment stage classification describes the known anatomic extent of disease based on complete histologic examination of a therapeutically resected specimen.[10] The same TNM definitions and stage grouping adopted for clinical staging of lung cancer, as discussed in detail in chapter 12 of this book, have been shown to be applicable to surgical staging.[1] Factors that argue for a favorable prognosis following definitive resection are as follows: (1) tumor size less than 3 cm in diameter, totally confined to the parenchyma of one lung; (2) a peripheral location or margination of malignancy at least 2 cm distal to the carina; (3) atelectasis or obstructive pneumonitis limited to a segment or a lobe with no pleural effusion; (4) no involvement of hilar or mediastinal lymph nodes; (5) no distant metastases; (6) a cell type other than undifferentiated small cell (oat cell) carcinoma. The probability of long-term survival is reduced in the presence of hilar lymph node metastases, and it is significantly lessened if the disease extends to the mediastinal nodes. Any major direct extension into the mediastinum, the presence of a pleural exudate or transudate containing malignant cells, or extension beyond the hemithorax of primary involvement are all factors of fatal consequence that preclude successful surgical therapy. If a lesion is less than 3 cm in diameter, hilar lymph node involvement is not a grave deterrent to successful outcome (stage I disease: T1 N0 M0, T1 N1 M0, T2 N0 M0). However, in the presence of a larger lesion, hilar lymph node involvement has a more deleterious effect (stage II, T2 N1 M0), particularly in adenocarcinoma and large cell carcinoma. Those factors responsible for the behavioral characteristics of each morphologic group are not well understood. However, the bidirectional effects of morphology and the extent of the disease in predicting survival are evident.[11] It is clear that the reporting of end results must include a stratification of experience according to stage and morphology if meaningful interpretations are to be realized.

PHYSIOLOGIC DETERMINANTS OF OPERABILITY

It is particularly true in lung cancer that host factors such as pulmonary reserve and cardiovascular function limit the feasibility of definitive surgical therapy. Common factors in the environmental background and the aging process that characterizes the lung cancer population are invariably associated with some degree of cardiopulmonary impairment. The essence of the preoperative physiologic evaluation is to determine which patients can reasonably be expected to survive the required surgery. To complicate matters, the preoperative surgical plan is largely judgmental and is often subject to change during the course of exploratory thoracotomy. Accordingly, what is planned as a lobectomy may frequently become a pneumonectomy. Clearly it would be desirable to have a specific set of rules that would delineate the individual physiologic risk for each surgical candidate. Unfortunately, such a set of rules does not exist, and an explicit index of physiologic risk has yet to be devised. However, the most important physiologic factors can be roughly quantified and projected in terms of surgical risk. In predicting a patient's ability to survive a pulmonary operation the severity of any observed impairment must be matched to the anticipated extent of resection. In view of the seriousness of the malignant process, physiologic criteria tend to be liberal.

The impact of reduced ventilatory function subsequent to pulmonary resection must be considered in terms of its interaction with other major organ systems. This is especially important in judging cardiac reserve. Moreover, during the course of general anesthesia pronounced physiologic changes occur that are unrelated to pulmonary resection. These may be reflected in a decreased minute ventilation and may be associated with varying degrees of hypoxemia.[12] The most common cause of arrythmias in patients with normal preoperative electrocardiograms probably relates to hypoxemia associated with induction of anesthesia.

A serious reduction in the patient's pulmonary ventilatory reserve and the presence of significant cardiovascular, hepatic, or renal disease are major general contraindications to resectional pulmonary surgery.[13] It is of much greater value to assess the patient's physiologic age than it is to rely rigidly on chronologic age. The presence of uncorrected dehydration, a poor nutritional status, or anemia adds to the risk of anesthesia, as with any other type of major surgery.[14] Abnormal electrolyte concentrations and acid–base imbalance may lead to serious cardiac arrhythmias. An excess of serum calcium or a deficiency of serum potassium tends to cause cardiac irritability and can potentiate the effects of digitalis.[15]

The most common causes of postoperative morbidity and mortality relate to cardiac and respiratory complications. It is vital that the reserve capacity of these interrelated organ systems be carefully evaluated. The cardiac complications most frequently encountered are arrhythmias, myocardial failure, myocardial infarction, and cardiac arrest.

Pulmonary insufficiency resulting from the loss of functioning lung tissue at one time accounted for about 40 percent of operative deaths. With the general availability of more reliable methods for assessing ventilatory function in recent years, and particularly with the introduction of ^{133}Xe scanning, this figure has been markedly reduced. Some degree of preexisting pulmonary insufficiency is a contributing cause of death in the majority of patients who develop pulmonary embolism, infection, and myocardial infarction.

In the total spectrum of physiologic assessment, the nature and extent of anomalies observed within the cardiopulmonary system lend themselves to more structured criteria of operability, as related to surgical hazard, than do other parameters. If a documentable myocardial infarction has occurred within the previous 3 months, thoracic surgery is contraindicated. Patients undergoing general anesthesia within 3 months following a myocardial infarction were reported on by Tarhan and associates.[16] Within the first postoperative week 37 percent of the group had recurrent myocardial infarction, with a mortality rate of 54 percent. A contraindication to major resection is explicitly implied by evidence of pulmonary hypertension, as might be shown on the electrocardiogram, by cardiac catheterization studies, or by ^{133}Xe scanning. Uncontrolled

arrhythmia, such as multifocal premature ventricular contractions, is a manifestation of serious myocardial ischemia and carries a high risk factor. A history of angina is not by itself a contraindication to pulmonary resection if a Master's test or other stress tests are negative. Arteriography should be obtained in patients with significant coronary insufficiency when their tumors are classified as biologically favorable and are technically resectable by a conservative procedure. Where such coronary disease is surgically correctable, simultaneous tumor resection and coronary bypass may be considered. Overall, about 10 to 15 percent of all patients evaluated for lung cancer surgery will have definitive abnormalities by electrocardiography. Surgical intervention is not precluded by a bundle branch block. From the viewpoint of risk assessment, a right bundle branch block or a left anterior fascicular block carries the least risk for the patient. Left posterior fascicular blocks are intermediate in risk, and combination or bifascicular blocks hold the highest risk.

A complete pulmonary function evaluation should (1) indicate patients who are at high risk for simple thoracotomy, (2) suggest a ventilatory risk factor for pulmonary resection, (3) estimate the maximum tolerated extent of pulmonary resection, and (4) predict the postresection ventilatory capacity. Such studies are designed to detect irregularities of ventilation and perfusion and abnormalities in the interchange of oxygen and carbon dioxide between the alveoli and pulmonary capillary bed. Spirometric determinations of ventilatory function such as the vital capacity (VC), forced vital capacity (FVC), forced expiratory flow (FEF), and maximum voluntary ventilation (MVV) are familiar procedures.

In a study of the preoperative evaluation of dyspneic surgical candidates it was found that all of the patients with maximum breathing capacities of less than 40 percent prior to pulmonary resection had fatal cardiopulmonary impairment postoperatively.[17] In this same group 90 percent of patients having maximum breathing capacities greater than 40 percent survived. In our experience, however, measures of maximum air flow are the most reliable and most prognostically significant mechanical ventilatory indices of the patient's ability to tolerate pulmonary surgery. Provisional quantitative evaluation of patients may be made on the basis of the volume forcibly exhaled in the first second (FEV_1). It is possible to place patients into one of three categories according to this simple index: (1) if the FEV_1 is 2.5 liters or more the patient can tolerate pneumonectomy; (2) if the FEV_1 is less than 1 liter the patient cannot tolerate any loss of functional lung tissue; (3) if the FEV_1 lies between 1.1 and 2.4 liters of flow, both the risk of any resection and the estimate of the maximum tolerable resection remain judgmental or must be resolved by further study. The great limitation of simple indices of total function, even when supplemented by information from arterial blood-gas studies, is that the majority of lung cancer patients fall into the third group. A number of patients who appear to be marginal with respect to surgical risk may readily tolerate even extended resection if the burden of the ventilatory defect is in the tumor-bearing lung. In the presence of major shunting on the affected side, such patients may even be benefited by resection.

Weighing information obtained from split function studies will improve judgment, but superior data are derived from regional pulmonary function studies using ^{133}Xe gas. This technique has shown itself to be of great value in judging the degree of resection that can be tolerated. The percentages of ventilation and pulmonary blood flow between and within the two lungs may be determined. The value of this tool in predicting postoperative functional status has been demonstrated through studies that correlate the preoperative and postoperative determinations.[18] The technique and normal values have been described. Indices of regional functional distribution are presented as ratios of perfusion and ventilation to unit volume. An example of preoperative and postoperative regional pulmonary function evaluations is shown in Fig. 14-2. This example of a patient with bilateral apical emphysema illustrates the excellent correlation observed between regional function and structural disruption.

Pneumonectomy is functionally tolerable if the percentage of ventilation to the non-tumor-bearing lung when multiplied by the FEV_1 equals 1 liter or more of flow. In defining the adequacy of ventilation, the level of arterial CO_2 is particularly important. The loss of any functional pulmonary tissue probably cannot be tolerated by patients having any preoperative evidence of CO_2 retention. Pneumonectomy is similarly tolerable if the percentage ventilation and perfusion within the unaffected lung are normal by ^{133}Xe scan and there is a normal rising gradient from apex to base with no major defect observed. The volume of the non-tumor-bearing lung should not exceed its ventilation by more than 5 percent; there is a

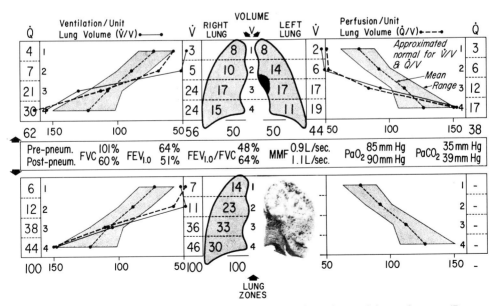

Fig. 14-2. Regional pulmonary function study: Patient with bilateral upper lobe emphysema. (Reproduced by permission from Ali MK, Mountain CF, Miller JM et al: Regional pulmonary function before and after pneumonectomy using ^{133}xenon. Chest 68:293, 1975.)

great chance of postpneumonectomy ventilatory failure if the volume exceeds the ventilation by more than this amount. In this group of patients, ranging from borderline to operable, zonal functional defects within the non-tumor-bearing lung are common. The occurrence and severity of these defects increase as the FEV$_1$ decreases, indicating that the loss of regional function is the result of chronic obstructive lung disease. Within the tumor-bearing lung functional impairment probably is related to the proximity of the tumor to the hilum.[19] There were no deaths from respiratory failure in the reported study, which confirms the value of the method in rejecting bad-risk cases.

If a minor prepneumonectomy defect exists in the non-tumor-bearing lung, it will persist and usually become worse following resection. If the lung is initially healthy, as indicated by regional function studies, it usually remains healthy following surgery, and the volume and ventilation ratios remain stable. Our current practice, which provides an entirely adequate and satisfactory preoperative evaluation of pulmonary function,

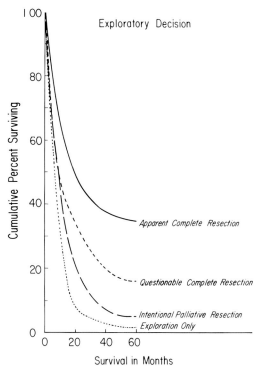

Fig. 14-3. Survival in lung cancer: Relationship of exploratory decision to survival.

employs combined studies of mechanical lung function, arterial blood-gas analysis, and regional function by ^{133}Xe gas.

TECHNICAL DETERMINANTS RELATED TO RESECTABILITY

The current criteria of surgical resectability and the proportion of long-term survivors following definitive surgical therapy are relatively uniform throughout urban areas of the United States. The mortality rate of surgery will vary between 4 percent and 10 percent. The end-result experience of an individual surgeon will be conditioned by his judgment in assessing physiologic operability and by the proportion of his patients that fall into each morphologic-anatomic stage group. Differences in technical competence among the majority of surgeons performing lung cancer surgery appear to be small. Accordingly, this factor plays a lesser role in the final outcome of management. Among the general population of patients with lung cancer, it is estimated that 43 percent will undergo thoracotomy. Approximately 33 percent will have definitive resection, 5 to 8 percent will be explored for diagnosis or evaluation of disease extent, and 5 percent will have a palliative procedure or there will be known residual tumor. Regional cancer centers and other institutions specializing in cancer therapy will see a higher proportion of far-advanced and inoperable cases. Their incidences of diagnostic and exploratory thoracotomy may be less, and their rates of resectability will be somewhat higher. The relationship between the preoperative intent of the surgeon and survival is shown in Fig. 14-3. The surgeon's judgment regarding the probable extent of tumor, as based on exploratory findings, and its relationship to survival are shown in Fig. 14-4.

The selection of the appropriate surgical procedure in resectable patients is influenced by the size of the tumor, its topographic extent, and the physiologic status of the patient. While the planned extent of surgery should be carefully assessed preoperatively, the actual extent of resection remains a matter of surgical judgment based on the findings at exploration. The surgeon should select and follow a procedure that will encompass all known disease and offer the patient the optimum opportunity for long-term survival if such a plan is technically and physio-

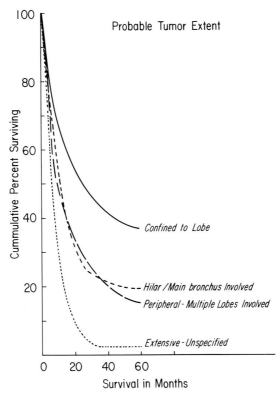

Probable Tumor Extent

— Confined to Lobe

--- Hilar /Main bronchus Involved

— Peripheral - Multiple Lobes Involved

...... Extensive - Unspecified

Fig. 14-4. Survival in lung cancer: Relationship of exploratory findings to survival.

logically feasible. In general, the procedure of choice is the one that provides the greatest opportunity for complete ablation of the malignant condition and also allows for the maximum conservation of lung tissue. Among patients of equivalent disease status where conservative pulmonary resection is both technically and biologically feasible, it has been repeatedly noted that the average disease-free interval is equal to that obtained with more extensive procedures.[20-22] Predictably, there are less morbidity and mortality associated with the more limited surgery. However, as noted by Brock,[23] the chance for cure should never be endangered by an overly conservative policy. In the final act of surgery, therefore, it is mandatory that an individualized approach be taken that accounts for all determinants discussed.

The terms pneumonectomy, lobectomy and bilobectomy, and segmental and wedge are commonly used to denote the type and extent of pulmonary resection. Wedge resections disregard segmental anatomy and may involve a portion of one segment, but more commonly they transgress segmental planes. The terms sleeve resection and sleeve lobectomy, more recently introduced, refer to removal of a main bronchus, with the tracheobronchial continuity reestablished. Procedures for peripheral tumors invading the thoracic cage are referred to as en bloc chest wall resections. In our own practice, to better understand the analysis of end results, we use the modifying terms standard, extended, and radical to more fully designate the extent of lobectomy and pneumonectomy. The standard lobectomy or pneumonectomy encompasses all of the regional lymph nodes in the vicinity of the bronchial transection. In the extended procedure a major effort is made to remove all lymph nodes accessible within the mediastinum. The classification of radical pneumonectomy is reserved for those cases in which an intrapericardial ligation is undertaken. Unfortunately, surgeons do not widely subscribe to any convention with respect to definition of such modifying terms. If there is no evidence of residual disease the procedure is classified as "apparently complete," as previously defined. When residual disease is known to be present following resection, it should be recorded in the description of the operative procedure.

In operable patients with non–oat-cell carcinoma, surgeons unequivocally agree that definitive resection in stage I and stage II disease is the treatment of choice. Pneumonectomy, lobectomy, and in uncommon circumstances even segmental or wedge resections may be undertaken. When there is an option in the matter, increasing numbers of surgeons are electing to perform lobectomy, in view of the high correlation between advancing age and postoperative mortality following pneumonectomy. In the uncommon circumstance of a patient with poor pulmonary reserve, negative lymph nodes, and a lesion 3 cm or less in diameter lying at the periphery of the lung, resection may be limited to a wedge excision or segmentectomy. Recent reports in the literature indicate that the results of such a conservative approach may be equivalent to those of lobectomy.[20,22] It must be remembered, however, that such series are very highly selected, and such limited resections may not prove advisable as a general rule. Lobectomy is indicated for lesions totally confined within a lobe, so as to permit at least 1 cm of normal lobar bronchus proximally. There should be no gross evidence of lymph node involvement central to the origin of the lobar bronchus. Meticulous attention should be paid to en bloc dissection of the regional lymph nodes, and frozen-section studies should be available during the course of surgery as a guide to the adequacy of resection. Pneumonectomy is indicated in the presence of more extensive involvement. There is some evidence to suggest that survival is improved following extended procedures, as compared to standard lobectomy and pneumonectomy.

Within stage III disease there are several categories of disease extent in which tumors remain technically resectable and for which definitive surgery remains a valid option. With appropriate selection of cases there is significant potential for long-term survival, which is particularly evident in epidermoid carcinoma. This includes superior sulcus tumors with painful apical syndrome, other peripheral tumors with direct chest wall invasion, small central tumors amenable to tracheal bronchial resection or sleeve lobectomy and epidermoid and large cell carcinomas with limited mediastinal lymph node extension.

Opinion is divided on recommending surgery in the face of x-ray or biopsy evidence of mediastinal node involvement. Indeed, many physicians consider pulmonary resection to be contraindicated in these circumstances. Such attitudes are derived from the understanding that in the general lung cancer population any evidence of mediastinal lymph node metastasis portends a grave clinical outcome. In evaluating a series of 634 unselected cases with such involvement (stage III, N2) we found an overall cumulative 5-year survival rate of only 3 percent. However, the literature indicates that approximately 10 percent of these patients will survive 5 years following surgical resection. This is very consistent with our own overall experience in resecting these N2 cases, as demonstrated in Fig. 14-1. Definitive resection was carried out in 21 percent of these cases, and it was thought that all tumor had been removed. When these survival data were stratified by cell type, as shown in Table 14-3, it is seen that the surgical survival rate appreciably exceeds the surgical mortality rate in both epidermoid carcinoma and undifferentiated large cell carcinoma.

The overall contribution of surgery to survival in lung cancer, following apparent complete

Table 14-3
Survival in Stage III Lung Cancer with Positive Mediastinal Nodes following Apparent Complete Resection: Surgical Classification of Disease Extent

Cell Type	Cumulative Percentage Surviving 5 Years
Epidermoid carcinoma	13
Large cell carcinoma	11
Adenocarcinoma	2

Table 14-4
Survival in Lung Cancer following Apparent Complete
Resection by Postsurgical Stage

Cell Type	Cumulative Percentage Surviving 5 Years		
	Stage I	*Stage II*	*Stage III*
Epidermoid carcinoma	54	36	22
Adenocarcinoma and undifferentiated large cell carcinoma	51	21	12
Undifferentiated small cell carcinoma	0	0	0

resection, is summarized in Table 14-4 according to morphology and stage of disease. Attention is directed to the fact that the 5-year surgical survival rates in both stage I and stage II are considerably higher than generally perceived by the medical community.

Within stage I disease, small lesions with no lymph node involvement (T1 N0 M0) have a somewhat better prognosis than large lesions with negative nodes (T2 N0 M0). Either group will do better than small tumors with positive regional nodes (T1 N1 M0). Each of these subsets, however, shows a significantly better prognosis than does stage II disease. The results of resection in stage III epidermoid and large cell carcinoma with positive mediastinal nodes are hardly outstanding, but they are far superior to the results that would be achieved by other primary treatment modalities. Ongoing studies indicate that the survival rate is further improved if patients are selected, on the basis of mediastinoscopy, to include only those in whom the metastatic extent of disease is limited to the ipsilateral nodes of the tracheobronchial angle and/or subcarinal region. Our current surgical policy is derived from these observations, as supported by the published studies of others.[5-7,9,24] In physiologically able patients with stage III epidermoid or large cell carcinoma, extended pneumonectomy is recommended where the primary lesion is technically resectable with negative margins and the extent of nodal involvement is limited to the ipsilateral tracheobronchial angle or subcarinal space. We continue to resect in similar cases with more cephalad extension to the ipsilateral peritracheal nodes, but only if the capsules are intact. The biologic rationale for such surgery remains to be

justified. The presence of a positive inlet node is regarded as a contraindication, and we see no basis for definitive surgery in the presence of any contralateral peritracheal lymph node involvement. In patients with adenocarcinoma we regard the finding of positive mediastinal nodes as a contraindication to surgery, except in investigational therapeutic trials of adjunctive modalities, because survival doesn't equal operative mortality. The poor survival rate in patients undergoing intentional palliative resection, as shown in Fig. 14-3, severely limits the indications for such a procedure. In any resected stage III patient the probability of recurrent and/or metastatic disease is so high that some form of adjunctive therapy appears mandatory.[25] On the basis of the national prospective clinical trial of preoperative irradiation therapy,[26] we are forced to conclude that there is no benefit to be obtained from general application of this treatment strategy. We are currently investigating irradiation therapy in epidermoid carcinoma and polychemotherapy in adenocarcinoma and large cell carcinoma as postoperative adjuvants. With respect to epidermoid carcinoma, the report of Kirsh et al. is extremely encouraging. In patients with positive mediastinal nodes, extended pneumonectomy with postoperative radiotherapy has produced a 23.1 percent 5-year survival rate. This compares favorably with the 31 percent survival of patients in which nodal extension is limited to the hilar region.[27] In most reported series preoperative irradiation has been utilized as an adjunct to sleeve lobectomy or tracheobronchial sleeve resection. These procedures may be selected when the primary tumor involves a mainstem bronchus and an adjacent portion of lobar bronchus or when it is limited to a small area of trachea and carina. The indications for either procedure are very limited, but they have definite applicability, and a 5-year survival rate of approximately 30 percent may be expected with appropriate case selection.[28,29]

Superior sulcus tumors comprise a somewhat unique subset of the lung cancer population. Although locally invasive and frequently accompanied by incapacitating pain, these tumors tend to remain regional, and they are more radioresponsive than other bronchogenic carcinomas. Even in advanced stages the hilar, mediastinal, and supraclavicular nodes may be found negative for metastatic disease. It is important to distinguish between superior sulcus tumors associated with Pancoast's syndrome and superior sulcus tumors with painful apical syndrome; this is another instance where exact definition of regional extent is paramount in considering end results. The former group contains those cases with lytic lesions of adjacent bony structures, usually the second rib posteriorly and/or the adjacent vertebrae. Preoperative irradiation therapy with radical resection has been advocated in both categories of disease, with 5-year survival rates reported as high as 31 percent for combined groups.[30] In our own experience the patients with painful apical syndrome have an 18 percent 5-year survival rate, while those with Pancoast's syndrome have less than a 12 percent survival rate. We are currently evaluating the comparative salvage rates following Co^{60} irradiation in conjunction with high-energy neutron beam therapy in the presence of lytic lesions associated with superior sulcus tumors. In other peripheral lesions invading the chest wall the 5-year cumulative survival rate is 17 percent following en bloc chest wall resection and appropriate lung resection in association with adjunctive irradiation therapy postoperatively. The comparative survival dynamics for the various types of resection are demonstrated in Fig. 14-5.

In our own studies of apparent complete resections in non–oat-cell carcinoma, lobectomy provided a 5-year cumulative survival rate of 48 percent. Of those who survived more than 30 days from the time of operation, 13 percent died with recurrent or metastatic disease within the first 12 months, and the median survival for the group was 51 months. When stratified by cell type, 52 percent of the patients with epidermoid carcinoma survived 5 years (median survival 69 months) and 50 percent of the patients with adenocarcinoma survived 5 years (median survival 50 months). Survival expectation in large cell carcinoma following lobectomy was somewhat less, with 38 percent surviving 5 years (median survival 29 months). Following pneumonectomy the 5-year survival rate was 36 percent overall with a median survival of 20 months. Patients with epidermoid carcinoma are, again, in a clearly advantaged position, with 43 percent surviving 5 years (median survival 29 months), as compared to the 23 percent 5-year survival in adenocarcinoma and large cell carcinoma (median survival approximately 15 months). The unexpectedly high survival following radical pneumonectomy (40 percent at 5 years) undoubtedly reflects the biases introduced by patient selection and the disproportionate number of patients with epidermoid carcinoma falling into this resection category. However, our results are consistent with those reported by Brock in 1975.[23]

The optimist will find much that is encouraging in the contributions of surgical therapy and in its potential for cure in lung cancer. In an apparently localized state, about 60 percent of patients

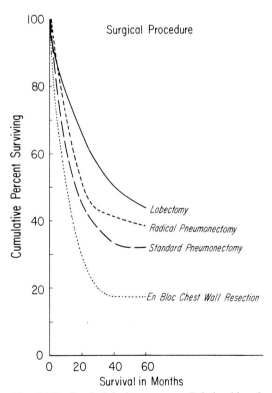

Fig. 14-5. Survival in lung cancer: Relationship of surgical procedure to survival.

will survive beyond 5 years, and at least 1 in 3 of those undergoing definitive surgical resection will have a similar long-term survival. The realist, however, must point out that far too few patients are diagnosed at an early stage of disease and that two-thirds of the patients undergoing curative surgery eventually die of local recurrence and/or disseminated metastatic disease. This relates to our inability to accurately measure the total tumor burden. The most common cause for the failure of definitive surgery to cure is the presence of undetected subclinical disease that is not manifest at the time treatment is instituted. In a study of similar patients by Matthews et al., half of those with epidermoid carcinoma had recurrent disease within the mediastinum, while those with adenocarcinoma and undifferentiated large cell carcinoma had distant metastatic foci of disease within 30 days of curative surgery.[31] Accordingly, it would appear that the best hope for improving the survival rate for resectable patients is through therapeutic strategies of regional and/or systemic treatment. A strong and rational theoretical basis exists for this concept, and in light of our current understanding it is imperative that we explore new methods. In view of the results of surgery alone in stage I disease, such adjunctive treatment will have to have a special ease of administration and exceptional safety with relative freedom from side effects. These restraints will be progressively less rigid as we pass through stage II and on to stage III disease. Of current interest is the possible role of immunotherapy in the multimodality scheme. The relationship between nonspecific immunocompetence and prognosis has recently been established (see Chapter 16). Preliminary clinical investigations of nonspecific agents such as intrapleural BCG and levamisole have shown promise for their use as surgical adjuvants in stage I disease.[32,33] Prospective randomized clinical studies of adjuvant specific immunotherapy and nonspecific immunotherapy are now in progress and should provide new directions for surgical treatment planning.

SUMMARY

In each individual case of lung cancer the therapeutic decision should involve a weighted balance between various biologic, physiologic, and technical factors. The decision-making process in selecting the surgical patient depends on the clinical biologic nature of the important morphologic patterns of this disease and their interrelationships with carefully defined physiologic parameters. The immediate future clearly lies with multimodality adjunctive therapy, and surgeons must be ready to utilize applicable developments as soon as they can be confirmed efficacious and safe.

REFERENCES

1. Mountain CF: Assessment of surgery in the control of lung cancer. Ann Thorac Surg (submitted for publication)
2. Hansen HH, Muggia FM, Selawry OS: Bone marrow examination in 100 consecutive patients with bronchogenic carcinoma. Lancet 2:443, 1971
3. Mountain CF, Carr DT, Anderson WAD: A system for the clinical staging of lung cancer. Am J Roentgenol Radium Ther Nucl Med 120:130, 1974
4. Mountain CF: The data base for the AJCS system for the clinical staging of lung cancer. (unpublished)
5. Baker RR: The clinical management of bronchogenic carcinoma. Johns Hopkins Med J 121:401, 1967
6. De Larue NC, Starr J: A review of some important problems concerning lung cancer. II. The importance of complete preoperative assessment in bronchogenic carcinoma. Can Med Assoc J 96:8, 1967
7. Nohl HC: The present position relating to cancer of the lung. A three-year follow-up of classified cases of bronchogenic carcinoma after resection. Thorax 15:11, 1960
8. Reynders H: The value of mediastinoscopic study in ascertaining the inoperability of pulmonary carcinoma. J Int Coll Surg 39:597, 1963
9. Shah HH, Lambert CJ, Paulson DL, et al: Cervical mediastinal lymph node exploration for diagnosis and determination of operability. Ann Thorac Surg 5:15, 1968
10. American Joint Committee for Cancer Staging and End Results Reporting: Clinical Staging System for Carcinoma of the Lung. Chicago, 1973
11. Mountain CF: The relationship of prognosis to morphology and the anatomic extent of disease:

Studies of a new clinical staging system, in Israel L, Chahinian P (eds): Lung Cancer. New York, Academic (in press)

12. Baker RR, Stitik FP, Summer WR: Preoperative evaluation of patients with suspected bronchogenic carcinoma. Curr Probl Surg: 1–48, 1974

13. Mountain CF: Surgical complications and their treatment, in Bucalossi P, Veronesi U, Emanuelli H, et al (eds): I Tumori Polmonari. Milan, Italy, Casa Editrice Ambrosiana, 1975, pp 175–179

14. Tarhan S, Moffitt EA: Principles of thoracic anesthesia. Surg Clin North Am 53:813, 1973

15. Messick JM Jr, Dawson B: Trends in anesthesia for surgical treatment of acid peptic disease. Surg Clin North Am 51:993, 1971

16. Tarhan S, Moffitt EA, Taylor WF, et al: Myocardial infarction after general anesthesia. JAMA 220:1451, 1972

17. Miller RD: Preoperative pulmonary evaluation of the dyspneic surgical candidate. Surg Clin North Am 53:805, 1973

18. Ali MK, Mountain CF, Miller JM, et al: Regional pulmonary function before and after pneumonectomy using ^{133}xenon. Chest 68:288, 1975

19. Ali MK: Preoperative pulmonary function evaluation of the lung cancer patient, in Clark RL Jr, Howe CD (eds): Cancer Patient Care at M. D. Anderson Hospital and Tumor Institute. Chicago, Year Book, 1976, pp 224–231

20. Jensik RJ, Faber LP, Milloy FJ, et al: Segmental resection for lung cancer: A 15-year experience. J Thorac Cardiovasc Surg 66:563–572, 1973

21. Jensik RJ: Primary lung cancer, in Conn HT (ed): Current Therapy 1975. Philadelphia, WB Saunders, 1975, pp 101–105

22. Shields TW, Higgins GA: Minimal pulmonary resection in treatment of carcinoma of the lung. Arch Surg 108:420, 1974

23. Brock R: Survival after operation for lung cancer. Br J Surg 62:1, 1975

24. Brock R: Thoracic surgery and the long-term results of operation for bronchial carcinoma. Ann R Coll Surg 35:195, 1964

25. Mountain CF: Surgical prospects and priorities for clinical research. Cancer Chemother Rep 4:19, 1973

26. Mountain CF (collaborative report): Preoperative irradiation of cancer of the lung. Cancer 23:419, 1969

27. Kirsh MM, Rotman H, Argenta L, et al: Carcinoma of the lung: Results of treatment over 10 years. Ann Thorac Surg 21:371, 1976

28. Jensik RJ, Faber LP, Milloy FJ et al: Sleeve lobectomy for carcinoma. A ten-year experience. J Thorac Cardiovasc Surg 64:400, 1972

29. Paulson DL, Urschel HC Jr, McNamara JJ, et al: Bronchoplastic procedures for bronchogenic carcinoma. J Thorac Cardiovasc Surg 59:38, 1970

30. Paulson DL: The importance of defining location and staging of superior pulmonary sulcus tumors. Ann Thorac Surg 15:549, 1973

31. Matthews MJ, Kanhouwa S, Pickren J, et al: Frequency of residual and metastatic tumor in patients undergoing curative surgical resection for lung cancer. Cancer Chemother Rep 4:63, 1973

32. McKneally MF, Maver CM, Kausel HW: Regional immunotherapy of lung cancer with intrapleural BCG. Lancet 1:377, 1976

33. Study Group for Bronchogenic Carcinoma: Immunopotentiation with levamisole in resectable bronchogenic carcinoma: A double blind controlled trial. Br J Med 3:461, 1975

Oleg Selawry

15
Chemotherapy in Lung Cancer

Chemotherapy is indicated in close to 90 percent of all patients with lung cancer: in the 50 percent of patients who have distant metastases at the time of diagnosis and in an additional 40 percent who have progressive disease after surgery or after radiotherapy.[1] But actual use of chemotherapy lags behind potential use. A given patient might be moribund or might have major complications that prevent effective use of chemotherapy. Or the physician might think that the expected toxicity of chemotherapy would outweigh the potential benefit. Moreover, in the fast-moving field of chemotherapy it is becoming increasingly difficult to stay abreast of the most recent information on which drug or drug combination to choose for an individual patient. Therefore an attempt will be made to adapt presently available knowledge to the needs of the practicing physician. It is assumed that the reader is familiar with the basic concepts of chemotherapy. Detailed information on drug dosages, schedules, and toxicity is therefore omitted unless the drugs are used in an unusual way.

The subject is conveniently divided under the headings of general aspects, chemotherapy with single agents, drug combinations, and use of chemotherapy in connection with surgery, radiotherapy, and immunostimulation. The discussion is based on published data covering more than 15,000 patients and on the author's own experience as a practicing oncologist.

GENERAL ASPECTS

Indications

The most widely accepted indication for chemotherapy of lung cancer is the need for palliation of the progressively symptomatic patient, when symptoms occur within a previously irradiated area or when the symptoms are related to disseminated progressive disease beyond the control of radiotherapy. Such symptoms can be local (e.g., cough, pain, dyspnea) and/or systemic (e.g., tiredness, anorexia, weight loss). Alternatives to tumor-inhibiting chemotherapy include symptomatic measures such as analgesics for pain and for irritative cough and oxygen-air for dyspnea. These latter measures might be used concomitantly. They might be preferred in the terminal patient.

Much experimental evidence points to substantially higher efficacy of chemotherapy against early disease with small tumor masses; small

This work was supported in part by NIH Grant CA14395 and by a donation from Mr. Sanford Chobel.

The excellent secretarial help of Ms. Josie Sanchez is gratefully acknowledged.

199

lesions are likely to have an adequate blood supply, thus permitting drugs to reach the tumor cells, while large tumor lesions often contain poorly vascularized or even necrotic areas. Small tumor lesions harbor a higher proportion of actively dividing cells (Chapter 2); hence, drugs such as methotrexate, with predominant activity against actively dividing cells, have been shown to be more active against early disease when used at 3- to 4-day intervals.[2,3] Finally, chemotherapy (as radiotherapy) results in "proportionate cell kill", raising hopes for complete eradication of very small lesions of highly sensitive tumors.[4]

For lung cancer, suggestive evidence of the superiority of early chemotherapy of the asymptomatic patient is limited to small cell carcinoma, and no convincing evidence is available for the other cell types.[5,6]

Extension of the concept of early treatment to the adjuvant use of chemotherapy in connection with radiotherapy and with surgery, in the hopes of better palliation or cure, shows some promise for small cell carcinoma, and this will be discussed later.

Choice of Drugs

The choice of drugs or drug combinations depends foremost on the cell type of bronchogenic carcinoma, because the efficacy of drugs in general depends greatly on the cell type, as will be discussed later. Therefore, diagnosis by cell type is very helpful in making the choice of chemotherapy. Great care must be exercised in the choice of the therapeutic regimen, because the patient without prior chemotherapy has the best chance (and in many situations the only chance) for response.[7]

When equally effective drugs are available, the obvious choice is for the agent with the most easily controllable side effects and the agent with which the physician is most familiar.

Drug combinations should be used only when they are clearly superior to single drugs; currently available combinations will control lung cancer for a limited time only. Thus the physician who uses most of the effective drugs at once will have expended his resources needlessly and will have little in reserve if additional chemotherapy is required for progressive disease. Moreover, most chemotherapeutic agents have overlapping toxicity. Therefore, the dosages of most component agents must be decidedly reduced in combination

chemotherapy, and these agents are not usually used to full effect, except when combinations are synergistic. The effective combination with the smallest number of drugs is the combination of choice.

Patients who fail to respond or who relapse after initial response usually have a lower response rate than previously untreated patients.[7] Their diseases might be more advanced, their tumors might be more resistant, or their dose-limiting normal tissues (e.g., hematopoietic cells, oral mucosa) might be more vulnerable. In this situation the most effective non-cross-resistant drugs are chosen.

Intensity of Treatment

Experimental evidence points to an optimal dosage for treatment. Suboptimal dosage results in insufficient control of disease, while overdosage leads to shorter survival because of toxicity.[2] Clinical evidence points in the same direction. This is exemplified by a double-blind comparative clinical trial where patients were allocated at random to receive either placebo or methotrexate at a low dosage of 0.2 mg/kg or methotrexate at a high dosage of 0.6 mg/kg twice weekly for 4 months[8] (longer in case of response). The formulations of methotrexate and placebo were indistinguishable to the physician and to the patient. Patients with leukopenia lived longer than patients without leukopenia. This held true in all three treatment groups, including the placebo group and including the entire patient population, irrespective of tumor regression. The same held true for patients with oral ulcerations on methotrexate. Data for methotrexate at 0.6 mg/kg are presented in Table 15-1. It is recommended, therefore, that one start chemotherapy at standard dosage and adjust the dosage upward or downward to the individual tolerance of each patient, inducing moderate, readily reversible toxicity, such as leukopenia between 3000 and 4000 cells/mm^3 and/or occasional oral ulcerations.

Duration of Treatment

Once chemotherapy is started, it should be given an adequate chance to act. It usually takes between 3 and 6 weeks to induce dose-limiting toxicity. Treatment should be stopped when progressive disease occurs in the presence of dose-limiting toxicity.

Table 15-1

Relation of Toxicity to Median Survival in Patients with Lung Cancer on Methotrexate 0.6 mg/kg Twice Weekly i.m.

Condition	Survival, Median Months	No. of Patients
No leukopenia; no oral ulcerations	1	19
Leukopenia < 4500 cells/mm³; no ulcerations	3	23
Leukopenia and ulcerations	5	31

Reproduced by permission of the author and publisher, from Selawry, OS et al: Methotrexate compared with placebo in the treatment of lung cancer. Cancer (in press).

In patients with objective response, chemotherapy is usually given for the duration of the response and/or for the duration of systemic response and symptomatic improvement. Continuation of a given treatment regimen beyond this point is undesirable because it is unlikely to retard progression. Instead, harm may be done to the patient if he experiences toxicity without therapeutic benefit. Moreover, toxicity will have to clear before a new chemotherapeutic regimen can be started.

Evaluation of Response

Everyone who treats lung cancer is aware of the difficulties in measuring tumor regression and progressive disease. The most widely accepted criteria for objective response include tumor regression by 50 percent or more of the product of the longest diameter and the widest perpendicular diameter of lesions regarded to be measurable by palpation or on chest films. Evaluable but nonmeasurable poorly outlined lesions are responding when regression is estimated to exceed 75 percent. Occurrence of new lesions or tumor progression of 50 percent or more elsewhere negates response and indicates progressive disease.[7] Response, as defined here, includes partial regression and complete regression. The latter signifies complete disappearance of all recognizable tumor masses.

These criteria are used throughout this chapter; but in some of the older literature referred to "partial regression" is not distinguished from "improvement," defined as 25 to 50 percent regression of well-outlined and usually palpable tumor lesions. Static disease with arrest of tumor growth (change of less than ±50 percent) after clear-cut tumor progression is rated by some authors as response and might prove valuable in the practice of oncology.[9]

The acuity of measurement can be augmented by endobronchial observation,[10,11] especially in areas where radiologic evaluation is obscured by pneumonitis and fibrosis following radiotherapy.[12]

On occasion the distinction between radiation pneumonitis or radiation fibrosis and progressive tumor involvement can pose a serious problem, as it did in one of the author's patients with small cell carcinoma. He was admitted with fever of 101.4°F and markedly increased shortness of breath. The chest film showed changes compatible with radiation pneumonitis in the rectangular field of previous radiotherapy over the left lung; a small infiltrate in the right lung was compatible with bronchopneumonia. Cultures were taken, and broad-spectrum antibiotics were administered. Prednisone was given, hopefully to counteract pneumonitis. All this occurred in the presence of almost complete regression of cervical lymph node metastases while on chemotherapy.

The day after admission the patient went into respiratory failure. Heroic efforts to save the patient (because of apparent response to chemotherapy) failed. The autopsy showed extensive lymphangitic tumor growth in the radiation field of the left lung and less pronounced lymphangitic spread in the right lung.

Table 15-2
Relation of Tumor Regression to Survival

Drugs	Cell Type	Survival, Median Months		No. of Patients		$p \leqslant 0.05$	Reference
		Resp.	*Nonresp.*	*Resp.*	*Nonresp.*		
Adriamycin	All types	7.3	6.3	11*	12*	0	15
CCNU, methyl-CCNU		12.6	2.3	6	79	+	16
Mechlorethamine		7.0	3.5	8	13	†	17
Thiotepa		17.3	7.9	5	43	†	43
Methotrexate	Epidermoid	8.3	4.7	10	61	†	19
	Adeno.	8.0	4.3	4	24	†	
	Large cell	8.0	4.0	5	24	†	

*Previously untreated patients.
†No statement on significance.

Other criteria for response are worth following on a research basis. Sputum cytology might give clues for response,[10,11] and marker substances (Chapter 3) have shown some correlation to response, while correlation to progressive disease has been less reliable. It should be pointed out, however, that markers as the sole criterion for tumor response can be misleading. This is illustrated in one of the author's patients with bronchogenic adenocarcinoma who was followed with serial determinations of CEA. CEA level before thoracotomy was 12 ng/ml. Thoracotomy revealed nonresectable tumor. CEA after surgery was 11.4 ng/ml. Subsequent CEA levels increased gradually to above 60 ng/ml, while the patient underwent combined radiotherapy to the tumor bed and chemotherapy and while follow-up with chest films, tomograms, transverse tomography, etc., showed no evidence for progressive disease. Within 1 month after radiotherapy the CEA fell to 14 ng/ml. Two weeks later a subcutaneous metastasis was noted and proven by biopsy. In the meantime a second lesion occurred elsewhere.

Symptomatic improvement and systemic improvement in terms of ambulation, increased appetite, and weight gain are usually (but not always) associated with objective response. The duration of response is commonly defined as the time from onset of objective tumor regression to the first sign of progressive disease, as defined above. The time from onset of treatment to the onset of progressive disease is usually a yardstick for evaluation of chemotherapy as adjuvant to surgery. In both cases, progressive disease might

or might not be preceded by nonspecific symptoms such as malaise and weight loss or by symptoms or signs related to local progression of disease (Chapter 6).

Under certain circumstances survival becomes an important additional measure of response. Thus objective regression might be too transient or might have been achieved at too high a price in terms of toxicity to be of therapeutic value. Therefore, improved survival of responders over nonresponders is a desirable criterion of response. Illustrative examples are given in Table 15-2. In all but one study there is a strong correlation between objective response and longevity, with responders living two to four times as long as nonresponders.

Conversely, mean or median survival as the sole criterion of response initially appeared foolproof as a reliable measure[13,14] for the evaluation of chemotherapy. However, detailed analysis of these data indicates that the median survival for successive cohorts of 60 or more patients treated with placebo by the same physicians varied by more than 50 percent, despite staging of patients with inoperable regional disease limited to one hemithorax with or without ipsilateral cervical lymph node involvement, as opposed to patients with more extensive disease.[13,14]

A special case is included in this general discussion—the case of cerebral metastases. There is no hard evidence for or against a blood-brain barrier for cerebral metastases that would make them less accessible to chemotherapy. Nevertheless, there is a widely held impression that at least the non-lipid-soluble drugs do not reach cerebral metastases. This is based on the observation that progressive cerebral metastases can develop in patients with continued systemic tumor response. Occurrence of cerebral metastases as the only sign of progressive disease is therefore not usually regarded as a failure of systemic chemotherapy.

EFFECTS OF SINGLE DRUGS

The effect of chemotherapy varies considerably with cell type. Therefore the usefulness of single drugs will be described under the headings of the major cell types of lung cancer.

The response rates for each drug are derived from a review of the literature. They represent averages, and they may serve as general guidelines, with the understanding that the relative ranking may change as new data become available, especially where the number of observations is small.

Epidermoid Carcinoma

Epidermoid carcinoma (Table 15-3) is relatively resistant to chemotherapy. Hard evidence for the superiority of polychemotherapy over monochemotherapy is lacking. It is useful, therefore, to consider chemotherapy with single agents for palliation of the symptomatic patient. The list is headed by methotrexate, followed by three alkylating agents, dibromodulcitol, cyclophosphamide, and mechlorethamine (HN_2, nitrogen mustard); all of them have comparable response rates of 21 to 25 percent.

The popularity of each drug as expressed in the number of patients treated adds an interesting dimension. Cyclophosphamide appears to be the

Table 15-3

Objective Response of Epidermoid Carcinoma of the Lung to Single Drugs

Drug	Percentage Responding	Patients Treated	References (3 and the following)
Methotrexate	25	83	8
	16*	157	19
Dibromodulcitol	23	39	21
Cyclophosphamide	22	280	22–25
Mechlorethamine (HN_2)	21	183	26
Vinblastine	16	20	
Adriamycin	14†	125	15
Fluorouracil	14	14	24
Procarbazine	13	55	
Hexamethylmelamine	12	68	
Bleomycin	12	278	18,27–29
CCNU	12	82	16,28,30,31
Methyl-CCNU	12†	112	32
Emetine, dehydroemetine	9†	34	33–36
BCNU	6	34	37
ICRF-159	6	15	38
Mercaptopurine	0	16	
Mitomycin C	0	22	

*Includes low-dose methotrexate and partial overlap with other data.
†Includes complete regressions.

most widely used drug, probably because of its ease of administration, when compared to the cross-resistant and equally effective mechlorethamine. Cyclophosphamide can be given directly i.v., whereas mechlorethamine is administered into the side arm of a rapidly running i.v. infusion. The drug is commonly given every 3 weeks. Thrombocytopenia, which could aggravate hemoptysis, is decidedly less common than with mechlorethamine or dibromodulcitol, which permits combination with other myelosuppressive agents.

The therapeutic margin for cyclophosphamide is wider than for dibromodulcitol with its potentially dangerous delayed marrow suppression. Thus the only advantage for dibromodulcitol might be seen in its better lipid solubility and hence its potential to affect cerebral metastases.

Methotrexate has a similar level of efficacy, but it requires adequate renal function. It rarely causes nausea or vomiting. Thrombocytopenia is uncommon with twice weekly oral dosage; instead, mucositis and oral ulcerations may develop, but they are readily reversible. Moreover, leucovorin (citrovorum factor) remains a readily available antidote in case of undue toxicity.

The combination of ultrahigh doses of methotrexate (1–18 g/dose) followed by leucovorin has been claimed to be superior to standard regimens of methotrexate.[20] This interesting research approach requires resources for the monitoring of serum levels of methotrexate and the monitoring of renal function, as well as the availability of blood components in case of toxicity. The future will show whether such expensive efforts are rewarded by superior response and survival.

Several other drugs can be considered for patients who fail to respond to methotrexate or cyclophosphamide, because they show no apparent cross-resistance. Two antibiotics, adriamycin and bleomycin, are commonly considered. Both are useful, but they have potentially hazardous cumulative toxicity for heart and lungs, respectively. Adriamycin offers the convenience of spaced dosage at 3-week intervals. Bleomycin is only mildly myelosuppressive and lends itself to weekly dosage. Vinblastine, fluorouracil, procarbazine, hexamethylmelamine, and CCNU or methyl-CCNU might be occasionally useful. Emetine, with a borderline response rate of 9 percent, is added to the list as a nonmyelosuppressive experimental agent that might lend itself

to combination chemotherapy. The remaining drugs in Table 15-2 are included as prominent negatives.

Small Cell Carcinoma

Small cell carcinoma (Table 15-4) is clearly the most chemosensitive cell type of lung cancer, possibly because it is the fastest growing, has the largest proportion of dividing cells (Chapter 2), and is rarely associated with central tumor necrosis, implying good vascularization (Chapter 4).

The rapid natural course of the untreated disease, the better response of the ambulatory patient to chemotherapy, and the better than 50 percent response rate to combination chemotherapy make small cell carcinoma the domain of elective polychemotherapy, including the asymptomatic patient. Treatment is frequently combined with radiotherapy when there is no positive evidence for distant metastases.

Because of these developments it becomes increasingly difficult to obtain representative new data on the response rate to single drugs, because most patients with small cell carcinoma receive chemotherapy with single agents only after they have failed on one or two combination regimens, and at that time their disease might be more resistant and their bone marrow might be inhibited by past chemotherapy.

Against this background, Table 15-4 serves a threefold purpose: as a resource for the understanding of currently used drug combinations, as background for the design of new drug combinations, and as an aid for the choice of single drugs when patients fail on combination chemotherapy.

Several observations warrant emphasis. Two plant products, vincristine and epipodophyllotoxin-ethylidene-glucoside, are near the top of the list, with response rates of 38 and 35 percent, respectively; both drugs inhibit mitosis in early metaphase and both drugs are DNA inhibitors. The latter is an insufficient explanation of their efficacy because of the low-order activity of methotrexate.

Cyclophosphamide, adriamycin, hexamethylmelamine, procarbazine, and two-nitrosoureas are substantially more effective against small cell carcinoma than against epidermoid carcinoma and are frequently used for drug combinations.

Surprisingly, bleomycin is probably ineffective against small cell carcinoma despite its frequent use in drug combinations.

Table 15-4
Objective Response of Small Cell Carcinoma of the Lung to Single
Drugs

Drug	Percentage Responding	Patients Treated	References (3 and the following)
Mechlorethamine	39	80	
Vincristine	38	21	39
Epipodophyllotoxin	35	23	40,41
Cyclophosphamide	32*	307	23,25,26
Adriamycin	28*	64	15
Hexamethylmelamine	26*	54	42
Procarbazine	25	44‡	
BCNU	21*	19	
CCNU	21*	47	16,28,31
Methotrexate	21	109	8,19
Dibromodulcitol	20	15‡	
Methyl-CCNU	11	44	32
Emetine, dehydroemetine	"22"	9‡	33,35,36
Mercaptopurine	"11"*	9	
Vinblastine	"33"†	9	
Mitomycin C	9	11	
Bleomycin	0	29	28
Fluorouracil	0	4	24

*Includes complete regressions.
†3 patients surviving for 1+ years.
‡Includes large cell anaplastic carcinomas.

Adenocarcinoma

Mitomycin is the unusual drug, with an apparently relatively high response rate against adenocarcinoma (Table 15-5). More data would be desirable to substantiate the ranking of this antitumor antibiotic.

Methotrexate and cyclophosphamide are similarly effective against epidermoid carcinoma; procarbazine and fluorouracil are likewise useful drugs. The position of fluorouracil is somewhat controversial; the response rate of 18 percent is likely to apply to previously untreated patients, while preceding intensive chemotherapy results in drastic reduction of response rate.*

As for epidermoid carcinoma, and in contrast to small cell carcinoma and large cell carcinoma, the nitrosoureas are unrewarding when used as single agents.

*Personal communication from D. Carr.

The data of Table 15-5 do not apply to bronchioloalveolar carcinoma as a subgroup of bronchogenic adenocarcinoma. Here response rates seem to be considerably lower; unfortunately, no larger series are available for guidance in the choice of chemotherapeutic agents.

In the day-to-day management of bronchogenic adenocarcinoma, one might wish to choose single agents after failure of combination chemotherapy (see below), using a mutually non-cross-resistant agent such as mitomycin, methotrexate, procarbazine, or fluorouracil.

Large Cell Carcinoma

The list of effective agents for treatment of large cell carcinoma (Table 15-6) is headed by procarbazine, with a response rate of 35 percent of 17 patients. Enlargement of this series would be desirable. As in small cell anaplastic carcinoma, two-nitrosoureas are among the most effec-

Table 15-5
Objective Response of Adenocarcinoma of the Lung to Single Drugs

Drug	Percentage Responding	Patients Treated	References (3 and the following)
Mechlorethamine	28	86	43
Mitomycin C	27	11	
Methotrexate	24	42	8,19
Cyclophosphamide	19	54	22,25–26
Procarbazine	19	16	
Fluorouracil	18*	28	24,44,45
Hexamethylmelamine	15	39	
Adriamycin	13	99	15
Bleomycin	13	31	28
CCNU	12	67	16,28,30,46
ICRF-159	10	20	38
Methyl-CCNU	10*	83	16,32,47–49
Emetine, dehydroemetine	"9"	11	35,36
Epipodophyllotoxin	"17"	6	41,50
Vinblastine	"17"	6	
Dibromodulcitol	8	12	
BCNU	0	22	
Mercaptopurine	0	9	

*Including complete regressions.

tive agents, followed by hexamethylmelamine, adriamycin, and methotrexate. The low-ranking response rate of only 13 percent for the latter is surprising. Chemotherapy with single agents appears indicated in patients who have failed on combination chemotherapy, using the highest non-cross-resistant agent in Table 15-6 as treatment of choice.

Drugs with Insufficient Data for Response by Cell Type

A number of widely used drugs received attention for treatment of lung cancer without adequate mention of response by cell type. Some of these drugs, notably hydroxyurea and DTIC, are included in drug combinations. Response rates for some of these drugs are listed in Table 15-7.

Local Chemotherapy

Intraarterial chemotherapy of local-regional lung cancer has repeatedly been explored. Drugs have usually been given through the bronchial artery. Fluorouracil and mechlorethamine, meth-otrexate followed by leucovorin, and mitomycin have been tried, but none of these proved superior to intravenous therapy. Thus intraarterial chemotherapy remains an investigational technique without proven clincal value.[52]

Topical treatment by means of aerosols would appear to be an interesting alternative, especially for a synchronous or metachronous second carcinoma in situ and for a bronchiolar carcinoma with spread along bronchial linings. Indeed, aerosols with tantalum dust less than 8 μ in particle size have proved useful for bronchographic delineation of tumor lesions,[53] and aerosols of two double-stranded RNA preparations from mycophage have prolonged survival of mice with pulmonary carcinogen-induced fibrosarcoma, as compared to untreated controls.[54] No clinical chemotherapeutic studies are on record.

DRUG COMBINATIONS

The following discussion is based on selected drug combinations. Preference is given to controlled clinical trials, because studies of small

Table 15-6

Objective Response of Large Cell Carcinoma of the Lung to Single Drugs

Drug	Percentage Responding	Patients Treated	References (3 and the following)
Procarbazine	35	17	
Mechlorethamine	26	148	26
Methyl-CCNU	21	43	32,47–49
CCNU	20	49	16,28,30,46
Cyclophosphamide	20	35	25,26
Hexamethylmelamine	18	39	
Adriamycin	17	64	15
Methotrexate	13*†	105‡	8,19
Emetine	"100"	1	35
ICRF-159	"12.5"	8	38
Mitomycin C	"50"	2	
Streptonigrin	"14"	7	
Vinblastine	"100"	2	
BCNU	9	22	
Mercaptopurine	3	29	
Epipodophyllotoxin	0	2	41
Fluorouracil	0	10	24
Bleomycin	0	4	27–29

*Including complete regressions.
†Including 20 patients labeled as anaplastic.
‡Reference 19 contains an unknown factor of overlap with reference 8 and includes "low-dose" methotrexate.

Table 15-7

Objective Response of Lung Cancer to Single Drugs with Insufficient Data on Response by Cell Type

Drug	Percentage Responding		Patients Treated	References (3 and the following)
	All Patients	Range		
Cytarabine	0	—	19	
Dactinomycin	0	—	16	
Dichloromethotrexate	9	—	22	55
Hydroxyurea	16	0–26	88	56
Imidazole carboxamide, dimethyl-triazeno	11	10–25	132	57
Mercaptopurine	3	0–4	105	
Mithramycin	0	—	23	
Thiotepa	15	7–32	141	

Table 15-8
Objective Response of Epidermoid Carcinoma to Drug Combinations

Drug		Percentage Response	No. of Patients	References
1a	5-FU+PROC	55	11	59
b	PROC	12	8	
2	ADR+BLEO+CCNU+HN$_2$+VCR	34	50	60
3a	CTX+MTX+PROC+VRC simultaneously	27	52	61
b	Same sequentially	10	29	
4a	CTX+MTX+PROC+VCR	25	16	5
b	ADR+CTX+CCNU+PROC+Hydroxyurea+MTX+VCR	11	19	
5a	CCNU+HN$_2$+MTX	12	17	20,62
b	HN$_2$+MTX	11	19	
6a	BLEO+CCNU	12	17	28
b	BLEO alone or CCNU alone	0	23	
7a	ADR+CCNU	11	19	63
b	ADR+CTX	3	15	
8a	CTX+Me-CCNU+VCR+BLEO	5	20	58
b	CTX	4	27	
9a	CCNU+HN$_2$	3	39	26
b	HN$_2$	10	41	

ADR = adriamycin, BLEO = Bleomycin, CTX = cyclophosphamide, 5-FU = Fluorouracil, HN$_2$ = mechlorethamine, Me-CCNU = methyl-CCNU, MTX = methotrexate, PROC = procarbazine, VCR = vincristine.

uncontrolled series of patients have led to unfounded optimism in the past. For example, a highly reputable group of investigators conducted a pilot study with COMB, a combination of the four drugs cyclophosphamide, vincristine (Oncovin), methyl-CCNU, and bleomycin. The choice of drugs was based on the apparent superiority of cyclophosphamide plus nitrosoureas over either drug alone in two experimental tumors and in small cell carcinoma, as well as on cell kinetic observations obtained in cell cultures implying that the sequential use of vincristine followed by bleomycin resulted in greater antitumor effect. The group reported an overall response rate of 38 percent in 12 evaluable patients with lung cancer, including partial tumor regression in 40 percent of 5 patients with epidermoid carcinoma.[47] The advantageous response rate for patients with epidermoid carcinoma continued when additional patients were added. The members of a cooperative study group (Working Party for Therapy of Lung Cancer) decided, therefore, to compare the new drug combination with cyclophosphamide as a standard control for treatment of patients with metastatic epidermoid carcinoma; only 20 of 33 patients assigned to COMB were deemed evaluable, and only 1 of these 20 patients responded.

Twenty-seven of the 31 patients assigned to cyclophosphamide (1100 mg/m^2 i.v. every 3 weeks) were evaluable. Again, only 1 patient responded (Table 15-8). Thus the regimens were equally ineffective, while COMB resulted in considerably more toxicity.[58]

Smaller uncontrolled series of patients are presented for illustration of general trends.

Combinations are described by cell type and ranked in order of reported response rates; as in the case of single agents, this ranking does not imply quantitative intercomparability of different studies.

Epidermoid Carcinoma

Only one of eight controlled clinical trials in epidermoid carcinoma (Table 15-8) offers any hope for superiority of a drug combination over the use of single drugs; fluorouracil plus procarbazine appears to be superior to procarbazine alone. Either drug alone has a response rate below 15 percent (v.s.). There is no background information implying more than an additive effect of these two drugs. Therefore confirmation of the data in a large group of patients would be desirable.

It is recommended, therefore, to consider the use of single drugs such as methotrexate at a starting dosage of 20 mg/m² twice weekly p.o. for treatment of the individual symptomatic patient with epidermoid carcinoma until such time as reliable information on the superiority of drug combinations becomes available.

Small Cell Anaplastic Carcinoma

The following discussion of small cell anaplastic carcinoma (Table 15-9) is based on 12 clinical trials, 7 of them controlled, including a total of 549 patients. Eleven of the 12 studies include objective responses in 52 to 92 percent of the patients. Between 3 and 7 of every 10 responders had complete tumor regression. Median durations of response (from onset of treatment) range between 3 and 10 months. The median survival of the treated patients ranges from 6 to 13 months, compared to approximately 2 months for untreated patients.[13,14]

No hard data are currently available on the quality of life of the treated patients. It appears, however, that the majority of patients are ambulatory while on treatment, with normal or close to normal performance status, except for 1–3 days at 3- to 4-week intervals when drugs like adriamycin, cyclophosphamide, and CCNU might cause nausea or vomiting. Most patients require weekly follow-up visits, with exceptions in either direction. The occasional patient with objective response might require hospitalization because of drug toxicity. This is rather uncommon in the hands of the experienced oncologist. Thus treatment is clearly worthwhile. Ambulatory patients, and those without recognizable distant metastases, have the highest response rates. Therefore, treatment is best started as soon as possible.

The choice of a particular drug combination depends on factors such as the efficacy of the treatment regimen per se, the experience of the oncologist with a given drug combination, and the functional status of the organ systems related to drug tolerance and to drug excretion. Several observations can be made on the efficacy of the treatment regimens per se:

1. Two controlled clinical trials (studies 6 and 12, Table 15-9) showed clear superiority of drug combinations over a single drug (cyclophosphamide) alone. The range of response rates of

patients on drug combinations is decidedly higher than the range of response rates of single agents. Hence the use of drug combinations is superior to the use of single drugs.

2. Only one controlled clinical trial showed superiority of three drugs (cyclophosphamide, CCNU, and methotrexate) over two drugs (cyclophosphamide and methotrexate) (study 9, Table 15-9).

3. There is no apparent correlation between the number of drugs used and response or median survival: two-drug combinations head the list and conclude the list of effective drug combinations. Moreover, the combination of two drugs (cyclophosphamide and methotrexate) that elicited a response rate of only 31 percent with a median survival of 6 months in study 9b, Table 15-9, resulted in a 91 percent response rate and a median survival of 13 months in pilot study 1 of Table 15-9. Contributing factors included the following: Stage of disease: both study 1 of Table 15-9 and study 9 included patients with extrathoracic metastases. However, the presence of extrathoracic metastases is usually associated with decreased survival. Dose schedule: both studies included intravenous administration of cyclophosphamide at 3-week intervals and oral dosage of methotrexate twice weekly. In study 1 methotrexate was given in courses, starting 1.5 weeks after each dose of cyclophosphamide, in the hope of hitting those cells that recovered from the widely spaced doses of cyclophosphamide. Study 9 included continuous twice-weekly administration of methotrexate. Inclusion of these cell kinetic considerations might have contributed to the success of study 1. The intensity of treatment varied greatly. The experienced investigator of study 1 was able to adjust his drug regimen to the individual tolerance of each patient, keeping the patient's leukopenic level safely at or below 3000 cells/mm³ and at the same time achieving higher dose levels of drugs. Patients on treatment 9b experienced much less hematologic toxicity.

4. Intensity of treatment: greater intensity of treatment (higher doses and more toxicity) results in higher response rates. This is best illustrated in a comparison of response rates for the three-drug combination of cyclophosphamide, CCNU, and methotrexate in studies 2, 4, and 9 of Table 15-9. The dose schedules were the same for studies 2 and 9, including administration of CCNU at 6-week intervals, cyclophosphamide every 3 weeks, and methotrexate twice weekly; in study 4

Table 15-9
Objective Response of Small Cell Carcinoma to Drug Combinations

	Drugs	Response Overall (%)	CR (%)	No. of Patients	Survival, Median Months	References
1	CTX→MTX	91	(64)	11	13	64
2a	CTX+MTX+CCNU, high dose	92	25	24		65
b	Same, standard dose	45	0	9		
3	ADR+CTX+DTIC+OH-Ur+MTX+VCR	92	(38)	13*		66
4a	CTX+MTX+CCNU+VCR	83		49	9	67
b	CTX+MTX+CCNU	75		47	6.5	
5a	ADR+CTX+CCNU+PROC→OH-Ur+MTX+VCR	81		26		5
b	CTX+MTX+PROC+VCR	68		22		
6a	ADR+CTX+DTIC	77		13		68
b	CTX	17		12	8	
7	ADR+BLEO+CTX+VCR	76	(21)	29	(6 CR=12+)	6
8	CTX+VCR	61		23	6	69
9a	CTX+MTX+CCNU	57		31	8.5	20,62
b	CTX+MTX	31		23	6	
10	CTX+Me-CCNU+VCR	54	(18)	22	9	70
11a	CTX+MTX+PROC+VCR simultaneously	52	(16)	25	9.5 resp.	61
b	Same sequentially	29	(6)	14	2 nonresp.	
12a	CTX+CCNU	45		83		26
b	CTX	28		88		

ADR = adriamycin, BLEO = Bleomycin, CTX = cyclophosphamide, MTX = methotrexate, OH-Ur = hydroxyurea, Me-CCNU = methyl-CCNU, PROC = procarbazine, VCR = vincristine.
*Includes at least 4 large cell carcinomas.

CCNU is started with 4-week cycles. Yet the response rates vary: 92, 75, and 57 percent. This is best explained by more intensive treatment. In study 2, patients were assigned at random either to standard dosages of drugs on an open ward or in an ambulatory care clinic (response rate 45 percent) or to substantially higher dosage while on intensive antibiotic treatment within or outside laminar air flow reverse isolation units. In the latter case methotrexate was given parenterally in order to circumvent malabsorption of the drug, and the response rate increased to 95 percent of 24 patients. As for study 4, it was conducted by the same investigator who played a major role in the conduct of study 9; he achieved a response rate of 75 percent of 47 patients, based on more intensive treatment. Hence the best clinical management includes adjustment of drug dosage to definite, safely reversible toxicity. This depends on the experience of the oncologist with a given drug combination.

The functional status of the patient's organ systems will modify the choice of drugs; a few illustrative examples include increased toxicity of methotrexate in the presence of renal failure and in the presence of effusion or edema, decreased tolerance to adriamycin and to vincristine with impaired hepatic excretory function, and the inadvisability of giving bleomycin to patients with preexisting, diffuse, debilitating pulmonary fibrosis.

The author's own current approach includes initiation of treatment with cyclophosphamide 1100 mg/m^2 i.v. at 3-week intervals, CCNU 50 mg/m^2 p.o. at 6-week intervals, and methotrexate 15 mg/m^2 twice weekly p.o. starting on day 8 after each dose of cyclophosphamide. Responding patients might receive radiotherapy to the bulk of residual tumor masses. Nonresponders or patients who escape response are treated with a non-cross-resistant drug combination such as adriamycin, procarbazine, and vincristine.

Adenocarcinoma

The paucity of data on adenocarcinoma (Table 15-10) leaves little middle ground. There is proof for superiority of the triple combination of cyclophosphamide, CCNU, and methotrexate over cyclophosphamide and methotrexate when given to comparable groups with moderate, readily reversible toxicity (study 5 in Table 15-10). Modification of the two-drug combination of cyclophosphamide and methotrexate, and intensification of treatment as described previously, led to a substantially improved response rate (study 1, Table 15-10) without corresponding

Table 15-10

Objective Response of Adenocarcinoma to Drug Combinations

		Percentage Response	No. of Patients	Survival, Median Months	References
1	CTX→MTX	63	8	7	64
2a	5-FU+PROC	83	6		59
b	5-FU	0	5		
3	CTX+MTX+PROC+VCR	71	7		61
4	BLEO→CTX+5-FU+MTX+VCR	35	17	8.5 resp. 3 nonresp.	71
5a	CTX+CCNU+MTX	30	20	8	
b	CTX+MTX	6	17	4.5	20,62
6	ADR+BLEO+VCR	25	8	5	38
7	ADR+CTX+CCNU+PROC+OH-Ur+MTX+VCR	0	7		5
8	ADR+miscellaneous other drugs	0	17		72
9	ADR+either CTX or CCNU	0	13		63
10a	CTX+CCNU	5	21		26
b	CTX	15	26		

ADR = adriamycin, BLEO = Bleomycin, CTX = cyclophosphamide, 5-FU = fluorouracil, PROC = procarbazine, MTX = methotrexate, VCR = vincristine, OH-Ur = hydroxyurea.

improvement of survival. Similarly good responses occurred with the combination of fluorouracil plus procarbazine in a randomized pilot study (study 2, Table 15-10). Surprisingly, drug combinations including adriamycin were unrewarding, with only 2 responders among 45 patients (studies 6–9, Table 15-10). The uniquely negative results with cyclophosphamide plus CCNU (study 10, Table 15-10) are puzzling in view of the above-stated superiority of cyclophosphamide plus CCNU when combined with methotrexate.

Making recommendations on treatment is admittedly arbitrary. Among the available options one might consider cyclophosphamide, 1100 mg/m^2 i.v. at 3-week intervals, followed by methotrexate, 20 mg/m^2 p.o. twice weekly, starting on day 8 after each dose of cyclophosphamide (in slight modification of an earlier regimen[64]). Alternatively, one might start with cyclophosphamide, CCNU, and methotrexate or with fluorouracil, 600 mg/m^2/week i.v. and procarbazine 100 mg/m^2 per day p.o. for the first 2 weeks of each month of treatment, in modification of another regimen.[59] Lack of response or relapse calls for use of a non-cross-resistant single drug.

Every oncologist and every chest physician encounters patients with bronchioloalveolar carcinoma as a less common subgroup of adenocarcinoma. Treatment is notoriously difficult, espe-

cially in the presence of bilateral pulmonary involvement. Occasional objective responses and subjective improvement have been reported with single drugs and with drug combinations, but no larger studies are available for guidance. In this situation it appears reasonable to limit chemotherapy to the symptomatic patient, using single drugs such as methotrexate or procarbazine, or the above-mentioned drug combinations, to moderate toxicity.

Large Cell Carcinoma

Large cell carcinoma (Table 15-11) has response characteristics of its own. For large cell carcinoma, as well as for small cell carcinoma (and in contrast to epidermoid carcinoma and adenocarcinoma), combinations including adriamycin are promising; there was an overall response rate of 61 percent of 23 patients who received a variety of additional drugs, as listed in Table 15-11.

For large cell carcinoma and epidermoid carcinoma (and in possible contrast to small cell carcinoma and adenocarcinoma) combinations of CCNU and an alkylating agent (mechlorethamine) are no better or worse than single agents (studies 4 and 5, Table 15-11). At first glance this is surprising, because CCNU as a single agent has comparable low-grade activity against all four cell

Table 15-11
Objective Response of Large Cell Carcinoma to Drug Combinations

	Percentage Response	No. of Patients	Comments	References
1 CTX+MTX	71	7	Including 2 complete regressions; median survival 12 months	64
2 ADR+other drugs	61	23	Summary of several papers	72
3 CTX+MTX+PROC+VCR simultaneously nonrandom	32	16		61
Same simultaneously randomized	33	9		
Same sequential randomized	14	7		
4 CCNU+HN$_2$	6	19		26
HN$_2$	16	17		
5 CCNU+HN$_2$+MTX	11	9		20,62
HN$_2$+MTX	8	13		

CTX = cyclophosphamide, ADR = adriamycin, VCR = vincristine, HN$_2$ = mechlorethamine, MTX = methotrexate, PROC = procarbazine.

types. Mechlorethamine is at least equal to cyclophosphamide in all cell types and was given preference over cyclophosphamide in these combinations because of its apparent superiority as a single agent for treatment of epidermoid carcinoma[13] and because pathologists in some of the cooperating institutions tended to assign poorly differentiated epidermoid carcinomas to the large cell category.[73] Whether the low order of activity of CCNU plus mechlorethamine was due to lack of synergism with this particular alkylating agent or whether thrombocytopenia (a common side effect of both mechlorethamine and CCNU) resulted in decreased tolerance remains an open question.

As for small cell carcinoma and large cell carcinoma, the sequential use of cyclophosphamide followed by methotrexate bears promise.

Thus the treatment of an individual patient with large cell carcinoma might be initiated with cyclophosphamide and methotrexate, keeping a non-cross-resistant combination such as adriamycin, procarbazine, and vincristine in reserve, or vice versa.

COMBINATIONS OF CHEMOTHERAPY WITH OTHER TREATMENT MODALITIES

Combinations of chemotherapy with other modalities of treatment can be divided into two major categories: (1) combination with other modalities of systemic treatment, such as immunologic manipulations, hyperthermia, fever, ultrasound, or nutritional factors (interaction between chemotherapy and immune factors is discussed elsewhere in this book); larger pilot studies on the other systemic treatment modalities are not presently available; (2) combination with surgery and/or with radiotherapy as a means of local treatment; this type of multidisciplinary approach is (or should be) the basis for the planning of treatment for each patient. The development of a multidisciplinary team takes time, effort, and patience. Participants include thoracic surgeons and internists, radiotherapists, chemotherapists, immunotherapists, and representatives of the diagnostic sciences (foremost, pathologists, cytopathologists, and radiologists). The time and effort are rewarded in more effective management and, hopefully, better end results.

The following discussion is intended to update current knowledge on multidisciplinary treatment. The focus is on well-controlled clinical trials as the basis for adaptation to the needs of individual patients.

Chemotherapy as Adjuvant to Surgery

The most common motivation for the surgical adjuvant use of chemotherapy (Tables 15-12, 15-13, and 15-14) is the attempt to eradicate micrometastases. The concept is supported in animal models; chemotherapy induces proportionate cell kill.[4] Hence chemotherapy might well be able to eradicate micrometastases containing 100, 1000, or even 100,000 cells. But the larger the cell population the smaller the cure rate. Indeed, removal of the primary tumor permitted cure of small metastatic lesions in experimental animals[74] and significantly prolonged survival of animals with incomplete resection of the primary tumor.[75] Translation of this principle into clinical medicine resulted in marked postsurgical delay of recurrent or metastatic breast cancer,[76] even with suboptimal chemotherapy[77] at or below the range of active treatment regimens from bronchogenic carcinoma. It might be expected, therefore, that surgical adjuvant chemotherapy of lung cancer is firmly established. The past seven major controlled clinical trials, including over 5000 patients, failed to confirm this notion, with two possible exceptions.

The first possible exception falls short of statistically significant proof because of the small number of patients (Table 15-12). A major cooperative study included random allocation of resected patients either to placebo or to cyclophosphamide in courses of 7.8 mg/kg/day for 5

Table 15-12

Surgical Adjuvant Treatment of Small Cell Carcinoma with Cyclophosphamide

Survival	Patients Surviving, Treatment with	
	CTX	Placebo
2 years	28%	11%
4 years	16%	4%
5 years	9%	4%
Number of patients	32	26

Table 15-13

Comparison of Levamisole with Placebo as Surgical Adjuvant

Parameter	Levamisole	Placebo	p
Patients, No.	50	59	no
Epidermoid, No.	37	34	no
% relapse	16	32	
Tumor diameter ≤ 3 cm, No.	18	22	no
% relapse	17	14	
Tumor diameter 4–6 cm, No.	19	18	0.09
% relapse	21	50	
Tumor diameter > 6 cm, No.	7	17	0.03
% relapse	14	73	

Reproduced by permission of author and publisher, from Selawry OS et al: Methotrexate compared with placebo in the treatment of lung cancer. Cancer (in press).

days every 5 weeks for 18 months.[78,79] This study showed no advantage for cyclophosphamide over placebo. Evaluation of a small subgroup of patients (the 58 resected patients with small cell carcinoma) gave suggestive evidence for superiority of cyclophosphamide because the proportion of surviving patients remained consistently two to four times higher than for placebo-treated counterparts.

The second possible exception relates to levamisole, a tetrahydro-6-phenyl-imidazole-thiazole derivative that is widely used as an anthelmintic, in this country for animals and in Europe for man as well. Levamisole is used experimen-

Table 15-14

Negative Surgical Adjuvant Chemotherapy Studies

	Drugs	Dose Pulses q 1–4 Months	Schedule Cont. q 1–7 Months	Short Term	Duration (years)	No. of Patients	References
1	Cyclophosphamide	+			1.5	504*	78
	Placebo	+			2	621	
2	Cyclophosphamide	+			2	70	82,83
	Placebo	+				69	
3	Cyclophosphamide		+		2	259	84
	Busulfane		+			254	
	Placebo		+			249	
4	Cyclophosphamide	+				96	79
	Cyclophosphamide +MTX	+			1.5	103	
	Placebo	+				110	
5	CTX+5-FU+MTX+VIB	+			4	55	85
	Placebo	+				27	
6	Mechlorethamine			+	—	620	78
	Placebo			+		623	
7	Mechlorethamine			+	—	588	86
	Placebo			+		604	
8	Vinblastine			+	0.25	68	87
	Placebo			+		61	

*Excluding patients in Table 15-12.

tally for the restoration of depressed T-cell function and depressed T-cell numbers.[80,81] Direct antitumor effect in experimental tumors is very limited. This compound was used in a double-blind trial at doses of 50 mg t.i.d. p.o. for 3 days prior to surgery and every fortnight thereafter. The distribution of patients to the two treatment programs was comparable for most prognostic factors, except for a disproportion of patients with epidermoid carcinoma (75 percent of 68 patients in the levamisole group, 54 percent of 79 patients in the placebo group).

An interim report of this study shows significant superiority of levamisole over placebo for large primary tumors and suggestive superiority for patients with epidermoid carcinoma (Table 15-13). This superiority is limited to a delay in the occurrence of distant metastases. The rate of local relapses is not affected. The data are preliminary, the study is current, and further results will be followed with interest.

The data for negative studies are summarized in Table 15-14. The reasons for the failure of these surgical adjuvant studies are many. Continuous treatment periods or prolonged courses of treatment could have resulted in suppression of host defenses. This is particularly implied in study 2 of Table 15-14, where patients on cyclophosphamide had a significantly shorter median time to recurrent disease. The trend persisted throughout the 5-year observation period, with 54 percent of the 86 control patients and 32 percent of the 86 treated patients surviving free of disease. Cyclophosphamide was given in 8- to 9-week courses of 12 mg/kg/week i.v. Repeat courses were given every 4 months for 2 years.[82] Short, spaced intensive-treatment courses at 3- to 4-week intervals might be a worthwhile alternative, possibly combined with immunostimulation. Chemotherapy of very short duration around the time of surgery is probably insufficient to result in meaningful cell kill. The choice of drugs should be adjusted to the cell type. Cyclophosphamide and mechlorethamine were overemphasized, accounting for almost 90 percent of all patients (including corresponding placebo patients).

Cell-cycle-phase-sensitive single agents or kinetically designed drug combinations would be worth trying for control of micrometastases, which are likely to have a high proportion of actively dividing cells. Small cell carcinoma might be a worthwhile target for surgery plus radiother-

apy[88] plus chemotherapy, i.e., surgery for local debulking, radiotherapy for regional proportionate cell kill of lymphatic micrometastases, chemotherapy for proportionate cell kill of systemic micrometastases, and immunoadjuvant treatment to counteract the immunosuppressive effects of surgery, radiotherapy, and chemotherapy. One such controlled clinical trial is in progress. It should be stressed, however, that chemotherapy is not currently indicated for elective treatment of the individual patient with resection for cure.

Combination Chemotherapy and Radiotherapy

The combination of chemotherapy and radiotherapy (Tables 15-15 and 15-16) was explored in 25 controlled clinical trials including 2275 evaluable patients with local-regional disease, including one hemithorax (T1–3, N0–2) with or without ipsilateral supraclavicular lymph node involvement (M1.11).

Statistically significant superiority of combination therapy over radiotherapy alone is stated for three studies (Table 15-15). Study 1 of Table 15-15 shows a survival gain from 7 to 10 months (median) for all patients and from 5 months to 10+ months for patients with small cell carcinoma. The most interesting observation of this study relates to the optimal duration of chemotherapy. Patients receiving four triweekly doses of cyclophosphamide over 3 months lived just as long as patients receiving twice as many doses over 6 weeks. Hence more attention should be paid to the optimal duration of chemotherapy. Study 2 of Table 15-15 shows superior tumor regression for combination therapy when endobronchial observation is added to serial chest films. Better tumor shrinkage was not reflected in clinical benefit or prolonged survival. Cyclophosphamide was given in daily increments of 200 mg p.o. on 5 of every 7 days, in contrast to the widely spaced doses of 1000 mg/m^2 in study 1. Thus the dose schedule of cyclophosphamide might be important in that widely spaced doses are less immunosuppressive. Study 3 of Table 15-15 is surprising. Chlorambucil alone induced objective tumor shrinkage in only 1 of 21 patients (Table 15-6). Yet combination with radiotherapy resulted in survival gain when the drug was adjusted to individual tolerance, as indicated by leukopenia of

Table 15-15

Combination Chemotherapy and Radiotherapy with Significant ($p < 0.05$) Advantage over Radiotherapy Alone

	Treatment	Objective Response (%)	Survival (months)	No. of Patients	References
1	RT 4000–5000 R/4–5 wk		7.2 med.	43	89
	RT+CTX 1 g/m² q 3 wk × 4		10.2 med.	38	
	RT+CTX 1 g/m² q 3 wk × 8			35	
2	RT 6000 R/6 wk	58(29)†	31% 1 yr	48(17)†	10
	RT+CTX 200 mg/day × 5 wk	70(78)	35%	46(18)	
3	RT 5000 R/5 wk	—	4.9 mean	15	90
	RT followed by chlorambucil,* 2–8 mg/day	—	7.6 mean	15	

*Dose adjusted to WBC 2000–4000 cells/mm³.

†Superior objective response when evaluated by chest film plus bronchoscopy.

2000–4000 cells/mm³. Thus giving effective chemotherapy might be an important precondition for success.

The remaining 22 controlled clinical trials showed no statistically significant advantage for combination chemotherapy (Table 15-16). Study 11 showed a suggestive survival gain for patients with adenocarcinoma using fluorouracil as adjuvant. In study 16 radiotherapy was preceded by methotrexate, with suggestive evidence for improved survival, especially in patients with small cell carcinoma. Study 21 implied superiority for adjuvant treatment with cyclophosphamide, methotrexate, and vincristine for small cell carcinoma. It appears from these observations that the choice of the chemotherapeutic regimen should be adapted to the chemosensitivity of each cell type.

Most studies showed neither advantage nor disadvantage for adjuvant chemotherapy. Studies 20 and 22 are examples of disadvantage for adjuvant chemotherapy with methotrexate in twice-weekly increments plus an alkylating agent (cyclophosphamide for small cell carcinoma and adenocarcinoma, mechlorethamine for epidermoid carcinoma and large cell carcinoma) at 3-week intervals. Impressively shortened survival in these studies speaks against the indiscriminate use of drugs as adjuvant to radiotherapy for the treatment of the individual patient. Reasons for the inferiority of combined use of chemotherapy and radiotherapy might include suppression of host defense mechanisms (possibly correctable by immunostimulation) or augmentation of the effect of ionizing radiation beyond an optimal dose. Such a possibility is implied in study 10 of Table 15-16, where combination of fluorouracil and 2000 R equalled the results of 4000 R alone, while addition of fluorouracil to 4000 R failed to result in improved tumor response.

Cautious generalization leads to the following considerations for the management of the individual patient with surgically or medically inoperable local-regional lung cancer confined to one hemithorax, with or without scalene, supraclavicular, or lower cervical lymph nodes: (1) Epidermoid carcinoma: Every effort should be made to shoot for maximum cell kill and possibly cure, because well-differentiated and moderately well-differentiated disease remains regional until death in close to 50 percent of patients. An option for chemotherapy includes cyclophosphamide, 1000 mg/m² i.v. every 3 weeks for 4 doses.[89] (2) Small cell carcinoma: High expectations are raised for long-term palliation or cure for small cell carcinoma using the best available drug combinations and radiotherapy. Reports of uncontrolled pilot studies flood the literature.

The following considerations might be of help. Emergencies such as superior vena caval obstruction might require immediate radiotherapy. All other patients might benefit from a short 2- to 3-week intensive course of polychemotherapy.

Patients with objective tumor regression and apparent local-regional disease receive adjuvant

Table 15-16
Combination of Chemotherapy and Radiotherapy:
Controlled Clinical Trials with Negative Results

	Adjuvant Drugs	Remarks	References
1	BCNU	185 mg/wk q 6 wk i.v.	91
2	Cyclophosphamide	20–40 mg/kg/dose	92
3		50 mg/kg, d1 + 35; increase median survival in small cell CA	93
4		80 mg/kg, q 5 wk	
5		400 mg i.v., then 100 mg/d	94
6		300 mg/m²/d i.v. × 5 d, then 200 mg/d p.o.; no adjuvant radiotherapy	91
7		200 mg/day p.o.	
8	Dactinomycin	—	52 (Hosley)
9	Fluorouracil	10–12 mg/kg/d × 5 + 2000 R superior to suboptimal 2000 R alone, but not to 4000 R alone; no difference in survival	52 (Hall)
10		Suggestive survival gain limited to adenocarcinoma	52 (Carr)
11	Fluorodeoxyuridine	—	52 (Cohen)
12	Mechlorethamine	Simultaneously or before radiotherapy	52 (Kraut)
13		Only 3 doses of drug	52 (Durrant)
14		Single dose before radiotherapy for superior vena caval obstruction	52 (Levitt)
15	Methotrexate	—	
16		Methotrexate before each radiotherapy treatment; median survival increased from 8 to 12 months; improved 1-year survival for epidermoid carcinoma from 12% to 42%	95
17	Procarbazine	—	96
18		Suggestive disadvantage for adjuvant radiotherapy	97
19	Vinblastine	—	98
20	Cyclophosphamide+methotrexate	CTX 1100 mg/m² q 3 wk, MTX 20 mg/m² p.o. twice weekly; no advantage for small cell carcinoma, disadvantage for adenocarcinoma	62
21	Cyclophosphamide+methotrexate +vincristine	Suggestive advantage for small cell carcinoma; 15 mg/m² q 3 wk + methotrexate 20 mg/m² twice weekly p.o.	69
22	Mechlorethamine	Disadvantage for epidermoid and large cell carcimonas	62

radiotherapy with intent to eradicate the tumor. This approach offers two advantages. First, small cell carcinoma is usually widely disseminated. Pretreatment with chemotherapy permits assessment of the efficacy of the treatment. Tumor shrinkage might permit the use of smaller fields of radiotherapy and might improve blood supply and hence oxygenation of the tumor, thus augmenting radiosensitivity. Second, split courses of radiotherapy, while apparently equally effective as extended courses, are particularly suitable for combination with chemotherapy, which is continued during the intervals and after radiotherapy.

REFERENCES

1. Cutler SJ: End results in cancer. Rep. #3. GPO, Washington, D.C., H.E.W., Public Health Service, 1968
2. Goldin A: Rationale of combination chemotherapy based on preclinical experiments. Cancer Chemother Rep 4:189–198, 1973
3. Selawry OS: Monochemotherapy of bronchogenic carcinoma with special reference to cell type. Cancer Chemother Rep 4:172–188, 1973
4. Skipper HD, Schabel FM: Quantitative and cytokinetic studies in experimental tumor models, in Holland JF, Frei ET (eds): Cancer Medicine. Philadelphia, Lea & Febiger, 1973, pp 629–650
5. Alberto P: Remission rates, survival and prognostic factors in combination chemotherapy for bronchogenic carcinoma. Cancer Chemother Rep 4:199–203, 1973
6. Einhorn LH, Fee WH, Farber MO, et al: Improved chemotherapy for small cell undifferentiated lung cancer. JAMA 235:1225–1229, 1976
7. Selawry OS: Initial therapeutic trials of new drugs in lung cancer. Cancer Chemother Rep 4:214–225, 1973
8. Selawry OS, Krant M, Scoho J, et al: Methotrexate compared with placebo in the treatment of lung cancer. Cancer (in press)
9. Israel L, Chahinian P, DePierre A: Response of 65 measurable epidermoid bronchogenic tumors of known spontaneous doubling time to four different chemotherapeutic regimens—strategic deductions. Med Ped Oncol 1:83, 1975
10. Brouet G, Flamant R, Hayat M: Results of a therapeutic trial of a combination of radiotherapy and chemotherapy in bronchopulmonary cancers. Eur J Cancer 4:437–445, 1968
11. Oka S, Sato K, Nakai Y, et al: Treatment of lung cancer with bleomycin—the third report. Sci Rep Res Inst Tohoku Univ 19:1–12, 1972
12. Pereslegin IA, Sarkisian RS, Savina EB: Bronchoscopic examination of patients with lung cancer after radiotherapy. Med Radiol 15:3–7, 1970
13. Green RA, Humphrey E, Close H, et al: Alkylating agents in bronchogenic carcinoma. Am J Med 46:516–524, 1969
14. Wolf J: Controlled studies of the therapy of nonresectable cancer of the lungs. Ann Thorac Cardiovasc Surg 1:25–32, 1965
15. Selawry OS: Response of bronchogenic carcinoma to adriamycin. Cancer Chemother Rep 6:349–351, 1975
16. Eagan RT, Carr DT, Coles DT, et al: A randomized study comparing CCNU and methyl-CCNU in advanced bronchogenic carcinoma. Cancer Chemother Rep 58:913–918, 1974
17. Karnofsky DA, Abelmann WH, Cravel LF, et al: The use of nitrogen mustards in the palliative treatment of carcinoma. Cancer 1:634–656, 1949
18. Blum RH, Carter SK, Agre K: A clinical review of bleomycin—a new neoplastic agent. Cancer 31:903–914, 1973
19. Vincent RG, Pickren JW, Fergen R, et al: Evaluation of methotrexate in the treatment of bronchogenic carcinoma. Cancer 36:873–880, 1975
20. Djerassi J, Rominger CJ, Kem JS, et al: Phase I study of high doses of methotrexate with citrovorum factor in patients with lung cancer. Cancer 30:22–29, 1972
21. Nyiredi G, Gevai E: Clinical experience with dibromodulcitol (DBD) in the treatment of cancer. Bronches 21:202–206, 1971
22. Batinov IN: Results of treatment of lung cancer with large single doses of cyclophosphamide. Moscow, unpublished thesis, 1970
23. Bodey GP, Lagakos SW, Gutierrez A, et al: Therapy of advanced squamous cell carcinoma of the lung. Cyclophosphamide versus "COMB" (in press)
24. Brugarolas A, Rivas A, Lacare AJ, et al: Fluorouracil compared with cyclophosphamide in bronchogenic carcinoma: A controlled clinical study. Cancer Chemother Rep 59:1025–1026, 1975
25. Cameron SJ, Grant IW, Crompton GK: Cyclophosphamide in disseminated bronchogenic carcinoma. Scott Med J 19:81, 1974
26. Edmonson JH, Lagakos SW: Combination chemotherapy for metastatic lung cancer. Proc Am Assoc Cancer Res 15:180, 1974
27. Blum RH, Carter SK, Agre K: A clinical review of bleomycin—a new neoplastic agent. Cancer 31:903–914, 1973
28. Hoogstraten B, Haas CD, Hant A, et al: CCNU and bleomycin in the treatment of cancer. Med Ped Oncol 1:95–106, 1975
29. Svanberg L: Clinical results of bleomycin treatment of bronchial carcinoma. London, Bleomycin International Symposium, 1972, pp 115–126
30. Goffin JC: Current state of treatment of primary bronchial cancer. J Belg Radiol 55:415–423, 1972
31. Israel L, Chahinian P, Accord JL, et al: Growth curve modification of measurable tumors by 75 mg/m² of CCNU every 3 weeks. Eur J Cancer 9:789–797, 1973
32. Tranum BL, Haut A, Rivkin S, et al: A phase II study of methyl-CCNU in the treatment of solid tumors and lymphomas. Cancer 35:1148–1153, 1975
33. Israel L, DePierre A, Chahinian P: Dehydroemetine in fifty disseminated carcinomas unresponsive to other drugs. Proc Am Assoc Cancer Res (Abstr) 15:42, 1974

34. Kane RC, Cohen MH, Broder LE, et al: Phase I-II evaluation of emetine in the treatment of epidermoid bronchogenic carcinoma. Cancer Chemother Rep 59:1171–1172, 1975

35. Panetiere F, Coltman CA: Phase I experience in emetine-hydrochloride as an antitumor agent. Cancer 27:835–841, 1971

36. Siddiqui S, Firat D, Olshin S: Phase II study of emetine in the treatment of solid tumors. Cancer Chemother Rep 57:423–428, 1973

37. Ramirez G, Wilson W, Graze T, et al: Phase II evaluation of BCNU (NSC 409962) in patients with solid tumors. Cancer Chemother Rep 56:787–790, 1972

38. Eagan RT, Carr DT, Coles DT, et al: ICRF-159 versus polychemotherapy in non-small cell lung cancer. Cancer Treatment Rep 60:947–948, 1976

39. Dombernowsky P, Hansen HH: Evaluation of vincristine as a single agent in small cell anaplastic bronchogenic carcinoma. Florence, XI International Cancer Congress, 1974

40. Eagan RT, Carr DT, Coles DT, et al: VP-16-213 versus polychemotherapy in patients with advanced small cell lung cancer. Cancer Treatment Rep 60:949–952, 1976

41. Falkson G, van Dyk J, van Eden EB, et al: A clinical trial of the oral form of 4'-demethyl-epipodophyllotoxin-beta-D-ethylene-glucoside. Cancer 35:1141–1144, 1975

42. Takita H, Didolkar MS: Effect of hexamethylmelamine on small cell carcinoma of the lung. Cancer Chemother Rep 58:371–374, 1974

43. Perevodchikova NI, Bychkov MB: Chemotherapy for lung cancer at the Institute of Experimental and Clinical Oncology Academy of Medical Sciences, U.S.S.R. Cancer Chemother Rep 4:251–255, 1973

44. Ahman DL, Moertel CG, Bisel HF, et al: A controlled evaluation of 5-fluorouracil utilizing a single injection technique. Oncology 29:166–171, 1974

45. Faulkner S, Adkins B, Reynolds VH: Chemotherapy of adenocarcinoma and alveolar cell carcinoma of the lung. Ann Thorac Cardiovasc Surg 18:578–583, 1974

46. Perloff M, Muggia F, Acherman C: Role of a nitrosourea (CCNU, NSC 79037) in advanced nonhematologic cancer. Cancer Chemother Rep 58:421–424, 1974

47. Bodey GP, Gottlieb JA, Livingston R, et al: New agents and combinations in the treatment of bronchogenic carcinoma. Cancer Chemother Rep 4:227–230, 1973

48. Richards F, Pajak TF, Cooper MR, et al: Study of methyl-CCNU (NSC 95441) in the treatment of lung cancer. Cancer Chemother Rep 57:419–422, 1973

49. Takita H, Brugarolas A, Mittleman A, et al: Phase II study of the effect of methyl-CCNU (NSC 95441) on bronchogenic carcinoma. Cancer Chemother Rep 4:257–260, 1973

50. Jungi WF, Senn HJ: Clinical study of the new podophyllotoxin derivative VP-16-213 in solid tumors in man. Cancer Chemother Rep 59:737–742, 1975

51. Bean R: Chemotherapy of lung cancer with apparent cure. Med J Aust 2:737–740, 1973

52. Selawry OS, Hansen HH: Lung Cancer, in Holland JF, Frei ET (eds): Cancer Medicine (ed 2). Philadelphia, Lea & Febiger, 1976

53. Gamsu G, Weintraub RM, Nadel JA: Clearance of tantalum from airways. Am Rev Respir Dis 107:214–224, 1973

54. Heyes J, Catherall EJ: Aerosol chemotherapy of lung neoplasia. Nature 247:485–487, 1974

55. Band P, Ross CA, Holland JF: Comparison of two dose schedule of dichloromethotrexate in lung cancer. Cancer Chemother Rep 57:79–82, 1973

56. Creasey WA, Capizzin RL, DeConti RC: Clinical and biochemical studies of high dose intermittent therapy of solid tumors with hydroxyurea (NSC 32065). Cancer Chemother Rep 54:191–194, 1970

57. Kingra GS, Comis R, Olsen KB, et al: 5-(3,3-dimethyl-1-triazeno) imizadole-4-carboxamide (NSC 45388) in the treatment of malignant tumors. Cancer Chemother Rep 55:281–283, 1971

58. Wilson H, Lagakos S, Bodey G, et al: Therapy of advanced epidermoid carcinoma: Lung. Proc Am Assoc Cancer Res 17:232, 1976

59. Bonadonna G, Monfardini S, Ordini W, et al: Sperimentazione clinical con procarbazina e fluorouracile nel carcinoma polmonare avanzato. Tumori 55:277, 1969

60. Livingston RB: Combination chemotherapy with bleomycin, adriamycin, CCNU, vincristine, and mechlorethamine in squamous cell lung cancer. Cancer Chemother Rep 6:361–362, 1975

61. Alberto P, Brunner K, Martz G, et al: Treatment of bronchogenic carcinoma with simultaneous or sequential combination chemotherapy, including cyclophosphamide, procarbazine and vincristine. Cancer 38:2208–2216, 1976

62. Hansen HH, Selawry OS, Simon R, et al: Combination chemotherapy of advanced lung cancer: A randomized trial. Cancer 38:2201–2207, 1976

63. Wolf S, Zelen M: Comparative trial of two drug combinations in pulmonary cancer. Proc Am Assoc Cancer Res 16:272, 1975

64. Straus MJ: Combination chemotherapy in advanced lung cancer with increased survival. Cancer 38:2232–2242, 1976

65. Cohen MH, Fossick BE, Creaven PJ, et al: Intensive chemotherapy of small cell bronchogenic carcinoma. Proc Am Assoc Cancer Res 17:273, 1976

66. Lowenbraun S: Cycle nonspecific preceding cycle

specific chemotherapy in metastatic lung carcinoma. Proc Am Assoc Cancer Res 15:162, 1974

67. Hansen HH, Hansen M: A comparison of three- and four-drugs combination chemotherapy for advanced small cell anaplastic carcinoma of the lung. Proc Am Assoc Cancer Res 17:129, 1976

68. Lowenbraun S, Kraus S, Smalley R, et al: Randomized study of cyclophosphamide alone versus cyclophosphamide, adriamycin, and DTIC in small cell lung carcinoma. Proc Am Assoc Cancer Res 16:246, 1976

69. Maurer LH, Tulloh M, Eagan R, et al: Combination chemotherapy and radiotherapy for small cell carcinoma of the lung. Cancer Chemother Rep 4:171–176, 1973

70. Taylor SG, Donovan MA, Sponzo RW, et al: Treatment of small cell carcinoma of the lung using methyl-CCNU combined with cyclophosphamide and vincristine in 3-week dose schedule. Cancer Chemother Rep 59:1127–1130, 1975

71. Lanzotti VJ, Thomas DR, Holoye PY, et al: Bleomycin followed by cyclophosphamide, vincristine, methotrexate and 5-fluorouracil for non-oat cell bronchogenic carcinoma. Cancer Treat Rep 60:61–68, 1976

72. Selawry OS: Polychemotherapy with adriamycin in bronchogenic carcinoma. Cancer Chemother Rep 6:353–359, 1975

73. Yesner R, Gerstl B, Auerbach D: Application of the World Health Organization classification of lung carcinoma to biopsy material. Ann Thorac Cardiovasc Surg 1:33–47, 1963

74. Mayo JG, Laster WR, Andrews CM, et al: Success and failure in the treatment of solid tumors. III. "Cure" of metastatic Lewis lung carcinoma with methyl-CCNU (NSC 95441) and surgery-chemotherapy. Cancer Chemother Rep 56:183–195, 1972

75. Straus MJ, Sege V, Choi SC: The effect of surgery and pre-treatment or post-treatment adjuvant chemotherapy on primary tumor growth in an animal model. J Surg Oncol 7:497–512, 1975

76. Bonadonna G, Brusamatino E, Varagussa P, et al: Combination chemotherapy as an adjuvant treatment in operable breast cancer. N Engl J Med 294:405–410, 1976

77. Fisher B, Carbone PP, Economou SG, et al: L-phenylalanine-mustard in the management of primary breast cancer: A report of early findings. N Engl J Med 292:117–122, 1975.

78. Higgins G: The use of chemotherapy as an adjuvant to surgery for bronchogenic carcinoma. Cancer 30:1383–1387, 1972

79. Shields TW: Status report of adjuvant cancer chemotherapy trials in the treatment of bronchial carcinoma. Cancer Chemother Rep 4:119–124, 1973

80. Amery WK: Double blinded levamisole trial in resectable lung cancer. NY Acad Sci 277:260–268, 1976

81. Swieringa J, Gooszen HC, Vanderschuerin RG, et al: Immunopotentiation with levamisole in resectable bronchogenic carcinoma. Br Med J 3:461–464, 1975

82. Brunner KW, Marthaler TH, Müller W: Effects of long-term adjuvant chemotherapy with cyclophosphamide for radically resected bronchogenic carcinoma. Cancer Chemother Rep 4:125–132, 1973

83. Brunner KW, Marthaler TH, Müller W: Unfavorable effects of long-term adjuvant chemotherapy with endoxan in radically operated bronchogenic carcinoma. Eur J Cancer 7:285–294, 1971

84. Miller AB (A Medical Research Council Working Party): Study of cytotoxic chemotherapy as an adjuvant to surgery in carcinoma of the bronchus. Br Med J 2:421, 1971

85. Karrer K, Pridun N, Zivintz E: Chemotherapeutic study of the Austrian Study Group. Cancer Chemother Rep 4:207–213, 1973

86. Slack NH: Bronchogenic carcinoma: Nitrogen mustard as a surgical adjuvant and factors influencing survival. Cancer 25:987–1002, 1970

87. Crosbie WA, Kamdar HH, Belcher JR: A controlled trial of vinblastine sulfate in the treatment of cancer of the lung. Br J Dis Chest 60:28–35, 1966

88. Bates M, Hurt R, Levison V, et al: Treatment of oat-cell carcinoma of the bronchus by preoperative radiotherapy and surgery. Lancet 1:1134–1135, 1974

89. Bergsagel DE, Genkins RDT, Pringle JF, et al: Lung Cancer: Clinical trial of radiotherapy alone versus radiotherapy plus cyclophosphamide. Cancer 30:621–627, 1972

90. Horowitz H, Wright TL, Perry H: Impressive chemotherapy in bronchogenic carcinoma. Am J Roentgenol Radium Ther Nucl Med 93:615–637, 1965

91. Kaung DT, Wolf J, Hyde L, et al: Preliminary report on the treatment of nonresectable cancer of the lung. Cancer Chemother Rep 58:359–364, 1974

92. Scheurlen H, Drings P, Vollhaber MM, et al: Strahlentherapie des inoperablen Bronchuskarzinoms in Kombination mit einer Endoxanbehandlung. Strahlentherapie 143:154–158, 1972

93. Tucker RD, Sealy R, van Wik C, et al: Clinical trial of cyclophosphamide and radiation therapy for oat cell carcinoma of the lung. Cancer Chemother Rep 4:159–160, 1973

94. Hoest H: Cyclophosphamide as adjuvant to radiotherapy in the treatment of unresectable bronchogenic carcinoma. Cancer Chemother Rep 4:161–164, 1973

apy for squamous cell carcinoma. Cancer Chemother Rep 4:157–158, 1973

96. Sandison AG, Falkson G, Fichardt T, et al: A statistical evaluation of the treatment of 215 patients with advanced bronchogenic cancer, managed by telecobalt therapy alone and in combination with various cancer chemotherapeutic agents. South Afr J Radiol 5:21–27, 1967

97. Landgren RC, Hussey OH, Samuels ML, et al: A randomized study comparing irradiation alone to irradiation plus procarbazine in inoperable bronchogenic carcinoma. Therapy Radiol 108:403–406, 1973

98. Coy, P.: A randomized study of irradiation and vinblastine in lung cancer. Cancer 26:803–807, 1970

Evan M. Hersh
Giora M. Mavligit
Jordan U. Gutterman

16

Immunotherapy and Lung Cancer

Because carcinoma of the lung is one of the three most common tumors and because it is one of the most aggressive, with a 5-year survival of approximately 5 percent,[1] improved modalities of treatment for this disease are urgently needed. Only a small portion of patients have operable disease at the time of diagnosis, and the recurrence rate, even in patients with operable disease, is greater than 50 percent.[2] There have been few advances in recent years in the surgery or radiotherapy of lung cancer.[2] Also, many of the newer chemotherapeutic agents that have markedly improved the prognosis for patients with diseases such as breast cancer and leukemia have had little impact on this disease, and the chemotherapy response rate is still well under 50 percent.[3] Conventional local therapies for carcinoma of the lung, namely surgery and radiotherapy, are severely limited in their effectiveness, because this disease is already widespread at the time of diagnosis in many patients.[4]

There are several reasons for believing that immunotherapy should have a profound impact on this grim situation. First, tumor antigens and tumor immunity have been identified in patients with lung cancer.[5] In many patients with lung cancer severe immunodeficiency exists, at least prior to surgery,[6] and in some individuals this immunodeficiency persists after surgical extirpation of disease. The patient receiving radiotherapy experiences additional and often prolonged compromise of his immune system.[7] Thus immunodeficiency, immunosuppression, and the presence of tumor antigens and associated tumor immunity provide a scientific basis and several targets for the development of immunotherapy of lung cancer.

During the last 10 years there have been major advances in immunotherapy both in animal models and in human malignant disease. In animals, several different types of experimental tumors metastatic to the lung have been found to be responsive to various immunotherapeutic approaches. In man, immunotherapy of acute leukemia, malignant melanoma, colon cancer, breast cancer, and head and neck cancer have established certain principles that can readily be applied to lung cancer.[8] Finally, during the last few years there have been several positive trials of immunotherapy of lung cancer itself, both after definitive surgery and for metastatic disease. These have involved one or more of the following approaches: nonspecific active, specific active, systemic, and local or regional immunotherapy.

Supported by Grant CA-05831 and Contract NO1-CB-33888 from the National Cancer Institute, National Institutes of Health, Bethesda, Md. Drs. Gutterman and Mavligit are recipients of Public Health Research Career Development Awards 1-K04-CA-71007-01 and 1-K04-CA-00130-01, respectively, from the National Institutes of Health, Bethesda, Md.

The results of these trials, even though they have been conducted in relatively small numbers of patients, are very encouraging and are described in detail below.

The time is at hand for large-scale trials of immunotherapy of lung cancer in man using established approaches, as well as for an intensive effort toward development of new and better techniques for immunotherapy of lung cancer. Based on the data to be outlined below, it is the opinion of the authors that all patients with lung cancer that is treatable by definitive surgery or radiotherapy should receive immunotherapy as prophylaxis against recurrence. Furthermore, in patients with metastatic disease, immunotherapy should be applied before chemotherapy and/or between courses of chemotherapy. Immunotherapy by the regional route, either intrapleural or intravenous (to reach the nodes or parenchyma) should be given particular attention. Finally, the immunosuppressive effects of conventional treatment, particularly radiotherapy, should be considered. This less-than-optimal modality of treatment for lung cancer should be carefully evaluated before it is administered, because there is little convincing evidence that adjuvant radiotherapy, given after surgery or in inoperable cases, provides any survival advantage to the patient.[9]

IMMUNOCOMPETENCE AND PROGNOSIS IN LUNG CANCER

One of the bases for developing approaches to immunotherapy in lung cancer is the relationship between immunocompetence and prognosis in cancer in general and in lung cancer specifically. Patients with good general immunocompetence usually have relatively good prognoses, while patients with poor general immunocompetence usually have relatively poor prognoses.[10] This phenomenon has been described in a variety of malignant tumors, including acute leukemia,[11] chronic lymphocytic leukemia,[12] chronic myelogenous leukemia,[13] malignant lymphoma,[14,15] and a variety of solid tumors[16] including malignant melanoma, breast cancer, colon cancer, and head and neck cancer. The relationship apparently holds at all stages of disease. Thus, both primary surgical patients and patients with advanced metastatic tumors show this relationship. It is interesting that this has also been demonstrated

using a variety of tests, including established delayed-type hypersensitivity to recall antigens,[17] primary delayed-type hypersensitivity to antigens such as DNCB,[18] in vitro lymphocyte blastogenic responses to mitogens and antigens,[19] and even the antibody response.[20] Most recently, T and B lymphocyte levels have shown this relationship.[21] In addition to the relationship between immunocompetence and prognosis, it must also be noted that all therapy for malignant disease is immunosuppressive. Thus surgery,[22] radiotherapy,[23] and chemotherapy[24] can all markedly suppress the immune responsiveness of the patient, sometimes for prolonged periods of time. These observations have important implications for immunotherapy. One must attempt to reverse the immunodeficiency associated with cancer, and yet one can attempt to devise regimens of conventional therapy that are less immunosuppressive. They are also important because they should determine the timing of the administration of immunotherapy.

The relationship between general immunocompetence and prognosis has also been demonstrated in lung cancer. Tests of the development of new or primary delayed-type hypersensitivity or of delayed-type hypersensitivity to recall antigens have been particularly useful. Several investigators have suggested that the response to immunization with DNCB can be used to identify and select those patients who will respond to surgery. Eilber and Morton observed that patients who could develop delayed hypersensitivity to DNCB had good prognoses after surgery.[18] This has recently been confirmed by another study.[25] In a population of patients in France, Israel and associates observed that a vigorous delayed-type hypersensitivity response to tuberculin was predictive of a good prognosis.[26] This was also observed by Steward.[6] The latter found that depressed tuberculin skin test reactivity in lung cancer patients was associated with a circulating serum factor that suppressed in vitro lymphocyte blastogenesis. Both tended to reverse after surgery, and those patients who had improvement in tuberculin reactivity and loss of the immunosuppressive serum factor had good prognoses. An immunosuppressive serum factor was also observed by Silk[27] and by Sample and associates.[28] Another recall antigen useful in evaluating immunocompetence and prognosis in lung cancer is streptokinase-streptodornase.[29] Patients with reactivity greater than 25 mm induration had good prognoses, while patients with reactivity under 5 mm induration had poor prognoses after surgery.

Recently the Working Party for Therapy of Lung Cancer conducted a large multi-institute study of immunocompetence and prognosis in lung cancer.[30] The approach utilized recall delayed-type hypersensitivity skin testing with a battery of antigens including dermatophytin, *Candida,* streptokinase-streptodornase, and mumps. Patients at all stages of disease were studied. Several skin test responses were useful in predicting prognosis. Patients with vigorous reactivity to *Candida* had prolonged survival, compared to very short survival in patients with negative *Candida* reactivity. Patients with vigorous mumps reactivity had a higher remission rate than patients with negative reactions. There were specific subclasses of patients in which these tests were useful and predictive. For example, *Candida* reactivity was predictive only in male patients, and both *Candida* and mumps reactivities were predictive only in patients with an intermediate performance status, while patients with normal or very poor performance status did not show this relationship. It was concluded that in vivo recall delayed-type hypersensitivity skin testing was useful in evaluating the prognosis of lung cancer patients.

In vitro lymphocyte function studies have also been useful in evaluating these patients. Thus a number of investigators have shown that lymphocyte blastogenic responses to a variety of mitogens and antigens are abnormally low in patients with lung cancer who have poor prognoses.[7] These responses decline further after radiotherapy,[31] but they tend to improve after surgical extirpation of tumor.[6] The relationship to circulating serum factors has already been mentioned. A number of investigators feel that the mixed lymphocyte reaction is the most useful in vitro test.[32] The immunosuppressive serum factor resides in the α_2-macroglobulin fraction[33] and has recently been described as being a low-molecular-weight polypeptide.[34]

Other investigators have observed poor local inflammatory responses in the skin of lung cancer patients as compared to normals.[35] This has been observed using the skin-window technique. It may be a contributing factor to the poor delayed-type hypersensitivity. Pisano and colleagues have described poor phagocytic and reticuloendothelial system function in lung cancer patients related to a deficiency in macrophage humoral recogni-

tion factor.[36] This is particularly important to the development of immunotherapy, because this factor can be restored by the administration of BCG. A poor antibody response has also been observed in patients with lung cancer and is also associated with a poor prognosis.

Recently, immunologists have focused their attention on peripheral blood levels of T and B lymphocytes. In lung cancer the levels of circulating T lymphocytes detected by rosette formation with sheep red blood cells were found to be markedly depressed as compared to normals.[37] The most depressed values were found in patients with advanced disease. Similarly, depressed levels of B lymphocytes were found to be associated with progressive disease in patients with a variety of solid tumors including lung cancer.[38] Patients with particularly low levels of B lymphocytes had poor prognoses, both in terms of remission rate and in terms of subsequent remission duration and survival after the time of the test.

An important factor in immunocompetence that is not measured by any of these tests is regional immunocompetence. Thus in vivo delayed cutaneous hypersensitivity, the levels of circulating T and B lymphocytes and monocytes, and in vitro studies of circulating peripheral blood lymphocytes tell us very little about host defense mechanisms within the lung parenchyma, within pulmonary tumor, or within the regional draining lymph nodes. Many investigators have demonstrated that regional lymph nodes are extremely important in host defense against cancer[39] and that the function of regional lymph nodes is not necessarily reflected by the function of peripheral blood lymphocytes.[40] Indeed, there is evidence that regional lymph nodes may show specific or general immunologic deficiency with regard to the tumor or to general host defense, respectively, while this may not be manifested in the peripheral blood.[41] Several studies of solid tumor patients that have included studies of patients with lung cancer have demonstrated this. For example, it is common that lymphocyte blastogenic responses to tumor cells may be vigorous among peripheral blood lymphocytes and depressed among lymph node lymphocytes, or the reverse.[41] Similar observations have been made for the mixed lymphocyte reaction. Lymphocytes extracted from tumors themselves usually have weak blastogenic responses, while lymphocytes from tumor-bearing lymph nodes may have either weak or vigorous blastogenic responses.[42] Obviously the situation is complex and warrants considerable further work. Approaches to augmentation of regional immunity must be investigated in animal models.

In conclusion, immunocompetence and prognosis are closely related in lung cancer. However, current methodology to evaluate this is insufficient because we have no useful clinical approaches to evaluating regional host defense mechanisms in lung cancer. This applies to host defense mechanisms within the tumor, within the lung parenchyma, or within the regional lymph nodes. Also, the etiology of the immunodeficiency associated with lung cancer is not clear. Etiologic factors that may play a role include exposure to carcinogens (cigarette smoke and air pollution), genetic factors in the immune response,[43] nutritional factors,[44] and production of immunosuppressive molecules by the tumor itself.[45] That this is an important mechanism is suggested by the finding of circulating immunosuppressive serum factors that disappear in some cases after the tumor is removed. The nature of these is poorly understood, but some are low-molecular-weight polypeptides in the α_2-macroglobulin region. They may also be circulating antigen–antibody complexes.[46] The antibody may be to tumor antigens or rheumatoid factor, anti-idiotypic antibody, or antibody to the hinge region of the immunoglobulin molecule. Each of these may result in complexes that might block cell-mediated immunity. While our knowledge is incomplete, the phenomena described in this section clearly indicate a number of useful directions for immunotherapy. Thus one might attempt to restore the deficient general immunocompetence of the patient, one might attempt to activate general or tumor-specific regional host defense mechanisms, or one might institute maneuvers that would clear circulating immunosuppressive factors including antigen–antibody complexes from the peripheral blood.

TUMOR ANTIGENS AND TUMOR IMMUNITY IN LUNG CANCER

Tumor antigens and specific tumor immunity to these antigens have been observed in a variety of animal and human tumors. Strong evidence for specific tumor antigens exists in acute leukemia,[47] melanoma,[48] colon cancer,[49] head and neck cancer,[50] and cancer of the cervix,[51] to mention a few. Methods that have been useful in detecting

specific tumor immunity to tumor antigens in man have included delayed-type hypersensitivity to tumor cells and purified tumor antigens, lymphocyte blastogenesis, generation of migration-inhibition factor, detection of leukocyte or macrophage migration inhibition, lymphocyte cytotoxicity, leukocyte adherence inhibition, and the presence of antibody detected by complement fixation, immunofluorescence, or cytotoxicity. Because of the non-inbred nature of man, the moral constraints on human experimentation, and the relative impurity and heterogeneity of most human tumor antigen preparations, the studies of tumor immunity and tumor antigens that have been most convincing have been those done in the autochthonous setting.

Relatively few studies of tumor antigens and specific tumor immunity have been done in lung cancer as compared to other tumors such as leukemia, breast cancer, melanoma, etc. Since lung cancer is one of the most common human tumors and carries one of the worst prognoses, this might be considered surprising. However, there are several likely explanations. First, pulmonary neoplasms are often contaminated with microorganisms because of their bronchial location and the frequent association of pulmonary obstruction. Second, the tumors are often small and provide little tissue for experimentation. Third, the tumors may be quite fibrous, and therefore the preparation of single-cell suspensions is difficult. Finally, long-term stable lines of human bronchogenic carcinoma are not currently available for the kinds of experiments that have been done in breast cancer, colon cancer, and melanoma.

In spite of these problems, there have been increasing numbers of relevant studies. Delayed-type hypersensitivity has been the most important method used, with either crude or purified tumor antigen preparations. Stewart found delayed hypersensitivity to crude autologous lung cancer extracts in 4 of 9 patients studied.[52] Wells and associates, using membrane extracts of lung cancer, normal lung, normal leukocytes, fetal lung, and fetal liver, carried out skin tests in a series of lung cancer patients.[53] In 6 of 16 immunocompetent subjects there was a positive response to tumor antigen and a negative response to normal lung and leukocyte antigen. It is interesting that in 5 of 16 there was a response to fetal lung but not to fetal liver. Mavligit and associates, using KCl-extracted antigens, demonstrated positive delayed hypersensitivity skin test to tumor antigen reactions in the majority of non-anergic patients tested.[54] Nordquist demonstrated a specific tumor antigen in human alveolar cell carcinoma.[55] The most important studies are those reported by Hollinshead and associates.[56] These investigators use a sequential technique involving membrane preparation by hypotonic lysis, low-frequency sonication, Sephadex G-200 column chromatography, and polyacrylamide gel electrophoresis to purify tumor-specific antigens. This has been done in several histologic types of lung cancer including oat cell carcinoma, adeno-carcinoma, and squamous cell carcinoma, and a specific tumor antigen has indeed been demonstrated using delayed hypersensitivity skin testing. This approach is particularly significant because this antigen, as will be discussed later, apparently has potent effects when used for active-specific immunotherapy. Finally, during active-specific immunotherapy with modified tumor cells, Takita and Brugarolas observed increasing delayed-type hypersensitivity reactions at immunization sites after repeated immunization.[57]

Using an in vitro colony inhibition assay that they pioneered, the Hellströms and their associates demonstrated relatively specific lymphocyte cytotoxicity in lung cancer.[58] However, Baldwin and associates were unable to confirm this observation,[59] and subsequently a variety of studies have indicated a lack of specificity and a high level of reactivity among normal subjects for allogeneic lymphocyte cytotoxicity to target tumor cells in man.[60] However, using autologous lymphocyte tumor cell mixtures, Mavligit and associates demonstrated lymphocyte blastogenic responses to tumor cells quantitatively similar to those manifested by normal subjects to recall antigens.[61] Patients with vigorous in vitro lymphocyte blastogenic responses had good prognoses, while patients with poor tumor-specific blastogenic responses to their own tumor cells had relatively poor prognoses. Using lymphocyte blastogenic responses to hypertonic KC1-extracted lung cancer antigen, Roth and associates observed positive in vitro blastogenic responses among 75 percent of lung cancer patients but only 19 percent of other cancer patients.[62] Cochran and associates observed that specific tumor immunity was depressed after surgery in lung cancer patients.[63] Finally, Richters and associates observed that special active lymphocyte/tumor cell interactions of several types, including clustering and emperipolesis, occurred in explants of

lung cancer tissue examined by sophisticated microscopic techniques. It is interesting that this was less marked in lung cancer than in other types of tumors.

In conclusion, while the data are not as strong for some other tumors, there is evidence for the presence of tumor antigens in a variety of histologic types of lung cancer and for the development of cell-mediated immunity to cells bearing these antigens or to the antigens themselves. Several techniques, particularly in vivo delayed hypersensitivity to tumor antigen and in vitro blastogenic responses to tumor cells or antigen, have been particularly convincing. In vivo delayed hypersensitivity responses to purified tumor antigens seem the most relevant tests for tumor-specific immunity that are currently available. Using the techniques developed by Hollinshead and associates, highly purified antigen preparations can be produced. Once scale-up of this technology has been achieved, we should have very useful reagents for immunodiagnosis, quantitation of tumor immunity, and immunotherapy. Since the level of tumor immunity appears to be related to prognosis, both in cancer in general and in lung cancer specifically, various maneuvers directed at boosting specific tumor immunity, such as active-specific immunization, should be useful in lung cancer.

IMMUNOTHERAPY OF CANCER IN GENERAL

There are six major approaches to immunotherapy in cancer.[8] These include active-non-specific immunotherapy, active-specific immunotherapy, immunotherapy of the adoptive type (that is, immunotherapy with lymphoid cellular products), passive immunotherapy, local or regional immunotherapy, and combinations of two or more of the above approaches. Active-nonspecific immunotherapy is the administration of a material that immunizes the host in such a way as to boost one or more components of his general immunologic competence and responsiveness. Active-specific immunotherapy refers to immunization with tumor cells, tumor antigen, or antigen cross-reactive with tumor antigen. These may either be intact or be modified chemically, physically, or otherwise. The objective of active-specific immunotherapy is to boost specific tumor immunity, particularly those components known to be involved in effective host control of tumor. Adoptive or lymphoid cellular product immunotherapy refers to the use of lymphoid cells, extracts of lymphoid cells, or the secreted products of lymphoid cells to confer the donor's specific tumor immunity or general immunocompetence on the tumor-bearing recipient. Products included in this category are transfer factor, immune RNA, thymosin, lymphokines, and interferon. Passive immunotherapy refers to the administration of either intact or modified antibody specific for antigens on the surface of tumor cells. This antibody might have direct cytotoxic action, it might opsonize or otherwise prepare the tumor cell for attack by phagocytic cells, it might be concerned in antibody-dependent cell-mediated cytotoxicity, or it might change the balance in antigen–antibody complexes so that blocking of cell-mediated immunity is ameliorated. It might also be the carrier of another cytotoxic material, such as a radioactive isotope or an antitumor chemotherapeutic drug. Local and regional immunotherapy refers to the administration of (usually) an active-nonspecific immunotherapy reagent directly into a tumor nodule or into the regional lymphatic drainage of a primary or metastatic tumor. This can result in tumor killing through a bystander effect of the delayed hypersensitivity reaction on the active-nonspecific reagent or by activation of macrophages and/or lymphocytes within or surrounding metastatic or primary tumor cell deposits. Combinations of these approaches are often more effective than any single approach alone. Thus active-nonspecific and active-specific, active-nonspecific and adoptive, and active-specific and adoptive immunotherapies have all proved useful, either in animal models or in man.

During the last 10 years considerable progress has been made in the field of immunotherapy. It may now be stated with considerable support that a fourth major modality of cancer treatment, namely immunotherapy, has taken its place among the major approaches to cancer treatment. Several principals of immunotherapy have been developed during this time: (1) At present, immunotherapy is to be considered additive to or synergistic with conventional therapy. (2) There are two main approaches to the application of immunotherapy. One is its administration after or concurrently with maximal conventional cytoreductive therapy in order to bring the patient to a state of no evident disease. The second is the application of immunotherapy between courses of chemotherapy for patients with metastatic disease who cannot be brought to a state of no evident disease by conventional treatment. A third approach, which is its early developmental phase, is the application of immunotherapy as the only modality of treatment, or at least the earliest treatment, before conventional therapy. While immunotherapy is considered additive or synergistic at present, it may become the primary therapy of the future as better immunotherapeutic reagents are developed. (3) Since cancer often spreads from the primary site to regional lymph nodes via lymphatics, and then to distant sites via the hematogenous route, approaches to immunotherapy must be tailored to the pattern of spread, to the extent of disease, to host characteristics, and to histologic type of tumor. This results in three broad objectives for immunotherapy. One, local immunotherapy may be given to control local disease. Two, regional immunotherapy may be given to prevent or suppress regional recurrence at a time when only microscopic foci of tumor cells are present in the regional drainage. Three, systemic immunotherapy may be given to heighten tumor immunity throughout the body in order to prevent development of or to suppress distant metastases. Certain approaches combine two or even three of these objectives. Thus intralesional therapy with BCG destroys the injected tumor, eliminates lymph node metastases, and induces vigorous systemic tumor immunity. (4) Maximum tumor burden reduction should precede, if possible, or certainly should be carried out concurrently with, the administration of immunotherapy, A large or increasing tumor burden may preclude any immunotherapeutic benefit. This principle is coming under renewed scrutiny because there is some evidence that patients with metastatic disease and a large tumor burden may still respond to immunotherapy alone. (5) The immunocompetence of the host should be related to the design of the immunotherapeutic intervention. Thus if the host is immunocompetent, immunotherapy is used to potentiate regional or systemic specific host defense mechanisms. This is referred to as immunopotentiation. However, if the host is immunoincompetent, we use immunotherapy to restore the level of general immunocompetence so that the patient can then respond to immunopotentiation. This approach is called immunoreconstitution. (6) Immunotherapy should not be administered during the period of immunosuppression induced by conventional therapy unless its specific objective is to prevent or reverse that immunosuppression. Since there is often a rebound or overshoot in immunocompetence after the period of therapy-induced immunosuppression, it is probably best to wait for that period before starting immunotherapy. Conversely, immunotherapy, at least of the active type, should not be given just prior to a course of chemotherapy or other treatment known to be immunosuppressive. It is likely that such a course of chemotherapy may abrogate the immune boosting effects of the immunotherapy. (7) The empiric nature of immunotherapy must be carefully considered. Thus the timing, frequency, and dose must be investigated in detail. Basically, the same principles that apply to the development of new chemotherapeutic agents should be applied to the development of new immunotherapeutic reagents. One wishes to deliver the maximally tolerated dose in the shortest period of time with the least toxicity. In the case of immunotherapy one also wishes to find the maximum immunopotentiating dose. (8) Immunotherapy, because of its developmental nature, must be monitored carefully immunologically, so that the immunologic consequences can be evaluated independently of the clinical effects. This is important because the desired clinical effects may be aborted by other factors, while the immunotherapy produces the desired immunologic effects. Monitoring should include both general immunocompetence and specific tumor immunity. (9) Immunotherapeutic procedures should be designed mainly to augment cell-mediated immunity selectively. This is because our present knowledge indicates that cellular host defense mechanisms mediated by T cells, B cells, K cells, or macrophages or combinations of these are more important than humoral host defense factors. In addition, certain levels of antitumor antibody may result in the development of blocking factors, presumably antigen–antibody complexes.

Finally, it must be emphasized that the principles outlined above must be considered tentative. Recent developments in immunology and in tumor immunobiology, as well as expiric clinical observations, may lead to effective new approaches that may violate some of the principles outlined above. For example, both Band and associates[64] and Israel and associates[65] have recently described regression of metastatic tumor in up to 40 percent of patients who receive daily intravenous *Corynebacterium parvum* (*C. par-*

vum) as the only modality of treatment. If this observation is further confirmed, it means that maximal tumor burden reduction may not be necessary for immunotherapeutic effect even in the immunoincompetent patient with far-advanced metastatic disease.

IMMUNOTHERAPY OF TUMORS OTHER THAN LUNG CANCER

During the last 9 years a significant number of trials of immunotherapy have yielded positive results in a variety of human tumors. Even prior to 1968 there were scattered reports of immunotherapeutic benefits using active-nonspecific or active-specific immunotherapeutic approaches. For example, in the early 1900s Coley[66] treated a variety of sarcoma patients who experienced remissions or apparent cures after treatment with an extract of "killing" hemolytic streptococci and *Serratia marcescens* (the so-called Coley's or mixed bacterial toxins). Over 40 years later Nauts and associates[67] described the long-term follow-up results of 30 inoperable patients treated with Coley's toxins, and 20 had survived for more than 20 years. This approach has only recently begun to be effectively followed up (see below). In the late 1950s and early 1960s the Grahams immunized gynecologic cancer patients with extracts of their own tumors in complete Freund's adjuvant.[68] Prolongation of survival was observed as compared to controls, particularly in patients who showed vigorous local reactions to immunization.

The modern era of immunotherapy in man began with a report by Mathé and associates, who administered either active-specific immunotherapy with allogeneic irradiated tumor cells or active-nonspecific immunotherapy with BCG by scarification or a combination of both to children with acute lymphocytic leukemia in remission after the termination of combination chemotherapy.[69] All three regimens resulted in prolongation of remission duration as compared to a simultaneous control in a small number of patients. This study was based on the principles that active-nonspecific immunotherapy would boost general immunity, that active-specific immunotherapy would heighten the already existing antitumor immunity, and that administration after the end of chemotherapy would take advantage of the minimal residual tumor burden and the lack of concurrent immunosuppressive treatment.

During the last 9 years these observations have been amply confirmed and extended. Active-nonspecific immunotherapy with BCG and other reagents has been proved to be effective. For example, in acute myelogenous leukemia, BCG administered between courses of chemotherapy, both alone and in combination with allogeneic irradiated tumor cells, has prolonged remission duration and survival.[70,71] BCG administered after surgery and radiotherapy has done the same in patients with malignant lymphoma.[72] In patients with malignant melanoma, postsurgical administration of BCG to patients with stage IIIB and IVA malignant melanoma has prolonged the disease-free interval and survival.[73] BCG administered between courses of chemotherapy for metastatic melanoma has increased the remission rate in areas regional to the BCG administration and has prolonged the remission duration and survival.[74] In Duke's class C colon cancer the administration of BCG by scarification, either alone or between courses of 5-fluorouracil (5-FU), has dramatically improved the disease-free interval and survival.[75] Only 2 of 83 patients studied died during a 30-month follow-up period, compared to approximately 25 percent of appropriate historical controls. In metastatic breast cancer, BCG administered between courses of remission maintenance (5-FU, methotrexate, and cyclophosphamide) or administered starting between courses of remission-induction therapy with 5-FU, adriamycin, and cyclophosphamide (Cytoxan) has prolonged the remission duration and the survival of remission patients.[76] Even more important, the survival of patients whose disease stabilizes but does not regress is also prolonged by the addition of BCG to combination chemotherapy. This, again, is evidence that immunotherapy may have beneficial effects, even in patients with far-advanced disease. In head and neck cancer the administration of BCG between courses of chemotherapy has resulted in prolongation of survival.[77]

While immunotherapy with living BCG administered by Heaf gun, multipuncture plate, or scarification has shown the efficacy described, there are several disadvantages to BCG immunotherapy. First, this is a living organism; therefore there is always a danger of systemic BCG disease. Luckily, this is an extremely rare complication. Second, also because this is a living

organism, great biologic variability including genetic drift can be anticipated. Indeed, in vitro biologic studies, as well as in vivo studies by Mackaness and associates, have shown that the efficacy of BCG immunotherapy depends on the strain, the dose, the route of administration, the numbers of viable organisms, the numbers of dead organisms, the proportion of viable organisms to dead organisms, and the amount of free soluble antigens in the BCG preparation.[78] Greatest efficacy is achieved by a fully viable preparation of the Pasteur or related strains with little or no free soluble antigen.

For these reasons efforts have been directed toward the development of nonviable, more standardized BCG products. The first of these is the methanol-extraction residue of BCG, or MER, developed by David Weiss. This is a partially delipidated particulate preparation consisting mainly of BCG cell walls and fragments.[79] Immunotherapy with MER has shown activity in two studies in acute myelogenous leukemia, in which it prolongs remission when administered between courses of chemotherapy.[80] Two groups have also shown that MER has immunopotentiating activity in man.[81,82] Further efforts at purification of the active components of BCG have been carried out successfully by Ribi and associates.[83] This group has prepared purified BCG cell walls, purified delipidated BCG cell wall skeletons (which are mainly carbohydrate, specifically arabinogalactan), and a lipoprotein fraction referred to as P3. These materials have been extensively studied in the guinea pig hepatoma model. In this model, tumor is implanted in the flank, and it metastasizes to the regional lymph nodes.[84] Intralesional BCG causes regression of the primary tumor and can cure the disease in the regional lymph nodes in approximately 60 percent of cases. When BCG cell wall skeleton and P3 are attached to oil droplets in oil-and-water emulsion, up to 90 percent cures can be achieved, even when the immunotherapeutic reagent is administered at a time when native BCG is no longer effective.[85] These materials are just beginning to be applied to man, and BCG cell walls attached to oil droplets have already shown activity in lung cancer (see below).

A number of other active-nonspecific immunotherapeutic reagents are under intensive investigation. Most of these are microbial products. Thus *C. parvum* administered subcutaneously between courses of combination chemotherapy for advanced metastatic solid tumors has led to a doubling of survival time from 5 to 10 months in a large group of patients.[86] *C. parvum* administered intravenously on a daily schedule has caused regression of hepatic and pulmonary metastases in the absence of any other therapy.[65] The presumed mechanism of action is activation of macrophages and perhaps also lymphocytes already resident in the tumor, followed by the cytotoxic effects of these on the tumor cells. Another important mechanism probably involves activation of macrophages with clearance of immunosuppressive antigen–antibody complexes. Finally, in a recent study the administration of *Pseudomonas* vaccine to patients undergoing remission-induction therapy for acute myelogenous leukemia has resulted in a prolongation of survival in the treated patients as compared to patients receiving chemotherapy alone.[87]

A very interesting agent that may be classified with the active-nonspecific immunotherapeutic reagents, but that really belongs in a separate class, is levamisole. Levamisole is a simple imidazole compound with potent anti-helminthic activity and some antiviral activity that was inadvertently discovered to restore cell-mediated immunocompetence in immunologically depressed animals and patients. For example, patients sensitized to DNCB, but who do not manifest delayed hypersensitivity on challenge with DNCB, convert to DNCB positive after the administration of several days of levamisole therapy.[88] The probable mechanism of action of levamisole is to increase the activity of granylcyclase in lymphocytes, thus improving their immunologic reactivity. This, then, must be considered an immunorestorative agent. Very recently two positive reports regarding immunotherapeutic benefit from levamisole have been published. In breast cancer[89] and lung cancer,[90] after surgical extirpation of the disease, the administration of levamisole significantly prolonged the remission duration and survival. If it is correct that the major action of levamisole is immunorestoration of deficient or depressed immune responses, then levamisole will be most useful in combination with other modalities of immunotherapy. Thus levamisole may increase the responsiveness to active-nonspecific immunotherapy or may increase the responsiveness to active-specific immunotherapy. It will also be important to determine if levamisole immunotherapy is active in combination with chemotherapy. Animal experiments indicate

that levamisole administered after chemotherapy that induces complete remission is indeed effective.[91]

A variety of experiments demonstrating that active-specific immunotherapy is effective in cancer have been conducted during the last few years. We have already referred to the pioneering experiments of the Grahams and the classic work of Mathé and associates. The largest number of studies have been done in leukemia. Thus immunization with tumor cells plus BCG has been investigated and shown to be effective in ALL,[92] AML,[70] and CML.[93] The tumor cells were usually allogeneic, histologic-type-specific, and irradiated. However, Sokal used a cultured lymphoblastoid cell line in the CML study. In malignant melanoma, allogeneic or autologous irradiated tumor cells, either alone or in combination with DTIC immunotherapy, have led to remissions in advanced metastatic disease.[94,95] In osteogenic sarcoma, prolongation of disease-free interval and survival was induced by immunization with autologous homogenized ultraviolet-irradiated tumor.[96] In soft tissue sarcoma, after definitive surgery, immunotherapy with a cultured sarcoma cell line mixed with BCG has recently been described as being effective.[97] These data indicate that active-specific immunotherapy can prevent a recurrence of microscopic subclinical disease after surgery and can actually induce a regression of evident metastatic disease. Again, this supports the concept that modulation of the immune response may be effective, even when the disease is extensive.

Adoptive immunotherapy is in a much earlier stage of development than the two modalities of immunotherapy already discussed. In an early study Nadler and Moore cross-grafted patients with melanoma and other solid tumors, and after rejection of the tumor grafts they cross-transfused patients with presumably immune lymphocytes.[98] A small fraction of patients achieved remission as a result of this approach. In a number of studies transfer of tumor-specific immunity from relatives manifesting tumor immunity to immunologically unresponsive tumor-bearing patients has been achieved with transfer factor.[99] However, at the moment, except for one small study in breast cancer,[100] there is no compelling evidence that transfer factor has major therapeutic activity in cancer. However, this may very well be due to inadequate studies performed to the present time. Similarly, immune RNA has been demonstrated to be active in animal tumor systems,[101] and in addition, immune RNA from xenogeneic sources has been shown to confer tumor immunity on human lymphocytes in vitro.[102] Preliminary studies are now under way, and presumably the efficacy of immune RNA will be demonstrated in the near future. Interferon has definitely shown antitumor activity in a variety of animal systems.[103] In addition, there is one positive clinical study with interferon.[104] However, there are a number of reports of immunosuppressive activity by interferon,[105] and immunotherapeutic trials with this material must be approached with caution.

Finally, an important new adoptive immunotherapeutic reagent is thymosin. Thymosin is a partially purified extract of calf thymus that can partially restore T-cell-mediated immune functions in thymectomized animals.[106] Thymosin has been demonstrated to have potent therapeutic effects in children with immunodeficiency diseases based on hyporeactivity of the thymus.[107] In addition, thymosin can boost lymphocyte blastogenic reactivity when added to lymphocytes in vitro, and when administered to cancer patients in vivo it can augment delayed-type hypersensitivity and in vitro lymphocyte blastogenesis as well as a number of circulating T lymphocytes.[108] Phase I and II clinical trials with thymosin are now beginning, and the role of thymosin should be clarified shortly.

In certain animal models described above, local immunotherapy by intralesional injection of BCG has been highly effective. Not only does the infected tumor nodule regress, but regional metastases never develop. Animals receiving such primary local immunotherapy have resistance to subsequent challenge with tumor at distant sites. Local immunotherapy was at first applied to man by intralesional injection of BCG[109] or by topical application of DNCB or PPD.[110] Local tumor nodule regression, usually with little evidence of regression of noninjected nodules, was observed in immunocompetent patients with metastatic disease. Immunoincompetent patients usually did not respond. The presumed mechanism of action is killing of tumor cells at the injection site by the bystander effect of the local delayed hypersensitivity reaction to the injected material. There is probably activation of macrophages and perhaps lymphocytes in the regional lymph nodes, with resultant killing of microscopic foci of tumor cells within the lymph node. In addition, the intimate contact between

BCG and tumor cells apparently has a potent active-specific immunotherapeutic effect because of the resistance, at least in animals, to subsequent tumor challenge. Recently, local immunotherapy for primary tumors has shown efficacy. Thus one group has treated primary malignant melanoma with intratumor inoculation of vaccinia followed by surgical removal of the primary.[111] Such patients had prolonged disease-free intervals after surgery. Another group has treated recurrent primary bladder cancers with intravesical BCG and has delayed the development of new primaries by this treatment.[112] Thus local immunotherapy in man may have as potent effects as those described in animal systems.

Finally, as already partially indicated, combination approaches to immunotherapy are most important. We have already observed that active-nonspecific plus active-specific immunotherapy is highly effective in a number of disease categories. More important will be the combination of immunorestorative and either nonspecific or tumor-specific immunopotentiating approaches to immunotherapy. Therefore BCG or purified BCG subcomponents or tumor cells or purified tumor antigens will be given to patients after immunorestoration with agents such as levamisole or thymosin or after transfer of specific reactivity with materials such as transfer factor or immune RNA.

Based on the data outlined, several approaches to the immunotherapy of lung cancer according to its biologic characteristics, immunologic characteristics, and natural history become evident. Thus because of the immunodeficiency often associated with lung cancer and its poor prognosis, the approaches in the broad category referred to as immunoreconstitution are appropriate. This would include active-nonspecific immunotherapy with agents such as BCG[74] and C. parvum[86] that can boost cell-mediated immunity and adoptive or related immunologic approaches directed at restoring general immunocompetence, including the use of thymosin[107] and levamisole.[88] Since primary and metastatic tumors are infiltrated with lymphocytes and macrophages,[42] and since these cells can directly or indirectly kill target tumor cells, approaches to their activation at the local site should be taken. This would include systemic administration of agents known to activate macrophages,[113] such as BCG, C. parvum, and other microbial adjuvants. Since regional host defense mechanisms are very important in cancer, and since in other tumors regional immunotherapy[74] or local immunotherapy[109] has proved itself to be important, regional approaches to lung cancer, either intrapleural or intravenous, with macrophage- and lymphocyte-activating reagents, should be taken. Since specific tumor immunity is important in lung cancer,[56] and since tumor antigens are becoming available, active-specific immunotherapy with tumor cells or antigens (preferably mixed with adjuvant) or adoptive transfer of specific tumor immunity with transfer factor or immune RNA should be important. Finally, since circulating immunosuppressive factors may play an important role in the poor prognosis of lung cancer patients,[46] approaches to clearing these factors either through administration of passive antibody or through activation of the reticuloendothelial system and clearance of immune complexes should be actively investigated.

A number of studies in animal models provide important guidance for the development of immunotherapy of human lung cancer. Although there is no true model for lung cancer in animal systems, a variety of tumors metastasize to the lungs after subcutaneous implantation, or artificial pulmonary tumors may be created by intravenous injection of tumor cells with subsequent lodgement of those tumor cells in the pulmonary parenchyma. Several examples will suffice. Using the intravenous injection of syngeneic methylcholanthrene-induced fibrosarcoma in C57 black mice, Milas and Mujagic demonstrated that pulmonary tumor nodule formation was markedly reduced by the intravenous injection of 1 mg of *C. parvum*.[114] Pretreatment 7 days before tumor inoculation reduced nodule formation over 95 percent. Of greatest interest was the fact that treatment even 14 days after tumor inoculation reduced the number of metastatic pulmonary nodules by 66 percent. Several investigators have demonstrated that this effect is not dependent on the development of immunity to either *C. parvum* or tumor cells,[115] and the effect is still present in T-cell-deprived mice.[116] This effect is also resistant to radiotherapy.[116] This suggests that the mechanism involves activation of pulmonary macrophages and macrophage cytotoxicity to tumor cells, and this has been demonstrated directly.

Similar studies have been carried out with BCG. Thus Baldwin and Pimm observed that complete depression of pulmonary tumor growth after intravenous injection of methylcholan-

threne-induced sarcoma cells in the rat could be achieved when BCG was administered as late as 7 days after tumor cell administration. The BCG was administered intravenously.[117] A similar immunotherapeutic effect could be achieved by immunization subcutaneously with BCG plus the appropriate specific tumor cells. Some effect was noted even 10 days after tumor cell inoculation. In a related study, Pimm and Baldwin treated intrapleurally administered rat fibrosarcoma with irradiated BCG organisms given intrapleurally, intravenously, subcutaneously, or intraperitoneally.[118] Only the intrapleural BCG was active again, thus strongly indicating the need for regional immunotherapy in lung cancer. In these studies it was also thought that the mechanism of BCG activity was macrophage activation.

Using another tumor model (the guinea pig hepatoma), Hanna and associates have unequivocally demonstrated that after intralesional BCG immunotherapy very vigorous macrophage activation with killing of tumor cells at a killer cell/target cell ratio of 10:1 occurs.[119] In contrast, the same killing is only seen at a killer lymphocyte/target cell ratio of 10,000:1. There is also direct evidence for the potential for activated macrophages in lung cancer. Fidler has treated pulmonary metastases of the 3LL tumor in mice with intravenous activated macrophages and has observed a significant therapeutic effect.[120]

An intriguing observation forms a powerful argument for the potential role of immunotherapy in lung cancer of man; there is a dramatic direct association between postoperative empyema in lung cancer patients undergoing resection and a good prognosis.[121] The recurrence rate is lower and the disease-free interval is longer in patients who suffer empyema after surgery than in those who do not. It is hypothesized that the empyema activates regional lymph nodes and that activated lymph node cells kill tumor cells resident in them, preventing their further dissemination. In analogy to the guinea pig hepatoma model, in which intralesional therapy confers systemic tumor immunity,[84] it may also be that the interaction of residual tumor cells and bacteria or bacterial components heightens effective systemic tumor immunity.

Since the subject was last critically reviewed approximately 2 years ago,[122] major advances have been made in the immunotherapy of lung cancer. Studies of lung cancer immunotherapy can be divided into active-nonspecific systemic, active-nonspecific regional, immunorestorative, adoptive, and active-specific. Positive studies have been reported with all of these approaches.

Villasor treated patients with far-advanced breast, lung, colon, thyroid, and prostate cancer with chemotherapy plus BCG vaccination.[123] There were 31 controls and 43 BCG-treated patients. The addition of BCG vaccination to chemotherapy increased the percentage of good responses in terminal cancer patients, including objective and subjective responses, from 38 to 74 percent. The percentage of 1-year survivors increased from 45 to 58 percent. At 2 years the percentage of survivors was 6.4 and 16 percent, respectively, in the two groups. Khadzhiev and Kavaklieva-Dimitrova reported a series of studies in which an aqueous extraction of the Russian strain of BCG was administered to patients with inoperable bronchogenic carcinoma, some of whom were receiving other treatment.[124] Regression of histologically and radiographically proven tumors occurred in 28 percent of the patients and was attributed to the immunotherapy. The survival rate of patients receiving immunotherapy was superior to that in an "untreated" group. The efficacy of BCG in prolonging the disease-free interval after surgery and radiotherapy as either a single dose or on repeated injection has apparently been confirmed in two studies.[125,126] Israel, in an important study, used treatment with *C. parvum* given subcutaneously in combination with a multiple-drug chemotherapy program for the treatment of metastatic bronchogenic carcinoma.[86] A striking improvement in response rate and survival was noted, as compared to randomized patients receiving chemotherapy alone. There was a doubling of survival from 5 to 10 months. There was better response in immunocompetent patients than in immunoincompetent patients, but the effects of the addition of immunotherapy were clear-cut in both groups. Recently Yamamura and associates treated 39 patients with BCG cell wall skeleton attached to oil droplets.[127] Of 15 cases with stage I and II lung cancer, none died at 15 months, compared to survival of 84 and 19 percent, respectively, in historical controls. In patients with more advanced disease the addition of immunotherapy to surgery plus radiotherapy increased the median survival from 8 months to 15+ months, and at 19 months there were 40 percent survivors in the treated group compared to 5 percent survival in the historical

controls. In patients with far-advanced metastatic disease, when this type of immunotherapy was added to chemotherapy there was 50 percent survival at 14 months, as compared to zero in the controls. This clearly represents very potent active-nonspecific immunotherapy.

Very exciting data are also being generated in the area of regional immunotherapy. Based on their observations that postoperative empyema was associated with a good prognosis and on the original observation by Morton that intralesional BCG immunotherapy caused the regression of local tumor nodules,[109] McKneally and associates have carried out a study of regional immunotherapy in lung cancer.[128] Sixty patients were randomized to receive a single dose of BCG intrapleurally during the postoperative period or to receive no treatment. Previous studies had shown that intrapleural BCG was safe in hamsters and did not interfere with healing of vascular and bronchial suture lines following pulmonary resection in dogs. A single intrapleural injection of 10^7 viable units of Tice-strain BCG was given through the chest tube just prior to its removal or by thoracentesis in patients undergoing pneumonectomy. Fourteen days after administration of BCG, isoniazid at 300 mg/day was started and was continued for a period of 12 weeks. Controls were treated with isoniazid alone. To date, there have been no recurrences in 17 stage I patients treated by this approach, as compared to 9 recurrences in 22 patients in the control group. Other than a mild flulike syndrome during the 48 hr following the BCG administration there have been no side effects. This is indeed a remarkable study.

Recently Israel and associates[65] and Band and associates[64] have treated patients with *C. parvum* given intravenously. Band treated 19 patients with various solid tumors for 10 days with doses ranging from 0.5 to 6 mg/m². While there were considerable systemic side effects, objective regressions were noted in 4 patients, including 1 patient with pulmonary metastases of osteogenic sarcoma. In Israel's study patients were given intravenous *C. parvum* (4 mg/day) for as long as it was tolerated. Forty percent of patients showed some response. Median time to response was 3 weeks. Of 6 patients with lung cancer, 3 stabilized and 1 showed partial regression. Presumably the mechanism of action here is activation of macrophages and perhaps also lymphocytes within tumor masses. Both of these studies indicate that *C. parvum* has activity in the lung as well as at other sites and is effective alone even in patients with advanced disease.

Another approach to regional immunotherapy has been the aerosol administration of BCG. This is based on the fact that the aerosol route of administration is effective in controlling pulmonary infectious disease. Garner and associates[129] and Cusumano and associates[130] have done phase I trials of aerosol BCG in man. In both studies slow conversion of PPD skin reactivity and relatively severe respiratory side effects have been observed, thus suggesting that this approach will be limited. Indeed, it seems that with the activity and lower toxicity associated with intrapleural or intravenous administration of immunoadjuvants, use of the aerosol route will be quite limited.

In the area of immunorestoration a very important study has just been completed. Amery has coordinated a cooperative study on immunorestoration of patients with resectable bronchogenic carcoma in a multicenter group.[90] Patients with operable primary bronchogenic carcinoma received either a placebo or 50 mg of levamisole three times daily, repeated every 2 weeks, starting 3 days before surgery. No other therapy was given unless evidence of recurrence was observed. Recurrence was suspected or proved in 10 of 51 patients in the levamisole group (with 7 deaths), while recurrence was suspected or proved in 23 of 60 patients in the control group (with 12 deaths). Significant differences favoring levamisole were observed in patients with primary tumors greater than 7 cm in diameter, where recurrences were seen in 1 of 7 treated and 8 of 11 controls. Distant recurrences were much less frequent in levamisole-treated patients. Presumably the mechanism of action of levamisole is the restoration of general immunocompetence and specific tumor immunity in the patients, with subsequent lymphocyte-mediated killing of residual nests of tumor cells. The correlation of the most active therapeutic benefit with a large size of the primary tumor suggests that there is an important interaction between the tumor burden and the efficacy of this immunotherapeutic reagent.

A number of investigators have explored adoptive immunotherapy for lung cancer or for pulmonary metastases of other malignancies. Frenster administered autologous lymphocytes previously activated in vitro with phytohemagglutinin intravenously.[131] In this study lung cancer patients were not treated. However, only metastatic disease in the pulmonary area was affected, and Frenster noted significant regression in a number of patients with pulmonary metastases. In Humphrey's studies in which adoptive immunotherapy was carried out by cross-immunization of patients with a tumor extract followed by cross-transfusion of leukocytes, 15 percent responses were observed among lung cancer patients.[132] No studies of adoptive immunotherapy with transfer factor, immune RNA, or thymosin have yet been reported in lung cancer.

There are several important studies of active-specific immunotherapy in human lung cancer. Takita has treated patients with inoperable, partially resectable lung cancer with a vaccine consisting of fresh autologous tumor cells coupled to highly antigenic foreign protein.[133] This vaccine was administered repeatedly in complete Freund's adjuvant. Another approach, also used by Takita, was the administration of a tumor cell vaccine consisting of autologous tumor cells coated with concanavalin A. In a small group of patients these approaches have been associated with prolongation of survival, as compared to an appropriate control group. This is another example of benefit of immunotherapy alone in patients with large tumor burdens.

Recently Stewart and his colleagues have done an important trial of active-specific immunotherapy.[134] Antigen was prepared by the method of Hollinshead, and 100 μg mixed with complete Freund's adjuvant were administered repeatedly to patients after surgical extirpation of stage I bronchogenic carcinoma. This was a three-group study in which patients were treated with high-dose methotrexate followed by citrovorum factor rescue or chemotherapy plus the immunotherapy described above or the immunotherapy alone. Survival has been excellent in all 3 groups. There have been no deaths among the patients treated with immunotherapy, either alone or in combination, and all three groups are statistically superior to historical controls at this time. The immunotherapy was well tolerated, and only local toxic side effects were noted at the injection sites.

The data described above indicate that a variety of approaches to immunotherapy are effective in lung cancer. It is encouraging that systemic active-nonspecific, regional active-nonspecific, immunorestorative, adoptive, and active-specific immunotherapy all have shown activity. It is also encouraging that immunotherapy alone apparently has been active, either in causing regression of disease or in prolonging survival, even in patients with advanced metastatic disease.

The observations made to date provide important guidelines for the future development of this field. First, it is clear that since the prognosis of this disease is so poor, all patients with lung cancer should receive immunotherapy. The most promising approaches at the moment are the regional immunotherapy described by McKneally and associates, the immunorestorative use of levamisole described by Amery and associates, and the active-specific immunotherapy with purified tumor antigens described by Stewart and associates. Presumably, after considerable empirical work, the optimal doses, schedules, timing, and routes of administration of these various approaches to immunotherapy will be worked out. Also, one would presume that combinations of these and perhaps other approaches will be more effective than the individual approaches alone. It is conceivable that for optimal effects patients will undergo restorative immunotherapy to boost general immunocompetence, regional immunotherapy to activate immune cells in and around tumor masses and nodules, and active-specific immunotherapy to heighten specific tumor immunity.

SUMMARY AND CONCLUSIONS

In this review we have attempted to outline the current status of immunotherapy in human lung cancer and to describe its scientific basis. The scientific basis includes consideration of the facts that many patients with lung cancer are immunoincompetent and that good immunocompetence and a good prognosis are related in this disease. Tumor antigens and specific tumor immunity have been described in lung cancer, and vigorous specific tumor immunity, particularly of the cell-mediated type, is associated with a good prognosis. There is wide experience with immunotherapy in a variety of animal tumor models and human malignancies that strongly suggests that most if not all solid tumors, as well as the leukemias and lymphomas, will respond to immunotherapy. In these various systems immunotherapy is active in the prevention of recurrence of disease after the patient has been brought to a state of minimal residual disease by surgery, radiotherapy, or chemotherapy. Immunotherapy is also active in patients with advanced metastatic disease in combination with chemotherapy. Of great recent interest is the observation that immunotherapy alone can either stabilize or induce regression of malignant tumors, even in the patient with advanced metastatic disease. In a number of animal models in which experimental pulmonary or pleural metastases have been produced, active-specific immunotherapy and active-nonspecific immunotherapy (the latter of either the regional or the systemic type) have caused a reduction in the number of pulmonary metastases or a reduction in the size of the experimental tumor nodules. In man there are now a series of studies using active-nonspecific systemic, active-nonspecific regional, adoptive, and active-specific immunotherapy, all of which have shown either prolongation of disease-free interval and survival or regression of metastatic disease. We can no longer state that immunotherapy is in its infancy. Rather, immunotherapy appears to be an established modality of treatment, and although it is not curative at this time, certainly it is of major clinical benefit and should be applied widely to the lung cancer patient population.

REFERENCES

1. Selawry OS, Hansen HH: Lung cancer, in Holland JF, Frei E III (eds): Cancer Medicine. Philadelphia, Lea & Febiger, 1973, pp 1473–1518
2. Mountain CF: Keynote address on surgery in the therapy for lung cancer: Surgical prospects and priorities for clinical research. Cancer Chemother Rep 4:19–24, 1973
3. Hansen HH: Keynote address on chemotherapy for lung cancer. Cancer Chemother Rep 4:25–28, 1973
4. National Institutes of Health, Biometry Branch: End results in cancer, Report 3, Publication 30. NIH, Bethesda, Md, 1968, p 8
5. Hollinshead AC, Stewart THM, Herberman RB:

Delayed hypersensitivity reactions to soluble membrane antigens of human malignant lung cells. J Natl Cancer Inst 52:327–338, 1974

6. Steward AM: Tuberculin reaction in cancer patients, "Mantoux Release," and lymphosuppressive-stimulatory factors. J Natl Cancer Inst 50:625–632, 1973

7. Thomas JE, Coy P, Lewis HS, Yeun A: Effect of therapeutic irradiation on lymphocyte transformation in lung cancer. Cancer 27:1046–1050, 1971

8. Hersh EM, Gutterman JU, Mavligit GM: Immunotherapy of human cancer. Adv Intern Med 22:(in press)

9. Cohen MH: Lung cancer: A status report. J Natl Cancer Inst 55:505–511, 1975

10. Hersh EM, Gutterman JU, Mavligit GM: Cancer and host defense mechanisms, in Ioachim HL (ed): Pathobiology Annual. New York, Appleton-Century-Crofts, 1975, pp 133–167

11. Hersh EM, Gutterman JU, Mavligit GM, McCredie KB, Burgess MA, Matthews A, Freireich EJ: Serial studies of immunocompetence in patients undergoing chemotherapy for acute leukemia. J Clin Invest 54:401–408, 1974

12. Cone L, Uhr JW: Immunological deficiency disorders associated with chronic lymphocyte leukemia and multiple myeloma. J Clin Invest 43:2241–2248, 1964

13. Hester JP, MCredie KB, Freireich EJ: Immunological evaluation in patients with chronic myelogenous leukemia. Proc Am Assoc Cancer Res 15:180, 1974

14. Eltringham JR, Kaplan HS: Impaired delayed-hypersensitivity responses in 154 patients with untreated Hodgkin's disease. Natl Cancer Inst Monogr 36:107–115, 1973

15. Hersh EM, Curtis JE, Harris JE, McBride C, Alexanian R, Rossen RD: Host defense mechanisms in lymphoma and leukemia, in: Oncology 1970: Diagnosis and Management of Cancer. General Considerations. Proceedings of the Tenth International Cancer Congress. Chicago, Yearbook Medical Publishers, 1971

16. Twomey PL, Catalona WJ, Chretien PB: Cellular immunity in cured cancer patients. Cancer 33:435–440, 1974

17. Hersh EM, Whitecar JP Jr, McCredie KB, Bodey GP Sr, Freireich EJ: Chemotherapy, immunocompetence, immunosuppression, and prognosis in acute leukemia. N Engl J Med 285:1211–1216, 1971

18. Eilber FR, Morton DL: Impaired immunologic reactivity and recurrence following cancer surgery. Cancer 25:362–367, 1970

19. Levy R, Kaplan HS: Impaired lymphocyte function in untreated Hodgkin's disease. N Engl J Med 290:181–186, 1974

20. Lee AKY, Rowley M, Mackay IR: Antibody-producing capacity in human cancer. Br J Cancer 24:454–463, 1970

21. Stjernsward J, Joudal M, Vanky F, Wigzell H, Sealy R: Lymphopenia and change in distribution of human T and B lymphocytes in peripheral blood induced by irradiation for mammary carcinoma. Lancet 1:1352–1356, 1972

22. Park SK, Brody JL, Wallace HA, Blakemore WS: Immunosuppressive effect of surgery. Lancet 1:53–55, 1971

23. Campbell AC, Hersey P, MacLennan ICM, Kay HEM, Pike MC: Immunosuppressive consequences of radiotherapy and chemotherapy in patients with acute lymphoblastic leukaemia. Br Med J 2:385–388, 1973

24. Hersh EM, Freireich EJ: Host defense mechanisms and their modification by cancer chemotherapy, in Busch H (ed): Methods in Cancer Research. New York, Academic, 1968, pp 355–451

25. Eilber FR, Nizze JA, Morton DL: Sequential evaluation of general immune competence in cancer patients: Correlation with clinical course. Cancer 35:660–665, 1975

26. Israel L, Mugica J, Chahinian PH: Prognosis of early bronchogenic carcinoma. Survival curves of 451 patients after resection of lung cancer in relation to the results of pre-operative tuberculin skin test. Biomedicine 19:68–72, 1973

27. Silk M: Effect of plasma from patients with carcinoma on in vitro lymphocyte transformation. Cancer 20:2088, 1967

28. Sample FW, Gertner HR, Chretien PB: Inhibition of phytohemagglutinin-induced in vitro lymphocyte transformation by serum from patients with carcinoma. J Natl Cancer Inst 46:1291–1297, 1971

29. Brugarolas A, Han T, Takita H, Minowada J: Immunologic assays in lung cancer. NY State J Med 73:747–750, 1973

30. Hersh EM, Lurie PM, Takita H, Ritts R, Zelen R: Immunocompetence and prognosis in lung cancer. Proc Am Assoc Cancer Res 17:58, 1976

31. Jenkins VK, Olson MH, Ellis HN: In vitro methods of assessing lymphocyte transformation in patients undergoing radiotherapy for bronchogenic cancer. Tex Rep Biol Med 31:19–28, 1973

32. Golub SH, O'Connell TX, Morton DL: Correlation of in vivo and in vitro assays of immunocompetence in cancer patients. Cancer Res 34:1833–1837, 1974

33. McLaughlin AP III, Brooks JD: A plasma factor inhibiting lymphocyte reactivity in urologic cancer patients. J Urol 112:366–372, 1974

34. Occhino JC, Glasgow AH, Cooperband SR, Mannick JA, Schmid K: Isolation of an immunosuppressive peptide function from human plasma. J Immunol 110:685–694, 1973

35. Southam CM, Levin AG: A quantitative Rebuck technique. Blood 27:734–738, 1966

36. Pisano JC, DiLuzio NR, Salky NK: Absence of macrophage humoral recognition factor(s) in patients with carcinoma. J Lab Clin Med 76:141–150, 1970

37. Gross RL, Latty A, Williams EA, Newberne PM: Abnormal spontaneous rosette formation and rosette inhibition in lung carcinoma. N Engl J Med 292:169–181, 1975

38. Hersh EM, Gutterman JU, Mavligit GM, Dyre SE, Lee ET: Circulating B-lymphocyte levels, extent of disease and treatment in human cancer. Proc Am Assoc Cancer Res 16:227, 1975

39. Hamlin IME: Possible host resistance in carcinoma of the breast: A histological study. Br J Cancer 22:383–401, 1968

40. Alexander P, Hall JG: The role of immunoblasts in host resistance and immunotherapy of primary sarcomata. Adv Cancer Res 13:1–37, 1970

41. Ambus U, Mavligit GM, Gutterman JU, McBride CM, Hersh EM: Specific and non-specific immunologic reactivity of regional lymph node lymphocytes in human malignancy. Int J Cancer 14:291–300, 1974

42. Hersh EM, Mavligit GM, Gutterman JU, Barsales PB: Mononuclear cell content of human solid tumors. Med Ped Oncol 2:1–9, 1976

43. McDevitt HO, Sela M: Genetic control of the antibody response. I. Demonstration of determinant-specific differences in response to synthetic polypeptide antigens in two strains of inbred mice. J Exp Med 122:517–531, 1965

44. Law KK, Dudrick SJ, Abdou NI: Immunocompetence of patients with protein-calorie malnutrition. The effects of nutritional repletion. Ann Intern Med 79:545–550, 1973

45. Scheurlen PG, Schneider W, Pappas A: Inhibition of transformation of normal lymphocytes by plasma factor from patients with Hodgkin's disease and cancer. Lancet 2:1265, 1971

46. Jose DG, Seshadri R: Circulating immune complexes in human neuroblastomas: Direct assay and role in blocking specific cellular immunity. Int J Cancer 13:824–838, 1974

47. Metzgar RS, Mohanatumar T, Miller DS: Antigens specific for human lymphocyte and myeloid leukemia cells: Detection by nonhuman primate antiserums. Science 178:986–988, 1972

48. Herberman RB, Hollinshead AC, Char D, Oldham R, McCoy J, Cohen M: In vivo and in vitro studies of cell-mediated immune response to antigens associated with malignant melanoma. Behring Inst Mitt 56:131, 1975

49. Hollinshead AC, Glew D, Bunnag B, Gold P, Herberman R: Skin-reactive soluble antigen from intestinal cancer-cell-membranes and relationship to carcinoembryonic antigens. Lancet 1:1191–1195, 1970

50. Aurelian L, Strnad BC: Herpesvirus type 2-related antigens and their relevance to humoral and cell-mediated immunity in patients with cervical cancer. Cancer Res 36:810–820, 1976

51. Hollinshead AC, Chretien PB, Lee O, Tarpley JL, Kerney SE, Silverman NA, Alexander JC: In vivo and in vitro measurements of the relationship of human squamous carcinomas to herpes simplex virus tumor-associated antigens. Cancer Res 36:821–828, 1976

52. Stewart THM: The presence of delayed hypersensitivity reactions in patients toward cellular extracts of their malignant tumors. Cancer 23:1380–1387, 1969

53. Wells SA Jr, Burdick JF, Christiansen C, Ketcham AS, Adkins PC: Demonstration of tumor-associated delayed cutaneous hypersensitivity reactions in patients with lung cancer and in patients with carcinoma of the cervix. Natl Cancer Inst Monogr 37:197–203, 1973

54. Mavligit GM, Gutterman JU, McBride C, Hersh EM: Tumor directed immune reactivity and immunotherapy in malignant melanoma: Current status. Immunology of Cancer. Prog Exp Tumor Res 19:222–252, 1974

55. Nordquist RE: Specific antigens in human alveolar cell carcinoma. Cancer Res 33:1790–1795, 1973

56. Hollinshead AC, Stewart THM, Herberman RB: Delayed hypersensitivity reactions to soluble membrane antigens of human malignant lung cells. J Natl Cancer Inst 52:327–338, 1974

57. Takita H, Brugarolas A: Adjuvant immunotherapy for bronchogenic carcinoma: Preliminary results. Cancer Chemother Rep 4:293–298, 1973

58. Hellström I, Hellström KE, Sjögren HO, Warner GA: Demonstration of cell-mediated immunity to human neoplasms of various histological types. Int J Cancer 7:1–16, 1971

59. Baldwin RW, Embleton MJ, Jones JSP, Langman MJS: Cell-mediated and humoral immune reactions to human tumours. Int J Cancer 12:73–83, 1973

60. Golub SH: Host immune response to human tumor antigens, in Becker FF (ed): Cancer: A Comprehensive Treatise (vol 4). New York, Plenum Press, 1975, p 259

61. Mavligit GM, Hersh EM, McBride CM: Lymphocyte blastogenesis induced by autochthonous human solid tumor cells: Relationship of stage of disease and serum factors. Cancer 34:1712–1721, 1974

62. Roth JA, Holmes EC, Boddie AW Jr, Morton

DL: Lymphocyte responses of lung cancer patients to tumor-associated antigen measured by leucine incorporation. J Thorac Cardiovasc Surg 70:613–618, 1975

63. Cochran AJ, Spilg WGS, Mackie RM, Thomas CE: Postoperative depression of tumour-directed cell-mediated immunity in patients with malignant disease. Br Med J 4:67–70, 1972

64. Band PR, Jao-King C, Urtasun RC, Haraphongse M: Phase I study of *Corynebacterium parvum* in patients with solid tumors. Cancer Chemother Rep 59:1139–1145, 1975

65. Israel L, Edelstein R, DePierre A, Dimitrov N: Brief communication: Daily intravenous infusion of *Corynebacterium parvum* in twenty patients with disseminated cancer: A preliminary report of clinical and biologic findings. J Natl Cancer Inst 55:29–33, 1975

66. Coley WB: A report of recent cases of inoperable sarcoma successfully treated with mixed toxins of erysipelas and bacillus prodigiosus. Surg Gynecol Obstet 13:174–190, 1911

67. Nauts HC, Fowler GA, Bogatko FH: A review of the influence of bacterial infection and of bacterial products (Coley's toxins) on malignant tumors in man. Acta Med Scand 276:1–103, 1953

68. Graham JB, Graham RM: Autogenous vaccine in cancer patients. Surg Gynecol Obstet 114:1, 1962

69. Mathé G, Amiel JL, Schwarzenberg L, Schneider M, Cattan A, Schlumberger JR, Hayat M, De Vassal F: Active immunotherapy for acute lymphoblastic leukaemia. Lancet 1:697–699, 1969

70. Powles RL, Crowther D, Bateman CJT, Beard MEJ, McElwain TJ, Russell J, Lister TA, Whitehouse JMA, Wrigley PFM, Pike M, Alexander P, Hamilton-Fairley G: Immunotherapy for acute myelogenous leukaemia. Br J Cancer 28:365, 1973

71. Gutterman JU, Rodriquez V, Mavligit GM, Burgess MA, Gehan E, Hersh EM, McCredie KB, Reed RC, Smith T, Bodey GP Sr, Freireich EJ: Chemoimmunotherapy of adult acute leukaemia prolongation of remission in myeloblastic leukaemia with BCG. Lancet 2:1405–1409, 1974

72. Sokal JE, Aungst W, Snyderman M: Delay in progression of malignant lymphoma after BCG vaccination. N Engl J Med 291:1226–1230, 1974

73. Gutterman JU, McBride C, Freireich EJ, Mavligit GM, Frei E III, Hersh EM: Active immunotherapy with BCG for recurrent malignant melanoma. Lancet 1:1208–1212, 1973

74. Gutterman JU, Mavligit GM, Gottlieb JA, Burgess MA, McBride CE, Einhorn L, Freireich EJ, Hersh EM: Chemoimmunotherapy of disseminated malignant melanoma with DTIC and BCG. N Engl J Med 291:592, 1974

75. Mavligit GM, Gutterman JU, Burgess MA, Khankhanian N, Seibert B, Speer JF, Jubert AV, Martin RC, McBride CM, Copeland EM, Gehan EA, Hersh EM: Prolongation of postoperative disease-free interval and surgery in human colorectal cancer by Bacillus Calmette-Guerin (BCG) or BCG plus 5-Fluorouracil. Lancet 1:871–875, 1976

76. Cardenas JO, Gutterman JU, Livingston RB, Blumenschein GR, Einhorn LG, Freireich EJ, Hersh EM, Gottlieb JA: 5-Fluorouracil, Adriamycin, Cyclophosphamide (FAC) with or without BCG maintenance, chemotherapy for metastatic breast cancer (manuscript in preparation)

77. Donaldson RC: Methotrexate plus Bacillus Calmette-Guerin (BCG) and Isoniazid in the treatment of cancer of the head and neck. Am J Surg 124:527, 1972

78. Hersh EM, Gutterman JU, Mavligit GM, Reed RC, Richman SP: BCG vaccine and its derivatives: Potential, practical considerations, and precautions in human cancer immunotherapy. JAMA 235:646–650, 1976

79. Yron I, Weiss DW, Robinson E, Cohen D, Adelberg MG, Mekori T, Haber M: Immunotherapeutic studies in mice with the methanol-extraction residue (MER) fraction of BCG: Solid tumors. Natl Cancer Inst Monogr 39:33–54, 1973

80. Weiss DW, Stupp Y, Many N, Izak G: Treatment of acute myelocytic leukemia (AML) patients with MER tubercle bacillus fraction: A preliminary report. Trans Proc 7:545–552, 1975

81. Richman SP: Phase I study of immunotherapy with methanol extraction residue of BCG (MER). Proc Am Assoc Clin Oncol (abstract 1025) 16:227, 1975

82. Moertel CG, Ritts RE, Schutt AJ, Hahn RG: A phase I study of MER (methanol extraction residue) fraction of BCG as an immunostimulant in patients with advanced cancer. Cancer Res 35:3075, 1975

83. Ribi E, Meyer TJ, Azuma I, Parker R, Brehmer W: Biologically active components from Mycobacterial cell walls. IV. Protection of mice against aerosol infection with virulent *Mycobacterium tuberculosis*. Cell Immunol 16:1–10, 1975

84. Zbar B, Bernstein ID, Bartlett GL, Hanna MG Jr, Rapp HJ: Immunotherapy of cancer: Regression of intradermal tumors and prevention of growth of lymph node metastases after intralesional injection of living *Mycobacterium bovis*. J Natl Cancer Inst 49:119–130, 1972

85. Gray GR, Ribi E, Granger D, Parker R, Azuma I, Yamamoto K: Immunotherapy of cancer: Tumor suppression and regression by cell walls of *Mycobacterium phlei* attached to oil droplets. J Natl Cancer Inst 55:727–730, 1975

86. Israel L, Halpern G: Le *Corynebacterium parvum* dans les cancers avances. Nouv Presse Méd 1:19–23, 1972

87. Clarkson BD, Dowling MD, Gee TS, Cunningham IB, Burchenal JH: Treatment of acute leukemia in adults. Cancer 36:775–795, 1975

88. Tripodi D, Parks LC, Brugmans J: Drug-induced restoration of cutaneous delayed hypersensitivity in anergic patients with cancer. N Engl J Med 289:354–357, 1973

89. Rojas AF, Mickiewics E, Feierstein JN, Glait H, Olivari AJ: Levamisole in advanced human breast cancer. Lancet 1:211–215, 1976

90. Study Group for Bronchogenic Carcinoma: Immunopotentiation with levamisole in resectable bronchogenic carcinoma: A double-blind controlled trial. Br Med J 3:461–464, 1975

91. Perk K, Chirigos MA, Fuhrman F, Pettigrew H: Brief communication: Some aspects of host response to levamisole after chemotherapy in a murine leukemia. J Natl Cancer Inst 54:253–256, 1976

92. Mathé G, Amiel JL, Schwarzenberg L, Schneider M, Cattan A, Schlumberger JR, Hayat M, De Vassal F: Active immunotherapy for acute lymphoblastic leukaemia. Lancet 1:697–699, 1969

93. Sokal JE, Aungst CW, Grace JT: Immunotherapy in well-controlled chronic myelocytic leukemia. NY State J Med 73:1180–1185, 1973

94. Laucius JF, Bodurtha AJ, Berkelhamer J, Prehn LM, Prehn RT, Mastrangelo MJ: Intradermal injection of autochthonous irradiated tumor cells plus BCG in the treatment of metastatic malignant melanoma. Proc Am Assoc Cancer Res 15:171, 1974

95. Currie GA, McElwain TJ: Active immunotherapy as an adjunct to chemotherapy in the treatment of disseminated malignant melanoma: A pilot study. Br J Cancer 31:143–156, 1975

96. Southam CM, Marcove RC, Levin AG, Buchsbaum HJ, Mike V: Clinical trial of autogenous tumor vaccine for treatment of osteogenic sarcoma. Proc VII Nat Cancer Conf. Philadelphia, Lippincott, 1973, pp 91–100

97. Townsend CM, Eilber FR, Morton DL: Skeletal and soft tissue sarcomas. JAMA 236:2187–2189, 1976

98. Nadler SH, Moore GE: Immunotherapy of malignant disease. Arch Surg 99:376–381, 1969

99. LoBuglio AF, Neidhart JA, Hilberg RW, Metz EN, Balcerzak SP: The effect of transfer factor therapy on tumor immunity in alveolar soft part sarcoma. Cell Immunol 7:159–165, 1973

100. Oettgen HF, Old LJ, Farrow JH, Valentine FT, Lawrence HS, Thomas LL: Effects of dialyzable transfer factor in patients with breast cancer. Proc Natl Acad Sci 71:2319–2323, 1974

101. Pilch YH, Ramming KP, Deckers PJ: RNA extracts in tumor immunity. Induction of anticancer immunity with RNA. Ann NY Acad Sci 207:409–429, 1973

102. Veltman LL, Kern DH, Pilch YH: Immune cytolysis of human tumor cells mediated by xenogeneic "immune" RNA. Cell Immunol 13:367–377, 1974

103. Gresser I, Bourali-Maury C: Inhibition by interferon preparations of a solid malignant tumour and pulmonary metastasis in mice. Nature [New Biol] 236:78–79, 1972

104. Blomgren H, Strander H, Cantell K: Effect of human leukocyte interferon on the response of lymphocytes to mitogenic stimuli in vitro. Scand J Immunol 3:697–705, 1974

105. Thorbecke GJ, Friedman-Kien AE, Vilcek J: Effect of rabbit interferon on immune responses. Cell Immunol 12:290–295, 1975.

106. Hooper JA, McDaniel MC, Thurman GB, Cohen GH, Schulof RS, Goldstein AL: Purification and properties of bovine thymosin. Ann NY Acad Sci 249:125–144, 1975

107. Wara DW, Goldstein AL, Doyle NE, Ammann AJ: Thymosin activity in patients with cellular immunodeficiency. N Engl J Med 292:70–74, 1975

108. Schafer LA, Washington ML, Goldstein AL: Thymosin immunotherapy—a phase I study. Proc Am Soc Clin Oncol (abstract 1051) 16:233, 1975

109. Morton DL, Holmes EC, Eilber FR, Wood WC: Immunological aspects of neoplasia: A rational basis for immunotherapy. Ann Intern Med 74:587–604, 1971

110. Klein E, Holtermann OA, Papermaster B, Milgrom H, Rosner D, Klein L, Walker MJ, Zbar B: Immunologic approaches to various types of cancer with the use of BCG and purified protein derivatives. Natl Cancer Inst Monogr 39:229–239, 1973

111. Everall JD, O'Donerty CJ, Wand J, Dowd PM: Treatment of primary melanoma by intralesional vaccinia before excision. Lancet 2:583–586, 1975

112. Eidinger D, Morales A: Treatment of superficial bladder cancer in man. Ann NY Acad Sci 277:239–240, 1976

113. Mansell PWA, Ichinose H, Reed RJ, Krementz ET, McNamee R, DiLuzio MR: Macrophage-mediated destruction of human malignant cells in vivo. J Natl Cancer Inst 54:571–580, 1975

114. Milas L, Mujagic H: Protection by *Corynebacterium parvum* against tumour cells injected intravenously. Rev Eur Etud Clin Biol 17:498–500, 1972

115. Bomford R, Olivotto M: The mechanism of inhibition by *Corynebacterium parvum* of the growth of lung nodules from intravenously injected tumour cells. Int J Cancer 14:226–235, 1974

116. Scott MT: *Corynebacterium parvum* as a therapeutic antitumor agent in mice. I. Systemic effects from intravenous injection. J Natl Cancer Inst 53:855–860, 1974

117. Baldwin RW, Pimm MV: BCG immunotherapy

of pulmonary growth from intravenously transferred rat tumour cells. Br J Cancer 27:48, 1973

118. Pimm MV, Baldwin RW: BCG therapy of pleural and peritoneal growth of transplanted rat tumours. Int J Cancer 15:260–269, 1975

119. Hanna MG Jr, Fidler IJ, Peters LC, Budmen M: manuscript in preparation

120. Fidler IJ: manuscript in preparation

121. Ruckdeschel JC, Codish SD, Stranahan A, McKneally MF: Postoperative empyema improves survival in lung cancer: Documentation and analysis of a natural experiment. N Engl J Med 287:1013–1017, 1972

122. Hersh EM, Gutterman JU, Mavligit GM: Perspectives for the immunotherapy of lung cancer. Cancer Treatment Rev 1:65–80, 1974

123. Villasor R: The clinical use of BCG vaccination in stimulating host resistance to cancer: Phase II. Immuno-chemotherapy in advanced cancer. J Philippine Med Assoc 41:619–632, 1965

124. Khadzhiev S, Kavaklieva-Dimitrova Y: Treatment of bronchial cancer patients with a water saline extract of BCG. Vopr Onkol 17:15–57, 1971

125. Edwards FR, Whitwell F: Use of BCG as an immunostimulant in the surgical treatment of carcinoma of the lung. Thorax 29:654–658, 1974

126. Pines A: A 5-year controlled study of BCG and radiotherapy for inoperable lung cancer. Lancet 1:380–381, 1976

127. Yamamura Y, Azuma I, Taniyama T, Sugimura K, Hirao F, Tokuzen R, Okabe M, Nakahara W, Yasumoto K, Ohta M: Immunotherapy of cancer with cell-wall skeleton of Mycobacterium bovis–Bacillus Calmette-Guerin: Experimental and clinical results. Ann NY Acad Sci 277:209–227, 1976

128. McKneally MF, Maver C, Kausel HW: Regional immunotherapy of lung cancer with intrapleural BCG. Lancet 1:377–385, 1976

129. Garner FB, Meyer CA, White DS, Lipton A: Aerosol BCG treatment of carcinoma metastatic to the lung: A phase I study. Cancer 35:1088–1094, 1974

130. Cusumano CL, Jernigan JA, Waldman RH: Aerosolized BCG (Tice strain) treatment of bronchogenic carcinoma: Phase I study. J Natl Cancer Inst 55:275, 1975

131. Frenster JH, Rogaway WM: manuscript in preparation

132. Humphrey LJ, Jewell WR, Murray DR, Griffin WO Jr: Immunotherapy for the patient with cancer. Ann Surg 173:47–54, 1971

133. Takita H, Minowada J, Han T, Takada M, Lane WW: Adjuvant immunotherapy in bronchogenic carcinoma. Ann NY Acad Sci 277:345–354, 1976

134. Stewart THM, Hollinshead AC, Harris JE, Belanger R, Crepeau A, Hooper GD, Sachs HJ, Klaassen DJ, Hirte W, Rapp E, Crook AF, Orizaga M, Sengar DPS, Raman S: Immuno-chemotherapy of lung cancer. Ann NY Acad Sci 277:436–466, 1976

Mark G. Janis
Marc J. Straus

17
Pleural Effusions

Pleural effusion and lung cancer are intimately related. Pleural effusion is the presenting sign or symptom of the neoplastic process leading to the initial diagnosis of lung cancer in approximately 1 percent of patients.[1] According to the TNM classification (see Chapter 12) the presence of pleural effusion is considered a T3 lesion, contraindicating surgical intervention.[2] Dyspnea, shortness of breath, chest pain, and cough are associated with significant effusions. In the patient with lung cancer, effusions can be the major incapacitating feature restricting the patient's activity, compromising the quality of life, and necessitating repeated hospitalizations. It is estimated that 50 percent of patients with lung cancer will have a pleural effusion during the course of their disease.[3] Thus the frequency of occurrence and the symptomatic severity of malignant pleural effusions indicate the importance of knowing how to treat this potentially reversible complication of lung cancer and prevent its recurrence.

PATHOPHYSIOLOGY

Normally the pleural space is fluid-free or contains only a few milliliters of low-protein fluid.[4,5] Pleural fluid is constantly being formed and absorbed, and the net balance of these processes determines the presence or absence of an effusion. The parietal pleural vasculature is derived from the high-pressure systemic circulation, and normally there is a net positive pressure of 9 cm H_2O tending to drive fluid into the potential pleural space. The visceral pleural vasculature is associated with the low-pressure pulmonary system, which under normal circumstances has a net pressure of -10 cm H_2O and promotes absorption of fluid from the pleural space. Lymphatic vessels are located in the subepithelial layer of both pleural surfaces, and they also participate in the absorption of fluid and protein from the pleural cavity. These lymphatics in turn drain into the hilar and mediastinal nodes.

Pleural infiltration with tumor cells can be secondary to direct extension from a parenchymal primary, particularly a peripherally situated adenocarcinoma, or secondary to lymphatic or vascular metastases. Increased capillary permeability results, and it is associated with increased production of pleural fluid and increased protein secretion. Effusions produced in this manner will most likely contain many neoplastic cells, yielding a positive pleural fluid cytology. The incidence of pleural involvement found at postmortem study reflects the tumor histology; in one study 34 percent of epidermoid carcinoma, 32 percent of oat cell carcinoma, and 60 percent of adenocarcinoma cases had pleural implants.[6] It should be noted that the mere presence of pleural metastases may not result in clinically detectable effusion, as only 60 percent of Meyer's patients had effusion, despite findings of pleural metastases at autopsy.[7] Capillary permeability may also be increased by pleuritis associated with obstructive pneumonitis secondary to tumor occlusion of a bronchus. In this situation tumor cells may not be noted in the pleural fluid because the pleural surfaces are not directly infiltrated by tumor. However, the protein content of the pleural fluid may be elevated secondary to the increased capillary permeability.

Pleural effusions may also result from decreased absorption of fluid from the pleural space. Tumors that infiltrate the mediastinal lymphatic system may lead to lymphatic obstruction[2,7] and increased hydrostatic pressure, which will decrease fluid and protein absorption.[4] These patients will also have a negative pleural fluid cytology unless concomitant pleural metastases are present. Pleural fluid protein will be elevated because of the decreased lymphatic protein absorption. Lymphatic absorption of pleural fluid may be further decreased by the presence of the pleural effusion itself because of diminished intercostal muscle activity and diaphragmatic excursion, which normally promotes lymphatic pleural fluid absorption by acting as a pumping mechanism.[4]

Less frequent causes of pleural effusion associated with lung cancer are (1) pericardial effusion, which can increase hydrostatic pressure; (2) superior vena caval obstruction, which is associated with an increased parietal pleural capillary pressure;[4,5] and x-ray therapy.[8]

Nonneoplastic causes of pleural effusion should also be considered, especially in older patients or patients with a history of heart disease. Congestive heart failure results in increased pressure in the pulmonary vascular system, resulting in fluid transudation and decreased pleural fluid reabsorption.[5] These effusions are often transudates and have a negative cytology. Hypoproteinemia, which may occur with repeated thoracentesis, increased catabolism, or decreased hepatic synthesis, will decrease osmotic pressure and may contribute to the recurrence of pleural effusion.[4]

PRINCIPLES OF TREATMENT

Pleural effusion may be present initially, or it can develop in the course of lung cancer. Effusions may be asymptomatic, an incidental radiographic abnormality, or they may be incapacitating. Small or asymptomatic effusions do not warrant immediate therapeutic intervention, unless it is necessary for diagnostic evaluation. Systemic treatment with multidrug chemotherapy or x-ray therapy, by effectively shrinking tumor masses, mediastinal or hilar nodes, or pleural metastases, may result in resolution of the pleural effusion. This may be the most effective mode of treatment with susceptible histologic classes such as small cell carcinoma, adenocarcinoma, and perhaps large cell carcinoma. It may eradicate the cause of the effusion and restore the normal pleural fluid dynamics. It should be considered as the initial mode of treatment for all patients with a reasonable chance of response, except in the presence of life-threatening pleural effusions. Simple thoracentesis can be used for symptomatic control in the interval before systemic response occurs.

Symptomatic effusions unresponsive to systemic chemotherapy will require local treatment, either by simple removal of fluid (thoracentesis or tube thoracostomy) or by instillation of a sclerosing agent (nitrogen mustard, Atabrine, or tetracycline) to obliterate the pleural space and to prevent fluid reaccumulation. Neither of these modalities will control systemic disease, but they may provide significant symptomatic relief and improve the quality of life if not prolong life. Thoracentesis should be used initially, but when fluid reaccumulation is rapid (i.e., within days) or after two or three taps a sclerosing agent should be used; repeated thoracentesis in this clinical setting will not prevent reaccumulation and may impair response to subsequent therapeutic modalities (see below).

Tube thoracostomy with instillation of a sclerosing agent will usually control these refractory effusions by producing a pleurodesis. Patients on a specific chemotherapy protocol for systemic disease or with significant bone marrow suppression should not receive nitrogen mustard because of systemic absorption from the inflamed pleura, and Atabrine or tetracycline may be preferred. Otherwise the ease of administration and rapidity of response make mustard the treatment of choice. Patients failing to respond to one sclerosing agent may be given a course of the other agents.

Nonneoplastic processes such as congestive heart failure, pneumonia, fluid overload, and hypoproteinemia should be ruled out and treated when present. From a review of the literature it is difficult to determine the pathogenic contribution of these processes, but it would seem to be minimal, as more than 70 percent of all pleural effusions associated with neoplastic processes had a positive cytology,[7,9-11] and 90 percent of effusions had either positive cytology or pleural biopsy. In the study by Anderson et al. only 13 of 125 effusions were noted in patients who were in congestive heart failure, and 10 of these patients had positive pleural fluid cytology.[10] Diuretics may reduce the size of the effusion in an occasional patient, but their role in therapy is peripheral and probably insignificant.[13]

THORACENTESIS

The simplest procedure is ordinary thoracentesis. Its effect is immediate, and it can be performed at almost any time; it usually does not require the patient to be hospitalized and does not require specialized services. Two liters or more can be removed,[5] with rapid relief of dyspnea or respiratory embarrassment. Unfortunately its effects are often of short duration. Lambert et al. noted 100 percent recurrence of effusions treated only with thoracentesis,[9] and Anderson et al. reported a 96 percent recurrence within 1 month, as only 4 of 97 patients were effusion-free for more than 30 days.[10] The average time to recurrence in the series of Anderson et al. was 4.2 days.[10] Repeated thoracentesis, especially the high-protein exudates, can contribute to the development of hypoproteinemia, and the subsequent reduction of osmotic pressure may contribute to reaccumulation of pleural fluid. Hypoproteinemia in these generally catabolic patients may also contribute to their general debility and malnutrition. Empyema, pneumothorax, bronchopleural fistulas, and fluid loculation are other frequently noted complications of repeated thoracentesis, and they may make subsequent therapeutic procedures technically more difficult by preventing pleural apposition and pleurodesis. Additionally, it is almost impossible to remove all accumulated fluid and obtain full lung expansion with simple needle aspiration.[14] Thus the role of simple thoracentesis should probably be restricted to (1) evaluation of the initial effusion to determine its etiology and tendency to reaccumulate, (2) relief of acute life-threatening respiratory embarrassment if tube thoracostomy is not practicable, and (3) palliation in the terminal patient whose life expectancy is only a few days. Some patients will not reaccumulate pleural fluid, and for this reason a more comprehensive initial procedure is not indicated.

SCLEROSING AGENTS

Once the recurrent nature of the malignant pleural effusion has been established and it is determined that systemic therapy either is ineffective or is not indicated, the most effective mode of treatment is the production of a sterile adhesive pleuritis with subsequent obliteration of the potential pleural space. Fusion of the pleural surfaces requires near-total reexpansion of the underlying lung and complete removal of pleural fluid so that the parietal and visceral pleural surfaces can be in complete apposition when the sclerosing agent is introduced. This is best accomplished by tube thoracostomy[3,9,10,14-16] with removal of all accumulated pleural fluid over a period of 24–48 hr. Chest x-ray can be used to determine lung reexpansion prior to introduction of the sclerosing agent via the indwelling tube. Failure to remove all the fluid or to reexpand the lung will prevent pleurodesis and render fluid reaccumulation more likely.[14,16,17]

Nitrogen Mustard

Following tube thoracostomy and pleural fluid drainage, nitrogen mustard instilled into the pleural cavity at a dose of 0.4 mg/kg (maximum dose 20 mg) results in a response rate of 55 to 87 percent.[3,9,10,14-20] Mustard alkylates proteins and nucleic acids rapidly. As soon as it has been instilled the patient must rotate through all postural positions at 1-min intervals (right side, back, left side, stomach) for approximately 15 min to ensure distribution of the drug throughout the entire pleural cavity.[3] The therapeutic effect of nitrogen mustard most likely is related to its vesicant action[20] rather than its antineoplastic properties. Postmortem studies have shown almost complete obliteration of the pleural space secondary to fibrinous serositis despite the presence of abundant tumor implants,[16] which may explain the therapeutic benefit noted in patients previously unresponsive to systemic administration of the mustard. The patient should be premedicated with an antiemetic to counteract the nausea and vomiting commonly noted within 6 hr of instilla- tion of the mustard. Virtually 100 percent of treat- ed patients develop fever. It begins within several hours of administration and may reach 103°F; it usually subsides within 48 hr. Local pleuritic chest pain necessitating analgesics frequently complicates the mustard instillation as well. Some patients may temporarily note rapid pleural fluid reaccumulation following mustard—a mus- tard-induced serositis.[3] For this reason it is rec- ommended that the chest tube be left in place following injection of the mustard to permit drain- age and not be removed until the pleura have fused.[10,21] Leukopenia is another of the reported complications following intrapleura mustard; it was found in 10 percent of the patients treated by Mark et al.[20] The usual recommendation is to reduce the dosage at least 50 percent in patients receiving concomitant systemic chemotherapy with preexisting bone marrow suppression or in patients who have had or are having a significant functional marrow area irradiated. Reexpansion is often noted within 48–72 hr.[10] Patients who fail to respond may have the treatment repeated in 2– 3 weeks if blood counts permit. With retreatment, subsequent side effects may not be as prevalent because of decreased systemic absorption due to the fibrosis from the initial treatment. The advan- tages of nitrogen mustard are relative ease of administration, inexpensiveness, rapid relief of symptoms, and relatively mild toxicity.

Atabrine

Atabrine (quinacrine hydrochloride) is the other frequently instilled sclerosing agent,[15,22–26] with a response rate of 64 to 88 percent reported. In vitro cytotoxic activity and antineoplastic activity have been described with Atabrine. Its primary therapeutic effect is inflammatory, with pleural fibrosis and adhesions and obliteration of the pleural space following its intrapleural instilla- tion.[22] The Atabrine is dissolved in 10 ml of saline and injected into the pleural space following thor- acentesis. Initially 50–100 mg are given to deter- mine individual sensitivity or idiosyncrasy. If significant pain, fever, hypotension, or hallucinations do not occur, 100–200 mg are given daily on days 2–5 until local pleuritis is produced, hallmarked by significant local pleural pain and fever. Toxicity consists of (1) local pleuritic pain, noted in 50 percent of patients, which begins several hours after treatment; (2) fever, seen in 100 percent of patients, with temperatures to

103°F or 104°F beginning 4–8 hr after treatment and lasting up to 10 days; (3) hallucinations noted in patients receiving high-dose Atabrine (more that 800 mg as a single dose); and (4) hypotension, also noted in patients receiving more than 800 mg as a single dose.[25] As a rule the frequency and severity of toxic reactions are dose-dependent and are less of a clinical problem when Atabrine is given in smaller dosage.[25] If one is willing to accept the increased side effects, a single dose of 800 mg of Atabrine via thoracostomy tube will control effusions in 70 percent of patients with malignant pleural effusions.[25] One must be care- ful in interpreting the chest x-ray in patients suc- cessfully administered Atabrine, as often a fibro- thorax develops that radiographically can be indistinguishable from a massive pleural effusion (i.e., an opacified hemithorax).[3] If the clinical situation dictates, a thoracentesis may be neces- sary to rule out recurrence of the pleural effusion. Response may take up to 3 months.[3] There is no marrow toxicity with Atabrine, and it may be the treatment of choice for patients with recurrent pleural effusions and concomitant hematologic suppression. Because of the more frequent thora- centeses required to administer the Atabrine, I would favor the initial use of nitrogen mustard, as both have similar success rates.

Tetracycline

Tetracycline has been utilized as a sclerosing agent.[27] It is highly acid in solution (pH 2.4) and is able to induce mesothelial destruction. Thorsrud demonstrated that tetracycline was more effec- tive in producing pleural symphysis, as compared to talc, nitrogen mustard, and thiotepa, in an animal model.[28] Closed-tube thoracostomy is per- formed with overnight drainage: 500 mg of tetra- cycline is diluted in 30 ml of saline and injected into the tube, followed by 10 ml of saline to clear the tube. The tube is clamped for 6 hr, with positional changes, and then is opened and hooked to low suction and permitted to drain for 24 hrs, followed by extubation when significant drainage has stopped.[27] In 4 patients who had failed to respond to either nitrogen mustard (3 patients) or thiotepa (1 patient), successful con- trol for 3–19 months was obtained without further thoracentesis. The only contraindication to the use of tetracycline is hypersensitivity. To date, too few patients have been treated to recommend tetracycline as the initial mode of therapy. How- ever, it is a promising modality, particularly in patients who are unable to receive mustard or have failed to respond to the other sclerosing agents.

Iodized Talc

Iodized talc is yet another agent capable of producing scrositis and pleurodesis and pleural space obliteration,[15,17,29-32] with success rates up to 90 percent reported. Unfortunately this mode of treatment requires submitting the patient to thoracotomy and general anesthesia. Postoperatively patients usually have significant local pain for at least 3–5 days. Considering the poor prognosis of most patients with metastatic lung cancer, it is too extensive a procedure and is best reserved for neoplastic processes with more favorable prognoses (i.e., certain patients with breast cancer).[15] It may become a more important therapeutic tool in the future as better systemic agents become available to control disseminated bronchogenic carcinoma.

RADIOTHERAPY

External-beam supervoltage x-ray has also been successfully utilized to control pleural effusions. [60]Co sources and linear accelerators have been used.[33] Three weeks are required to complete this course of treatment, which can be administered on an inpatient or outpatient basis. In one study the authors reported an 80 percent response rate in 17 patients with no evidence of bone marrow toxicity or radiation pneumonitis 3 months after treatment.[33] This mode of treatment is not well suited to the acutely symptomatic patient, but it may be helpful in the prophylactic treatment of high-risk patients (i.e., peripheral adenocarcinoma) or the asymptomatic patient with an incidentally noted effusion in order to prevent the development of symptomatic recurrent effusions. In those patients whose effusions are thought to be secondary to mediastinal node involvement or lymphatic infiltration, mediastinal irradiation may help prevent pleural fluid reaccumulation.

MISCELLANEOUS

Extensive experience with the instillation of intracavitary radioactive colloids (gold, chromic phosphate, and yttrium) has been report-ed.[3,34,35,37,38] Compared to the other available treatment modalities outlined above, their use is more expensive and technically more difficult; they are not universally available, and their clinical effectiveness is not sufficiently superior to recommend their use as primary therapy. Their use should be considered for the symptomatic problem patient unresponsive to the more standard therapies.

CONCLUSIONS

Recurrent pleural effusions often are the cause of marked symptomatic debilitation and a major limitation to the quality of life in patients with incurable carcinoma of the lung. The therapeutic goal is simple, rapid palliation with minimal toxicity. Systemic multidrug chemotherapy or radiotherapy to control the entire disease process should be the initial form of treatment when possible, except for life-threatening respiratory embarrassment. Initially, simple thoracentesis or tube thoracostomy may provide adequate symptomatic relief. With recurrence, tube thoracostomy with nitrogen mustard instillation in patients without marrow depression is the treatment of choice. Atabrine or tetracycline can be used for patients receiving systemic cytotoxic drugs or extensive radiotherapy involving functional marrow areas. Patients unresponsive to mustard may improve with Atabrine, tetracycline, or intracavitary radioisotopes. Mediastinal radiotherapy may help control recurrent effusions secondary to lymphatic obstruction.

Extensive or risky surgical procedures such as pleurectomy or talc pleurodesis should be discouraged, unless the patient has an unusually good prognosis, because of the greater morbidity and mortality of these procedures.

All refractory patients should be evaluated for congestive heart failure, pneumonia, or hypoproteinemia as contributing factors.

Except for patients who are moribund and terminal, treatment should not be withheld from any symptomatic patient. Repeated simple thoracentesis is to be discouraged, as it is painful and relatively ineffective and may do more harm than good. It is usually more humane to treat the patient with lung cancer and pleural effusion as outlined above than to allow him to suffer unnecessarily with potentially reversible respiratory embarrassment.

REFERENCES

1. Mayer E, Maier H: Pulmonary Carcinoma (ed 1). New York, NYU Press, 1956, pp 159
2. Brinkman GL: The significance of pleural effusion complicating otherwise inoperable bronchogenic carcinoma. Chest 36:152–154, 1959
3. Dollinger M: Management of recurrent malignant effusions. CA 22:138–147, 1972
4. Black L: The pleural space and pleural fluid. Mayo Clin Proc 47:493–506, 1972
5. Green R, Johnston R: Pleural inflammation and pleural effusion, in Baum G (ed): Textbook of Pulmonary Diseases (ed 2). Boston, Little, Brown, 1974, pp 959–983
6. Mathews M: Morphology of lung cancer. Semin Oncol 1:175–182, 1974
7. Meyer PC: Metastatic carcinoma of the pleura. Thorax 21:437–443, 1966.
8. Whitcomb M, Schwarz M: Pleural effusion complicating intensive mediastinal radiation therapy. Am Rev Respir Dis 103:100–107, 1971
9. Lambert CJ, Urschel HC, Paulson DL, et al: The treatment of malignant pleural effusions by closed trocar tube drainage. Ann Thorac Surg 3:1–5, 1967
10. Anderson CE, Philpott GW, Ferguson TB: The treatment of malignant pleural effusions. Cancer 33:916–922, 1974
11. Luse SA, Reagan JW: A histologic study of effusions. Cancer 7:1167–1181, 1954
12. Salyer WR, Eggleston JC, Erozan YS: Efficacy of pleural needle biopsy and pleural fluid cytopathology in the diagnosis of malignant neoplasm involving the pleura. Chest 67:536–539, 1975
13. Cline MJ, Haskell CM: Cancer Chemotherapy (ed 2). Philadelphia, WB Saunders, 1975, p 283
14. Kinsey DL, Carter D, Klassen KP: Simplified management of malignant pleural effusion. Arch Surg 89:389–392, 1964
15. Sutton ML: The management of malignant pleural effusion. Postgrad Med J 49:729–731, 1973
16. Leininger BJ, Barker WL, Langston HT: A simplified method for management of malignant pleural effusion. J Thorac Cardiovasc Surg 58:758–763, 1969
17. Jones Gr: Treatment of recurrent malignant pleural effusion by iodized talc pleurodesis. Thorax 24:69–73, 1969
18. Weisberger AS: Direct instillation of nitrogen mustard in management of malignant effusions. Ann NY Acad Sci 68:1091–1096, 1958
19. Levison VB: Nitrogen mustard in palliation of malignant effusions. Br Med J 1:1143–1145, 1961
20. Mark JB, Goldenberg IS, Montague AC: Intrapleural mechlorethamine hydrochloride therapy for malignant pleural effusion. JAMA 187:858–860, 1964
21. Farber LR: Correctable complications of neoplastic disease. III: Neoplastic effusion. Conn Med J 35:411–412, 1971
22. Dollinger MR, Krakoff IH, Karnofsky DA: Quinacrine (Atabrine) in the treatment of neoplastic effusions. Ann Intern Med 66:249–257, 1967.
23. Gellhorn A, Zaidenweber J, Ultmann J, et al: Use of Atabrine (quinacrine) in control of recurrent neoplastic effusions; preliminary report. Dis Chest 39:165–176, 1961
24. Ultmann JE, Gellhorn A, Osnos M, et al: The effect of quinacrine on neoplastic effusions and certain of their enzymes. Cancer 16:283–288, 1963
25. Borja ER, Pugh RP: Single dose quinacrine (Atabrine) and thoracostomy in the control of pleural effusions in patients with neoplastic diseases. Cancer 31:899–902, 1973
26. Council on Drugs: An agent for the palliative treatment of neoplastic effusions—Quinacrine hydrochloride (Atabrine). JAMA 195:1189, 1966
27. Rubinson RM, Bolooki H: Intrapleural tetracycline for control of malignant pleural effusion: A preliminary report. South Med J 65:844–849, 1972
28. Thorsrud GK: Pleural reaction to irritants; an experimental study with special reference to pleural adhesions and concresence in relation to pleural turnover of fluid. Acta Chir Scand [Suppl] 355:1–74, 1965
29. Pearson FG, MacGregor DC: Talc Poudrage for malignant pleural effusion. J Thorac Cardiovasc Surg 51:732–738, 1966
30. Roche G, Delanoe Y, Moayer N: Talc Poudrage of the pleura under pleuroscopy. Results, indications, technique. J Fr Med Chir Thorac 1:677, 1963
31. Camishion RC, Gibbon JH, Nealon TF: Talc Poudrage in the treatment of pleural effusion due to cancer. Surg Clin North Am 42:1521–1526, 1962
32. Şhedbalkar AR, Head JM, Head IR, et al: Evaluation of talc pleural symphysis in management of malignant pleural effusion. J Thorac Cardiovasc Surg 61:492–497, 1971
33. Strober JS, Klotz E, Kuperman A, et al: Malignant pleural disease; a radiotherapeutic approach to the problem. JAMA 226:296–299, 1973
34. Card RY, Cole DR, Henschke UK: Summary of 10 years of the use of radioactive colloids in intracavitary therapy. J Nucl Med 1:195–198, 1960
35. Ariel IM, Oropeza R, Peck GT: Intracavitary administration of radioactive isotopes in the control of effusions due to cancer. Cancer 19:1096–1102, 1966
36. Siegel EP, Hart HE, Brothers M, et al: Radioyttrium (Y^{90}) for the palliative treatment of effusions due to malignancy. JAMA 161:499–503, 1956
37. Walter J: Malignant effusions treated by colloidal radioactive yttrium silicate. Br Med J 2:1282–1284, 1960
38. Izbicki R, Weyhing BT, Baker L, et al: Pleural effusion in cancer patients. A prospective randomized study of pleural drainage with the addition of radioactive phosphorus to the pleural space vs. pleural drainage alone. Cancer 36:1511–1518, 1975

Robert J. Polackwich
Marc J. Straus

18
Superior Vena Caval Syndrome

Malignant disease is currently responsible for approximately 95 percent of all cases of superior vena caval (SVC) syndrome, with bronchogenic carcinoma accounting for 85 to 90 percent of all cases. Some 5000 to 15,000 new cases of SVC obstruction occur annually in the United States, with perhaps an additional 1000 cases caused by various other malignancies, primarily lymphoma.

Although the diagnosis of SVC syndrome is readily established by an essentially pathognomonic constellation of symptoms and signs, the cause of the obstruction is nearly always unknown at the time of presentation. The clinician who must treat his plethoric, edematous, and dyspneic patient is reminded that this represents the one "oncologic emergency." Consequently, mediastinal irradiation, the traditional treatment of choice, is instituted immediately, frequently in the absence of a histopathologic diagnosis. Because of the overwhelming likelihood that inoperable malignancy is present, little effort generally is expended in establishing a tissue diagnosis. Although mediastinal irradiation frequently affords the patient some symptomatic relief, he most often experiences an inexorable course to death, generally in 2–6 months.

The concepts of management in this disorder have evolved little, if at all, over the past 25 years. Radiotherapy remains the principal mode of treatment, and most patients are offered little additional diagnostic or therapeutic intervention.

This explains the fact that overall survival in this disorder has not improved appreciably since the early 1950s.[1-7]

HISTORY OF SVC SYNDROME

Hunter[8] is generally given credit for the initial description of SVC syndrome in 1757. The first major review was by Fischer in 1904,[9] in which he collected 252 cases from the literature. The majority were due to aortic aneurysms or fibrosing mediastinitis, presumably of syphilitic or tuberculous origin. Only 37 percent of his cases were attributed to malignant disease. McIntire,[10] in a review of the literature from 1904 to 1948, added only 48 additional histologically documented cases of SVC syndrome due to malignancy, and only 20 of these were secondary to bronchogenic carcinoma.

Only after 1950 did intrathoracic malignancy, particularly bronchogenic carcinoma, become established as the primary etiologic factor in SVC syndrome. A recent review[11] has suggested that as many as 97 percent of cases are currently secondary to thoracic neoplasia, with 90 percent of these due to bronchogenic carcinoma. The small remaining percentage is of benign etiology such as histoplasmosis, substernal thyroid enlargement, bronchogenic cysts, etc.[12-14]

249

SYMPTOMS AND SIGNS IN SVC OBSTRUCTION

The patient with SVC syndrome usually presents with symptoms and signs unlikely to be confused with those of any other disorder. Shortness of breath, headaches, cough, and hoarseness are frequent complaints, and these symptoms may be exacerbated during recumbency. Swelling of the neck, face, and upper extremities may be particularly troublesome, and the patient may describe the recent onset of difficulty in buttoning his collar. Increasing somnolence, lethargy, and forgetfulness are commonly observed.

On physical examination the patient is frequently in acute distress with marked shortness of breath. Chest and abdominal venous dilatation, a plethoric or cyanotic complexion, and edema of the face, neck, and upper extremities may be apparent. Auscultation and percussion of the chest may suggest the presence of a pleural effusion. Papilledema will occasionally be observed and nearly always reflects nonspecific increased intracranial pressure rather than metastatic brain disease. Abnormal mental status, as manifested primarily by somnolence and inattentiveness, may be noted. Finally, pathologic respiratory patterns, including Cheyne-Stokes or Biot respirations, are not uncommon, particularly in patients with severe symptomatology. Other signs and symptoms associated with thoracic neoplasia such as weight loss and hemoptysis may also be present (see Chapter 6).

All of these symptoms and signs reflect SVC or associated great vein obstruction with secondary venous hypertension and stasis in the cranium, upper extremities, and thorax.

Several bedside diagnostic maneuvers are available to confirm the diagnosis of SVC obstruction. Peripheral venous pressures are consistently elevated, generally from 150 to 500 mm of H_2O. In general, there is little difference in the pressures of the upper extremities, and more than 10 mm H_2O difference between the right and left should suggest increased obstruction on the side of the greatest pressure (i.e., in the innominate or subclavian veins). The astute observer may note that the peripheral venous pressure rises with inhalation and falls during exhalation, a finding that is normal in the inferior vena cava but abnormal in the superior vena cava or its tributaries. Hitzig[15] has suggested that this finding is indicative of SVC obstruction and azygos vein obstruction with extensive collateralization to the inferior

vena cava. This elevation of pressure during inhalation may also be seen in spinal fluid manometric recordings.[16]

An exercise test originally described by Veal,[17] in which the patient opens and closes his fist for 1 min while peripheral venous pressures are recorded in the ipsilateral arm, may reveal more than 10 mm H_2O elevation in pressure at the end of 1 min. This finding occurred in 18 of 18 patients with SVC syndrome described by Hussey.[16]

Simultaneous measurements of pressure in the superior vena cava and inferior vena cava have been helpful in at least one reported case in differentiating SVC syndrome from cardiac tamponade.[18] Pressure in the superior vena cava should be greater than concomitant inferior vena cava pressure in SVC syndrome but approximately the same in tamponade.

Finally, circulation times, which are uniformly prolonged in congestive heart failure or severe mitral stenosis, may be normal in complete obstruction of the superior vena cava.

These bedside diagnostic maneuvers, although generally unnecessary, may prove useful in marginal circumstances when the diagnosis remains in doubt after initial evaluation.

Several laboratory values are likely to be abnormal. The chest roentgenogram may reveal a widened mediastinum. The primary lesion in bronchogenic carcinoma will usually be observed in the right lung, particularly near the right hilum or in the right upper lobe. A pleural effusion will sometimes be present, frequently on the right. Hughes[19] recently described a radionucleotide "hotspot" on conventional technetium-99m liver-spleen scans in patients with SVC obstruction in the area of the gallbladder fossa. This was presumably due to increased blood flow from epigastric venous channels to remnants of the portal system in the ligamentum teres. Hyponatremia may occur, reflecting inappropriate antidiuretic hormone secretion.[20] Other nonspecific laboratory features of metastatic malignant disease, such as anemia and hypoalbuminemia may also be present.

PATHOPHYSIOLOGY

The pathophysiology of SVC syndrome involves three major phenomena: obstruction of the superior vena cava and/or associated great veins, marked increase in venous pressure distal to the obstruction, and subsequent development of venous collaterals.

In general, obstruction of the superior vena cava secondary to malignant disease is the result of direct caval invasion by tumor (Table 18-1). In approximately 68 percent of patients reported since 1945 who have come to postmortem examination, frank invasion of the superior vena cava has been found. Of those cases due to bronchogenic carcinoma in Failor's series,[24] 18 of 18 cases were due to direct invasion. Associated thrombus arising in areas of metastatic involvement is also frequently noted at postmortem examination.[4,24,25,28] The contribution of venous thrombosis in the production of SVC syndrome is

less clear, but it probably is important in many instances by further compromising venous return.

The lymph nodes of greatest importance in SVC obstruction are the right anterior mediastinal nodes and the right lateral tracheal nodes.[10] The latter receive most of the lymphatic drainage from the right lung. These mediastinal nodes are frequently the initial areas of metastatic involvement from right lung primaries. Because of the proximity of the superior vena cava to this area, the caval wall may become secondarily involved with tumor by direct extension from the nodes or may sometimes be compromised by extrinsic compression by the nodes.[2,23,24] Approximately

Table 18-1
Pathophysiology of SVC Obstruction by Malignant Disease in Autopsied Cases since 1945

Author and Year	Number of Autopsied Cases	Number due to Bronchogenic Cancer	Invasion of Vein	Extrinsic Compression of Vein
Hussey[16]				
1945	3	2	3/3	
Rosenbloom[22]				
1949	3	3	3/3	
Hinshaw[21]				
1949	1		1/1	
McCord[27]				
1951	3	3	3/3	
Schechter[23]				
1954	12	11	11/12	
Schechter[2]				
1955	18	17	17/18	
Szur[25]				
1956	23	23	4/17*	
Failor[24]				
1958	28	18	26/28	2/28
Hayt[26]				
1964	2	1	1/2	1/2
Salsali[4]				
1965	23	23	16/21†	5/21
Longacre[5]				
1968	37	37	7/21‡	14/21
Salsali[28]				
1968	28	?	6/16§	10/16
Totals	181	138+	98/145	47/145

*Six autopsied cases showed no obstruction.
†Two autopsied cases showed no obstruction.
‡Twelve cases had no description of the SVC, 7 of 25 were described as occluded and 4 of 25 as patent.
§Three cases described as partially obstructed, 1 as patent; 3 were occluded by thrombi; 1 graft was thrombosed; no description was given in 4 cases.

85 percent of primaries in SVC syndrome due to bronchogenic carcinoma occur on the right (Table 18-2), primarily in the right upper lobe or right mainstem bronchus.

Once the superior vena cava becomes occluded, venous pressure rises distal to the obstruction. Obstruction–pressure relationships cannot definitively be established in SVC syndrome because of the in vivo variability of many factors, including venous distensibility and collateralization. However, in the Hagen-Poiseuille equation for volume flow Q through rigid tubes of capillary diameter, $Q = (P_1 - P_2)r^4/8lh$, flow is proportional to the fourth power of the radius of the tube. Although this equation is not entirely applicable to flow through a large distensible vessel, the implication is that minor variations in the radius of the lumen of the vessel can have dramatic effects on venous pressure and flow.

The development of venous collaterals involves at least five major routes (Fig. 18-1): the azygos, vertebral, lateral thoracic, internal mammary, and portal veins. Of major importance is the azygos vein, since integrity of this vein enables blood from the head and upper extremities to reach the right atrium via direct circuit from the internal mammary and intercostal veins. When the azygos vein is also obstructed, venous return must proceed through more circuitous routes to the inferior vena cava and portal veins. Mikkelsen[30] has described the appearance of esophageal varices, predominantly of the upper esophagus, in SVC obstruction. These varices result from obstruction of cephalic blood flow to the azygos system with redirection of flow caudally to the portal vein.

Carlson[31] demonstrated the importance of the azygos vein in dogs by applying ligatures to the superior vena cava above and below the level of the azygos vein. A dog can survive the procedure if the ligature is applied above the azygos vein; but a ligature applied below the azygos vein could be tolerated only if done in two stages, allowing time for adequate venous collateralization to develop. Pleural fluid was found to accumulate in animals whose ligatures were placed above the azygos vein, presumably from high intrathoracic venous pressures; pleural fluid may be troublesome in humans similarly affected by neoplastic obstruction of the SVC.[16,32]

A breakdown of the malignant diseases that cause SVC syndrome is summarized in Table 18-3: 87 percent of cases were due to primary lung cancer, 6 percent to lymphoma, and another 7 percent to nonpulmonary metastatic disease (breast, thymoma, etc.).

The breakdown of cell type in cases secondary to bronchogenic carcinoma is given in Table 18-4. Obviously histopathology, as reported by various authors, was not standardized to today's familiar categorizations. For example, some series apparently did not distinguish between oat cell disease and undifferentiated or anaplastic cell types.[5,6,23,34,35] Nevertheless, at least one-third of the cases are due to oat cell disease, while another one-fifth are due to unspecified anaplastic lung cancers.

NATURAL HISTORY OF SVC SYNDROME

Obstruction of the superior vena cava per se carries little or no mortality. This is demonstrated by those patients with SVC syndrome secondary to benign diseases such as granulomatous disease, substernal goiters, benign mediastinal tumors, etc.[12–14,37,38] Ten such patients followed

Table 18-2

Selected Series of Right Lung Primaries in SVC Obstruction Secondary to Bronchogenic Carcinoma

Author and Year	Number of Cases with Right Lung Primaries
Rosenbloom[22]	
1949	8/9
Roswit[1]	
1953	30/38
Schechter[2]	
1955	15/18
Failor[24]	
1958	18/18
Skinner[3]	
1965	23/23
Salsali[4]	
1965	106/137
Hanlon[29]	
1965	46/46
Salsali[28]	
1968	61/72
Total	307/361
Percentage	85%

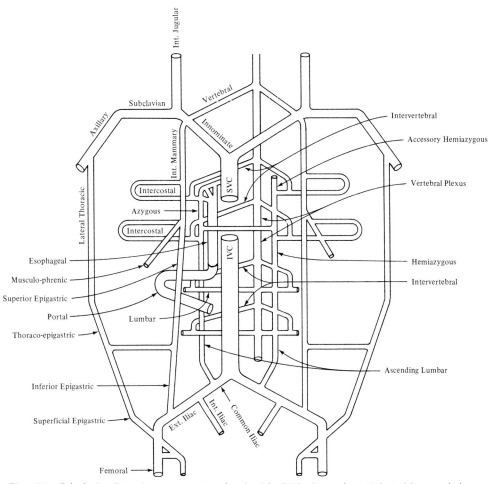

Fig. 18-1 Principal collateral venous systems involved in SVC obstruction. (Adapted by permission from McIntire FT, Sykes EM: Obstruction of the superior vena cava: A review of the literatture and report of two personal cases. Ann Intern Med 30:925–960, 1949.)

Table 18-3
Selected Series of Neoplastic Etiologies of SVC Obstruction Documented by Histopathology

References	Total Number of Cases	Number Secondary to Bronchogenic Carcinoma	Number Secondary to Lymphoma	Number Secondary to Nonbronchogenic Metastases
1–7,10,16,21–25,27–29,33–36	817	711	50	56
Percentage	100%	87%	6%	7%

Table 18-4

Selected Series of Histopathology in Bronchogenic Carcinoma Responsible for SVC Obstruction

Author and Year	Total Number of Cases	Squamous or Epidermoid	Small or Oat Cell	Adeno. or Alveolar	Undifferentiated or Anaplastic	Unclassified
Rosenbloom[22] 1948	8	3	3		2	
Roswit[1] 1953	38	29*	6	1		2
Schechter[23] 1954	18	4		7	4	3
Szur[25] 1956	69	12	27		30	
Rubin[34] 1963	14	3		1	10	
Holmes[35] 1963	13†		9			4
Skinner[3] 1965	23	5	5	2	7	4
Salsali[4] 1965	124‡	47	44	2		22
Urschell[36] 1966	29	13	8	2	6	
Howard[7] 1967	98	19	74	5		
Longacre[5] 1968	57	11		2	44	
Salsali[28] 1968	72§	24	24	7	13	
Levitt[6] 1969	23	9		2	12	
Total	586	179	200	31	128	35
Percentage	100%	31%	34%	6%	20%	6%

*Twenty-eight cases described as anaplastic epidermoid.
†Nine cases described as oat cell or anaplastic.
‡Nine cases described as terminal bronchiolar.
§Four cases described as terminal bronchiolar.

by Mahajan[12] for 1–10 years had no complications. Also, as noted previously, Carlson[31] found that dogs can survive surgical ligation of the superior vena cava both above and below the azygos vein.

There is little predictive value in the nature of the patient's presentation with SVC obstruction when it is caused by malignancy. Neither the duration of symptomatology prior to hospitalization nor the degree of severity of obstruction is correlated with survival time.[7] In addition, although obstruction below the azygos vein would theoretically carry greater morbidity and

mortality than obstruction above the azygos vein, no study has ever demonstrated this.

Rosenbloom[22] reported a series of 7 patients with SVC syndrome secondary to bronchogenic carcinoma who were untreated. The mean survival time was 6 weeks. However, no description was given regarding terminal events or the extent of metastatic disease at postmortem examination. Radiation therapy has allegedly increased survival to 2–6 months.[1–7] These short survival times, however, are comparable to those in patients with small cell carcinoma *without* SVC syndrome, both untreated[39] and treated with radiation therapy.[40] Since more than 50 percent of cell types responsible for SVC syndrome are due to small cell or anaplastic histopathology, the role of SVC syndrome in shortening survival in bronchogenic carcinoma is unclear.

No investigator has ever provided detailed clinical or autopsy findings indicating that SVC obstruction was the direct cause of death in patients with malignant disease. Do these patients die of laryngeal edema and asphyxiation, cerebral hemorrhage due to high intracranial venous pressures, recurrent pulmonary emboli from thrombi located in partially obstructed great veins, sepsis secondary to obstructed bronchi and pneumonia, respiratory center malfunction due to cerebral venous stasis, or distant metastases? Longacre[5] found that of 37 patients with SVC syndrome due to bronchgenic carcinoma who came to postmortem examination, 27 had pericardial involvement with tumor, 10 had direct myocardial involvement, and 25 had distant metastases. Szur[25] found evidence of extrathoracic metastases in 22 of 107 patients with SVC obstruction due to bronchogenic carcinoma at the time of presentation. Furthermore, these data were collected prior to the routine use of sophisticated scanning techniques or bone marrow biopsies. Schechter[2] concluded that 16 of 17 patients with SVC syndrome secondary to malignancy died as a result of progression of their disease.

Data regarding the natural history of SVC syndrome due to neoplasia are based on a very small group of patients who were reported in the late 1940s who received no specific therapy. There is no good evidence that these patients' survival times were significantly different from those of other patients with metastatic carcinoma not involving the superior vena cava, nor that patients with SVC obstruction die as a result of this obstruction. It seems much more plausible to attribute the short survival times in these patients to intrathoracic and extrathoracic metastases at the time of death.

INVASIVE DIAGNOSTIC MANEUVERS IN SVC SYNDROME

Considerable controversy exists in the literature regarding the safety and utility of venography in SVC syndrome.[11,41,42] The presumed risks of venography are excessive hemorrhage or hematoma formation at the venipuncture site,

intrathoracic hemorrhage caused by manipulation of catheters in dilated and obstructed great veins, iatrogenic chemical phlebitis that may augment obstruction and symptomatology, and exacerbation of the syndrome by increasing the intravascular volume distal to the obstruction by 30–100 ml of injected contrast material. The literature, however, suggests that venography carries little or no morbidity,[1,5,7,22,28,43–49] particularly when performed with flexible atraumatic catheters under fluoroscopy.[41]

Venography may provide useful information by defining the presence or absence of obstruction in marginal clinical cases and by establishing more precisely the extent and location of obstruction prior to radiotherapy so that ports can be tailored to each individual patient. Howard[7] found that venography influenced the technique of radiotherapy in 40 percent of his patients with SVC syndrome. Furthermore, the superior vena cava was involved singly in only 36 percent of cases, there being a high percentage of innominate and subclavian venous involvement. Venography may also reveal the extent of collateralization, which may be correlated with the patient's survival and response to radiotherapy.[7]

Since 1968 some centers have found technetium-99m scintiphotography to be a useful diagnostic tool in defining the location of venous obstruction.[50–53] The advantages of this method are that there need be injected only 1–2 ml of material intravenously and that technetium 99m can be used in patients sensitive to iodine. Both venous collateralization and radiation-induced relief of obstruction of the superior vena cava have been demonstrated with scintiphotography. The information gained by this technique, although not as detailed as that with conventional venography, may certainly be sufficient to establish a diagnosis in doubtful cases or to outline the extent of obstruction so that radiotherapy ports can be individualized.

Identification of cell type can be accomplished by several approaches discussed in greater detail elsewhere in this book. Bilateral posterior iliac crest bone marrow biopsies should be performed early. The high proportion of small cell and anaplastic cell types responsible for this syndrome makes this an especially useful procedure. Sputum cytologies, as discussed in Chapter 7, may frequently be diagnostic. Flexible fiberoptic bronchoscopy may be undertaken if the patient has been temporarily stabilized with the medical maneuvers discussed below.[54] Transvenous lung biopsy, which is occasionally used in some centers to establish histopathology, should be approached with caution. A single case report has already described exacerbation of SVC syndrome by the use of this technique.[55]

Supraclavicular or cervical node biopsy may be considered only if palpable nodes are present, although the physician should recall that thrombosed veins or edematous fat pads may mimic lymphadenopathy in SVC syndrome.[28] The most superficial nodes should be selected to minimize the risk of hemorrhage, which can be considerable because of high venous pressures. Except in rare circumstances mediastinoscopy and thoracotomy should not be attempted because of the well-documented high morbidity and mortality in SVC obstruction.[29,35,56−59]

Finally, as the patient's clinical condition begins to stabilize with medical management, he should undergo the routine workup to delineate the extent of extrathoracic metastatic disease. The presence or absence of disease in specific areas, of course, may have considerable therapeutic implications.

Vigorous attempts to identify the etiology of the obstruction of the superior vena cava should be undertaken whenever clinically feasible. In this way the occasional patient with benign disease will not be irradiated. In addition, identification of cell type may enable the physician to employ specific chemotherapeutic agents, when appropriate, either as primary therapy alone or as an adjunct to radiotherapy. The patient with SVC syndrome should not be denied the full evaluation and therapeutic considerations given to similar patients with nonobstructive metastatic disease.

TREATMENT AND SURVIVAL

As noted above, the presence of SVC obstruction secondary to neoplastic disease, except in rare circumstances, dictates inoperability.[29,35,56−59] Furthermore, if the syndrome is due to benign disorders, surgical relief of the obstruction will generally be unnecessary, since the patient's symptoms will gradually subside as venous collateralization develops.

Radiotherapy has been the principal treatment of this disorder since 1953, when Roswit[1] reported a large group of patients with SVC syndrome secondary to malignant disease, 76 percent of whom achieved symptomatic remission averaging about 14 weeks in duration. Of the 9 patients who failed to show any clinical improvement to radiotherapy, all died in less than 8 weeks. Although patients seemed to improve symptomatically with radiotherapy to the mediastinum, the question of whether survival was prolonged remained unanswered.[1] Nevertheless, radiotherapy has become the primary modality of treatment in the management of this disorder, most likely because of the frequently associated improvement in symptomatology.

Rubin[34] found that patients who received upwards of 400 rads per day for 10 days experienced more rapid clinical improvement than patients in whom radiation was delivered in lower dose schedules. Holmes[35] treated 172 patients with SVC obstruction secondary to neoplasia with a high-dose grid technique in which 4000 rads or more were delivered in a single session. Nevertheless, most radiotherapists currently treat SVC syndrome with the rapid high-dose schedule described by Rubin in 1963. Because of studies indicating that survival and duration of clinical response are related to the total radiation dose,[1,5,7] a minimum of 4000 rads is generally delivered to the mediastinum. Interestingly, there has been no reported association between cell type and the clinical response to radiotherapy or survival.[4,5,7]

Howard[7] has noted that the response to radiotherapy is significantly correlated with the degree of venous collateralization at the time of initiation of treatment. In his series of patients studied with venography, 9 of 10 patients with good venous collaterals had clinical remissions while undergoing radiotherapy, while 10 of 21 patients with poor venous collaterals failed to respond. Furthermore, of the 7 patients with good clinical responses who underwent repeat venography at the end of treatment, only 3 showed relief of the obstruction. These findings suggest that a substantial number of clinical "responses" to radiotherapy may actually be due to improvement in venous flow through collateral channels. Nevertheless, radiotherapy does seem to afford many objective clinical remissions; it probably prolongs survival in many instances, and currently it should be considered the principal mode of therapy.

Experience with chemotherapy in this syndrome has essentially been based on one substance, nitrogen mustard first used by Karnofsky in 1948,[60] with 6 of 9 patients demonstrating clinical improvement. Several studies have indicated that mustard yields shorter remissions and may be associated with greater morbidity than radiotherapy.[1,4,6,34] Combination chemotherapy, now employed extensively in the treatment of metastatic neoplasia, has never been adequately studied in SVC syndrome. Only a few case reports can be found in the literature regarding trials of combinations of drugs in the treatment of this disorder,[61] although these have been successful in inducing clinical remissions. We have treated 4 cases of SVC obstruction secondary to small cell carcinoma of the lung with combination chemotherapy, and all the patients had good clinical responses and objective remissions. Similar results have recently been reported by others.[62] It is our practice to treat patients initially with chemotherapy if their cell type is generally responsive (i.e., small cell carcinoma and perhaps adenocarcinoma) and if their symptoms are not severe.

Ancillary measures that can provide much relief to the patient with SVC syndrome are plentiful. Thiazide diuretics may be used both to lower the intravascular volume and to increase venous capacitance, and they have been shown to be remarkably effective in ameliorating symptomatology.[3,6,33] Fears of increasing viscosity and exacerbating symptomatology are unfounded. Phlebotomy of 200–300 ml of blood may be performed in the upper extremities and may rapidly improve abnormal mental status or respiratory patterns.[63] The patient should be given sufficient oxygen to correct hypoxemia and mild sedation to allay his intense discomfort and anxiety. The head of the bed should remain elevated to a minimum of 45 degrees, and all intravenous supplements should be administered via veins in the lower extremities whenever possible, both for technical facility and to ensure complete access to the general circulation. Correction of hyponatremia, if present, should be accomplished gradually, and hypertonic saline should be given only if the serum sodium is below 120 mEq/liter and the patient appears to be symptomatic from his low serum sodium. Otherwise, correction of hyponatremia will begin once therapy is directed at the primary neoplasm.[34] Thrombolytic agents have been used in a small group of patients with some success,[28] but additional studies are necessary to confirm their utility. Clinical studies employing anticoagulants and adrenocorticosteroids have not been done, and their use cannot currently be recommended.

SUMMARY

The patient who presents with SVC syndrome should be stabilized during the first 2 to 3 days of hospitalization with the ancillary medical maneuvers described above while vigorous attempts are made to identify the location and etiology of the obstructive process. Radiotherapy should be instituted as expediently as possible, particularly if the syndrome is advanced. Depending on the patient's cell type, combination chemotherapy should be considered and a search for extrathoracic metastases begun. By employing this systematic approach, patients with SVC syndrome secondary to neoplasia may begin to experience prolonged remission rates and survivals currently afforded similar patients with nonobstructing malignant disease.

REFERENCES

1. Roswit B, Kaplan G, Jacobson EG: The superior vena cava obstruction syndrome in bronchogenic carcinoma. Radiology 61:722–737, 1953
2. Schechter MM, Ziskino MM: The superior vena cava syndrome. Am J Med 18:561–566, 1955
3. Skinner DB, Salzman EW, Scannell JG: The challenge of superior vena cava obstruction. J Thorac Cardiovasc Surg 49:824–833, 1965
4. Salsali M, Cliffton EE: Superior vena cava obstruction with carcinoma of the lung. Surg Gynecol Obstet 121:783–788, 1965
5. Longacre AM, Schockman AT: The superior vena cava syndrome and radiation therapy. Radiology 91:713–718, 1968
6. Levitt SR, Jones TK Jr, Kilpatrick ST, et al: Treatment of malignant-superior vena cava obstruction. Cancer 24:447–451, 1969
7. Howard N: Mediastinal Obstruction in Lung Cancer. London, E&S Livingstone, 1967, pp 1–97
8. Hunter W: Medical observations and inquiries, 1757; quoted in McIntire FT, Sikes EM: Obstruction of the superior vena cava: A review of the

literature and report of two personal cases. Ann Intern Med 30:925–960, 1949

9. Fischer J: Über Verengerung und Verschliessung der Vena Cava Superior. Inaugural dissertation. Halle, Wischan & Burkhardt, 1904

10. McIntire FT, Sykes EM: Obstruction of the superior vena cava: A review of the literature and report of two personal cases. Ann Intern Med 30:925–960, 1949

11. Lokich JJ, Goodman R: Superior vena cava syndrome. JAMA 231:58–61, 1975

12. Mahajan V, Striman V, Van Ordstrand HS, et al: Benign superior vena cava syndrome. Chest 68:32–35, 1975

13. Rammohan G, Berger HW, Lajam F, et al: Superior vena cava syndrome caused by bronchogenic cyst. Chest 68:599–601, 1975

14. Silverstein GE, Burke G, Goldberg D, et al: Superior vena cava obstruction caused by benign endothoracic goiter. Dis Chest 56:519–523, 1969

15. Hitzig WM: On mechanisms of inspiratory filling of the cervical veins and pulsus paradoxus in venous hypertension. J Mt Sinai Hosp 8:625–632, 1942

16. Hussey HH, Katz S, Yater WM: The superior vena cava syndrome: Report of thirty-five cases. Am Heart J 31:1–26, 1946

17. Veal JR, Hussey HH: The use of "exercise tests" in connection with venous pressure measurements for detection of venous obstruction in the upper and lower extremities. Am Heart J 20:308–321, 1940

18. Callen JP, Gewertz BL: Letter to the editor. Lancet 2:229–230, 1974

19. Hughes FA III: The value of hepatic scintiangiography and static liver scans in superior vena cava obstruction: Case report. J Nucl Med 16:626–628, 1975

20. Dossetor JB, Venning EH, Beck JC: Hyponatremia associated with superior vena cava obstruction. Metabolism 10:149–161, 1961

21. Hinshaw DB: Obstructions of the superior vena cava. Am Heart J 37:958–969, 1949

22. Rosenbloom SE: Superior vena cava obstruction in primary cancer of the lung. Ann Intern Med 31:470–478, 1949

23. Schechter MM: The superior vena cava syndrome. Am J Med Sci 227:46–56, 1954

24. Failor HT, Edwards JE, Hodgson CH: Etiologic factors in obstruction of the superior vena cava. Meet Mayo Clin 33:671–678, 1958

25. Szur L, Bromley LL: Obstruction of the superior vena cava in carcinoma of the bronchus. Br Med J 2:1273–1276, 1956

26. Hayt DB: Roentgenographic signs of thrombosis of the superior vena cava and tributaries in neoplastic disease. Am J Roentgenol Radium Ther Nucl Med 93:87–98, 1965

27. McCord MC, Edlin P, Block M: Superior vena cava obstruction. Am J Dis Chest 19:19–27, 1951

28. Salsali M, Cliffton EE: Superior vena cava obstruction with lung cancer. Ann Thorac Surg 6:437–442, 1968

29. Hanlon CR, Davis RK: Superior vena caval obstruction. Ann Surg 161:771–777, 1965

30. Mikkelsen WJ: Varices of the upper esophagus in superior vena caval obstruction. Radiology 81:945–948, 1963

31. Carlson H: Obstruction of the superior vena cava. Arch Surg 29:669–677, 1934

32. Allansmith R, Richards V: Superior vena caval obstruction. Am J Surg 96:353–359, 1958

33. Bruckner WJ: Significance of superior vena caval syndrome. Arch Intern Med 102:88–96, 1958

34. Rubin P, Green J, Holzwasser G: Superior vena caval syndrome. Radiology 87:388–401, 1963

35. Holmes KS: The treatment of superior vena caval syndrome by high-dose grid technique. Radiology 81:402–405, 1963

36. Urschell HC, Paulson DL: Superior vena caval obstruction. Dis Chest 49:155–164, 1966

37. Murdock WR, Will G: Benign superior mediastinal syndrome. Scott Med J 5:37–41, 1960

38. Greenberg AG, Beal DD: Obstruction of the superior vena cava with 28 year survival. Ann Thorac Surg 1:444–447, 1965

39. Green RA, Humphrey E, Close H, et al: Alkylating agents in bronchogenic carcinoma. Am J Med 46:516–525, 1969

40. Bergsagel DE, Jenkin RDT, Pringle JF, et al: Lung cancer: Clinical trial of radiotherapy alone vs. radiotherapy plus cyclophosphamide. Cancer 30:621–627, 1972

41. Davidson KC: Letter to the editor. JAMA 233:420, 1975

42. Johnston RF: Letter to the editor. JAMA 233:420–421, 1975

43. Katz S, Hussey HH, Veal JR: Phlebography for study of obstruction of veins of the superior vena caval system. Am J Med Sci 214:7–22, 1947

44. Howard N: Phlebography in superior vena cava obstruction. Radiology 81:380–384, 1963

45. Hudson GW: Venography in superior vena caval obstruction. Radiology 68:499–505, 1957

46. Steinberg I, Dotter CT: Lung cancer. Arch Surg 64:10–19, 1952

47. Brown RC, Nelson CMB, Lerona PT: Angiographic demonstration of collateral circulation in a patient with superior vena caval syndrome. Am J Roentgenol Radium Ther Nucl Med 119:543–546, 1973

48. Okay NH, Bryk D: Collateral pathways in occlusion of the superior vena cava and its tributaries. Radiology 92:1493–1498, 1969

49. Howard N, Pick EJ: The value of phlebography in

superior vena caval obstruction. Clin Radiol 12:290–294, 1961

50. Son YH, Wetzel RA, Wilson WJ: ^{99m}Tc pertechnetate scintiphotography as diagnostic and follow-up aids in major vascular obstruction due to malignant neoplasm. Radiology 91:349–357, 1968

51. Maxfield WS, Meckstroth GR: Technetium-99m superior vena cavography. Radiology 62:913–917, 1969

52. Krishnamurthy GT, Winston MA, Weiss ER, et al: Demonstration of collateral pathways after superior vena caval obstruction with the scintillation camera. J Nucl Med 12:189–191, 1971

53. Krishnamurthy GT, Blahd WH, Winston MA: Superior vena caval syndrome: Scintiphotographic evaluation of response to radiation therapy. Am J Roentgenol Radium Ther Nucl Med 117:609–614, 1973

54. Snider GL: personal communication, 1976

55. Armstrong P, Hayes DF, Richardson PJ: Transvenous biopsy of carcinoma of bronchus causing superior vena caval obstruction. Br Med J 1:662–663, 1975

56. Scannell JG: Etiology and surgical approaches in superior vena caval obstruction. Radiology 81:378–379, 1963

57. Effler DB, Groves LK: Superior vena caval obstruction. J Thorac Cardiovasc Surg 43:574–584, 1962

58. Boruchow IB, Johnson J: Obstructions of the vena cava. Surg Gynecol Obstet 134:115–121, 1972

59. Schwartz SI: Principles of Surgery. New York, McGraw-Hill, 1969, p 539

60. Karnofsky DA, Abelman WH, Craver LF, et al: The use of nitrogen mustards in the palliative treatment of carcinoma. Cancer 1:634–656, 1948

61. Nitschke R, Acker S, Campbell D, et al: Letter to the editor. JAMA 233:1354–1355, 1975

62. Kane RC, Cohen MH, Broder LE, et al: Superior vena caval obstruction due to small-cell anaplastic lung carcinoma. JAMA 235:1717–1718, 1976

63. Waterfield R: Biot respiration in superior vena caval obstruction. Guys Hosp Rep 78:305–307, 1928

Marc J. Straus

19
Concepts of Lung Cancer Management

The individual chapters of this book have been concerned with diagnostic techniques, such as bronchoscopy and mediastinoscopy, and with approaches to the treatment of lung cancer. In this chapter we have briefly summarized in a narrative format, without further references, our approach to the workup of a patient suspected of having lung cancer and have reviewed the treatment of lung cancer. We then provide 8 cases that are discussed by Drs. Lee, Selawry, and myself; they illustrate the diagnostic approaches and treatment of specific situations. The case reports also focus on some differences of opinion in the treatment of lung cancer.

DIAGNOSIS

The therapy of lung cancer varies, depending on the cell type and the stage of disease. Proper staging of the disease necessitates a thorough workup. We have detailed in several chapters many of the diagnostic maneuvers and their roles in diagnosis and staging. In most cases a good history, physical examination, and chest x-ray suffice to raise a high index of suspicion for the presence of lung cancer. Generally a few days of diagnostic tests are indicated, but premature surgical exploration adds nothing to survival. The patient with a suspicious chest x-ray should undergo a workup aimed at determining the cell type and the stage prior to surgery.

Careful cytology entails multiple specimens obtained, if necessary, after nebulization; they must be properly and promptly collected (Chapter 7). Cell typing of cytologic specimens can be extremely accurate for well-differentiated lung cancer and small cell carcinoma. The great difficulties that exist in distinguishing the more anaplastic cell types cytologically may be no less of a problem with biopsy specimens. If cytology is absolutely diagnostic of small cell carcinoma, then bronchoscopy may be unnecessary.

Fiberoptic bronchoscopy can safely be performed in almost all patients, and it may provide the diagnosis from biopsies, brushings, or washings (Chapter 8). When properly done, it may yield the diagnosis in over 80 percent of patients with centrally located lung cancers. It is less effective in obtaining specimens from peripheral lesions, both because of location and because peripheral tumors are less likely to be endobronchial. Multiple lesions may sometimes be noted. In addition, bronchoscopy may obviate further consideration of surgery because of the location of the lesion close to the carina (Chapter 12).

The histopathology of *central lesions* in particular should be rigorously pursued, because they are most easily diagnosed and are likely to be epidermoid carcinoma or small cell carcinoma.

The former is the cell type that is most often resectable, and the latter is unresectable. *Peripheral lesions* are much less likely to yield positive results by cytology or bronchoscopy, and transbronchial or transthoracic biopsies are sometimes indicated. The presence of a pleural effusion warrants a diagnostic tap. An effusion in the presence of lung cancer automatically indicates a stage T3 lesion, and the tumor is usually considered unresectable (Chapter 12).

We order bone scans in almost all cases, since they are noninvasive and are fairly accurate in determining the presence of bone metastases. We have seen several patients, usually with primary lesions larger than 2 cm, who would have undergone surgery if not for positive bone scans. Liver chemistries are ordered routinely. However, unless the chemistries are obviously abnormal, a liver scan is optional unless the patient is on a study that requires it (Chapter 11). Abnormal liver function tests and even liver scans rarely can be taken as absolute evidence of metastatic disease. Sometimes, however, the findings are most persuasive, as in the case of a liver scan with a large defect. In these situations liver biopsy is indicated, but it is positive in slightly less than half the cases with liver metastases. Peritoneoscopy can provide more accurate information, and rarely a laparotomy should be undertaken. We have seen several cases in which the diagnosis of lung cancer was first established by liver biopsy; most of these patients had small cell carcinoma.

Brain scans, similarly, are not routinely ordered unless CNS symptoms are present. Bone x-rays will indicate the presence of metastatic disease in only an additional 3–4 percent of patients when bone scanning is done. The x-rays are obtained if there is a specific indication such as rib pain. Lung tomograms may provide a clearer picture of the shape and location of the lesion and may indicate the presence of more than one lesion.

If the cell type is in doubt and there is no evidence of metastatic disease, a bone marrow biopsy may be done. It is positive in over 40 percent of patients with small cell disease and may be the first diagnostic test that successfully identifies the cell type (Chapter 11). Scalene nodes are biopsied only if palpable.

The role of mediastinoscopy is primarily to determine the histology or to rule out surgery (Chapter 9). Centrally located lung cancers are usually diagnosed by cytology and/or bronchos-

copy. If they are not, and if the other tests are negative, mediastinal tomograms may be done to select patients likely to have positive nodes as shown by mediastinoscopy. Mediastinoscopy is usually confined to patients who still appear likely to have lung cancer that is probably unresectable. If the patient has compromised cardiac or pulmonary functions it may not be possible to perform thoracotomy, and mediastinoscopy may provide the histologic diagnosis. Central lesions and anaplastic lesions are more likely to metastasize to the mediastinal nodes. If the cell type has been established, then mediastinoscopy need not be done in patients with small cell carcinoma. If well-differentiated epidermoid carcinoma is present, then mediastinoscopy is positive in less than 20 percent of cases and should probably be omitted, with the investigation proceeding directly to thoracotomy. Mediastinoscopy in expert hands (Chapter 9) is associated with few problems, but it is otherwise very much an invasive procedure.

Occasionally open lung biopsy is necessary for diagnostic purposes, particularly in situations where a definitive resection may follow after frozen-section corroboration of lung cancer that is not small cell carcinoma.

Not all suspicious lesions necessitate the complete workup. If a small (<2.0 cm) peripheral lesion is seen, tomograms are justified, and perhaps cytology and bone scanning. However, bronchoscopy and mediastinoscopy are likely to be negative, and surgery is indicated.

Knowing the cell type can be very helpful. A well-differentiated epidermoid carcinoma has the lowest metastatic potential (Chapter 4) and the highest likelihood of surgical care. Especially in smaller lesions and in patients with a good performance status, thoracotomy with minimal workup is reasonable. We are, however, most vigorous in obtaining thorough workups in patients with poorly differentiated tumors, either epidermoid carcinoma, adenocarcinoma, or large cell carcinoma. The 5-year survival after surgery in these tumors is generally under 20 percent. Similarly, we usually do extensive workups to avoid unnecessary surgery in patients with large primary lesions.

Some patients present initially with symptoms of metastatic disease or with paraneoplastic syndromes (Chapter 6). In most cases the chest x-ray is abnormal and the history has helpful clues such as a long history of cigarette smoking. Inappropriate ADH syndrome or evidence of ectopic

ACTH production should make one suspect lung cancer. In a patient over 35 years of age, tomograms should be done if the chest x-ray is negative. Lung cancer associated with these syndromes will often be small cell carcinoma (Chapter 3) and will therefore often be resectable. Positive bone scans, skeletal x-rays, or liver scans in the absence of a positive chest lesion may necessitate bone or liver biopsy.

Between 1 and 3 percent of patients with lung cancer present initially with CNS symptoms. Brain scans and CAT scans will usually suffice to demonstrate a lesion. Most CAT scans will show multiple lesions. In most cases the chest x-ray will be positive.

The syndrome of superior vena caval obstruction connotes lung cancer in over 90 percent of cases (Chapter 18), and with few exceptions these patients have unresectable tumors.

In the presence of multiple chest lesions, greater consideration is given to metastatic disease of nonpulmonary origin. In the absence of a history or physical examination suggesting gastrointestinal disease, upper GI barium studies and barium enema are not usually done. If the chest lesion proves to be an adenocarcinoma, mucicarmine stain may be helpful. Lung cancers and GI cancers are generally positive, whereas renal carcinomas are generally negative.

Breast, thyroid, and renal cancers, and melanoma in particular, may present with lung lesions, and the primary disease is not apparent from history or physical examination. The histologic diagnosis of squamous cell cancer usually indicates that the primary lesion is of head and neck or lung origin. An adenocarcinoma may necessitate more extensive workup, including thyroid scans, intravenous pyelogram, and gastrointestinal barium series. We have occasionally treated patients with nonresectable cancer in the lung with unknown primaries.

TREATMENT

Certain precepts regarding the therapy of lung cancer have evolved in the past few years. Patients with cancer other than small cell carcinoma should undergo resection if the criteria outlined by Dr. Mountain (Chapter 14) have been met.

The 5-year survival in properly selected patients undergoing surgery with curative intent is 30–40 percent. For well-differentiated resectable epidermoid carcinoma the 5-year survival is over 50 percent. Various factors, such as location and size of the lesion, node involvement, associated symptoms or pulmonary abnormalities, are correlated with survival. The overall 5-year survival decreases to only 11 percent in cases apparently completely resected if mediastinal nodes are positive, and 13 percent for epidermoid carcinoma. Resection of stage N2 epidermoid carcinoma should be limited to only those cases with ipsilateral nodes in the tracheobronchial angle and/or subcarinal region. Postoperative radiation therapy may be valuable in these cases. Adjuvant chemotherapy may have a role in any resected stage III case. Currently there is no apparent advantage to surgically debulking an otherwise unresectable lung cancer.

The technical approach to surgery has been outlined (Chapter 14). When possible, lobectomy is generally performed in preference to pneumonectomy. The mortality rate of surgery varies between 4 and 10 percent, and the expected outcome must always be balanced against this factor.

Radiotherapy is administered at some point to most patients with lung cancer (Chapter 13). It is a regional treatment that is rarely curative but is highly effective in relieving certain symptoms. Radiotherapy is sometimes used in stage I and II lung cancers when surgery is contraindicated because of medical problems, and some of these patients, particularly those with epidermoid carcinoma, may be cured. We prefer radiotherapy, either alone or postoperatively, for epidermoid carcinoma with mediastinal node involvement. In stage III limited small cell carcinoma Dr. Lee advocates the use of curative radiation therapy and would add chemotherapy as well. We are currently using combination chemotherapy in all these patients plus radiotherapy in selected patients who are responding to drugs. Preoperative radiotherapy is the treatment of choice for superior sulcus tumors.

There is rationale for debulking some tumors by radiotherapy prior to chemotherapy. Certainly for many drugs the percentage cell kill is diminished when tumors are larger. We are more likely to choose radiotherapy and chemotherapy in stage III limited disease in cell types, such as small cell carcinoma, which is most sensitive to drug therapy. Diminishing the tumor burden may also enhance the effects of immunotherapy, but this has not been tested as yet. In extensive disease the benefits of radiotherapy are strictly palliative.

The doses and courses of radiotherapy have been detailed by Dr. Lee. We use a shorter split-course as he proposes. Patients must have adequate pulmonary function for radiotherapy, and side effects include a functional destruction of the irradiated area.

The major therapeutic change in lung cancer in the last few years is the more frequent use of chemotherapy (Chapter 15). More than 90 percent of patients will develop widespread disease. Chemotherapy is properly being directed more and more to the earlier cases of regional nonresectable disease and is also being used as surgical adjuvant therapy. As more studies have been conducted with single drugs, our armamentarium of effective agents has increased, and most treatments now include combination chemotherapy.

The rapid proliferative characteristics that make small cell carcinoma so quickly lethal also make it the cell type most responsive to cytotoxic chemotherapy (Chapter 2). A number of single agents provide reasonably high objective response rates but little meaningful increase in survival. Optimal therapy consists of aggressive combination chemotherapy. Response rates over 50 percent are common. In our study using high-dose cyclophosphamide (Cytoxan) followed by intermittent methotrexate, there were 11 objective responses in 12 patients with a mean survival over 1 year (Chapter 15). All but 1 patient had extensive disease. We believe that virtually all patients with small cell carcinoma should receive chemotherapy, as good remissions are noted even in very advanced cases. Studies are in progress to determine whether prophylactic irradiation of the brain, liver, or chest in patients with small cell carcinoma improves survival. It is not recommended, however, outside of a study setting. We and others are investigating the use of radiotherapy at specific times after chemotherapy has been initiated.

The objective response rates of adenocarcinoma and large cell carcinoma to chemotherapy are usually less than 50 percent, but increasingly it appears worthwhile to treat these cell types. However, patients with very extensive disease, and particularly those with poor performance status, rarely respond. In our series using Cytoxan and methotrexate over 75 percent of patients with adenocarcinoma and large cell carcinoma and a

good performance status responded, compared to under 25 percent for the sicker patients. The response rates thus far in epidermoid carcinoma are most discouraging—generally under 25 percent. Except in study programs, aggressive chemotherapy may be unjustified.

Chemotherapy as an adjunct to surgery has not been effective thus far in delaying recurrence or in increasing the 5-year survival. To achieve positive results we will have to treat patients with combinations of drugs that have been shown to be most effective in nonresectable disease. Such studies are under way, and they may yet change the cure rate, which has remained unaltered for the past 20 years. Adjuvant chemotherapy implies that some cured patients will be subjected to unnecessary toxicity, and it is currently limited to experimental use.

The newest method in the treatment of lung cancer is immunotherapy, and it is receiving wide attention (Chapter 16). There have now been studies in lung cancer showing remissions with nonspecific immunostimulants such as BCG and *C. parvum*. There are studies under way in nonresectable disease comparing standard chemotherapy with the addition of immunotherapy to chemotherapy. One such study by the Eastern Cooperative Oncology Group is comparing our Cytoxan and methotrexate regimen with or without C. parvum. Other studies have included the immunorestorative agent levamisole. Since it is thought that immunologic cell kill may be limited to small numbers of tumor cells, various studies are under way to test immunotherapy as a surgical adjuvant therapy. The results of a study using intrapleural BCG in stage I disease is very encouraging. There is no recommendation for the use of immunotherapy in lung cancer outside of a study setting.

Failure of one therapy or one modality no longer means that patients cannot benefit from alternative therapy. Ultimately we must use the four modalities in various combinations to achieve optimal results. In the future we may treat most surgical patients with chemotherapy and immunotherapy. The criteria for resection may change to include more stage III patients if adjuvant therapy proves effective. The treatment of nonresectable disease may include a combination of drugs and radiation given at times and doses that promote synergism. We need to know whether these relationships can be generalized for certain cell types or whether optimal therapy will necessitate a system for tailoring therapy to the individual patient (Chapter 2).

CASE REVIEWS

In the following section 8 cases will be concisely presented from the files at Boston University Medical Center. These cases are used to illustrate approaches to diagnosis and management. They are discussed by Drs. Robert E. Lee, Oleg S. Selawry, and Marc J. Straus.

Case 1

A 48-year-old male presented with a 2-month history of cough and dyspnea; history and physical examination were otherwise unremarkable. A small right perihilar mass was noted on chest x-ray. Sputum cytology was consistent with *small cell carcinoma*. Bronchoscopy demonstrated small cell carcinoma partially occluding right mainstem bronchus 3 cm from carina. Liver function tests, liver scan, bone scan, and bone marrow biopsy were normal. Performance status was good.

Lee: The operative mortality of small cell carcinoma exceeds the 5-year survival rate. The patient has disease limited to the right hemithorax; thus curative radiotherapy is to be considered providing pulmonary function in the left lung is satisfactory.

Megavoltage radiotherapy is preferred because it spares normal tissue (e.g., skin and bone) and allows simple field arrangement that spares the contralateral lung. I would favor radiotherapy aimed at cure, and because of the high likelihood of occult distant metastasis I would favor concurrent multiple-drug therapy (Chapter 15). I prefer radiotherapy with 4 MeV if the AP diameter of the chest (central axis) is 22 cm or less and 10 MeV if this diameter is 23 cm or more. We use an anterior and opposing posterior port to encompass the field: the primary with at least a 2-cm margin of apparently normal lung, and the mediastinum from suprasternal notch to at least 5 cm below the carina and to include 1 cm of contralateral lung, with a superior extension of the port to include the ipsilateral supraclavicular region. Both ports are treated daily; the midplane tumor dose is 2000 rads in five fractions over 5

days, then 3 weeks rest. If on reexamination the condition of the patient is satisfactory, I would give a second course of 2000 rads in 5 days. This dose is for unit-density material. During this radiotherapy an anterior and posterior cervical lead block over the larynx and spinal cord extends down to the level of the suprasternal notch. During the second course a posterior port is used to prevent overdosage of the spinal cord. This block is used for the number of days indicated from the maximum dosage to the spinal cord determined from a sagittal isodose plot of the patient. Roentgenograms are necessary to confirm the accuracy of the arrangement of the fields.[1,2]

Selawry: The only additional test I would suggest would be a brain scan. Radiotherapy alone would give an expected 5-year survival of approximately 5 percent. Instead, I would suggest giving a short course of radiotherapy of 1750 rads within 5–6 days followed by surgery because of an approximately 20 percent 4+-year survival rate following this treatment in an uncontrolled clinical trial reported by Bates. Because Bates' doses are not tumoricidal, except for very small tumor populations, I would be tempted to give further radiotherapy to tolerance within 2–3 weeks after surgery. Since approximately 85 percent of the patients would be expected to have distant metastases already, I would consider giving elective polychemotherapy even though there is no hard evidence to support this contention.[1,3]

Straus: Although this patient is classified as having regional disease, most of these patients have extensive disease. Small cell carcinoma would be the only cell type where we might include a brain scan in the absence of CNS symptoms. Despite the preliminary data of Bates, we prefer to treat all of these patients with systemic chemotherapy. If there are no immediate symptoms such as hemoptysis that might necessitate radiotherapy, we initiate treatment with cyclophosphamide (Cytoxan) and methotrexate, and we have noted an objective response rate of over 90 percent (Chapter 15). Aggressive therapy with combinations including adriamycin, CCNU, and vincristine in addition to Cytoxan may provide similar results. We are now seeing remissions with regional small cell carcinoma in excess of 1.5 years. Thus far, when disease recurs it invariably does so at the primary site. In some patients we have therefore instituted radiotherapy in a split course, similar to that described by Dr. Lee. The radiotherapy is given after remission is induced (6–9 weeks), and chemotherapy is continued in doses as high as are possible. Currently we are not prophylactically irradiating other organ sites.[3,4]

Case 2

A 58-year-old male presented with a 9-month history of cough and occasional hemoptysis. There was an area of dullness in the RLL; the physical examination was otherwise unremarkable. Chest x-ray showed a discrete 6-cm mass in the RLL. Cytology was consistent with *well-differentiated epidermoid carcinoma,* which was confirmed by bronchoscopy. Mediastinoscopy, bone scan, and liver function tests were normal. Liver scan showed multiple small areas of irregularity.

Lee: The workup should include a blind needle biopsy; if this is negative then peritoneoscopy and biopsy of the liver are indicated. If the biopsy is positive, then the patient has stage III extensive disease; if it is negative, he has stage II disease.

Surgery is the preferred treatment for stage II if the physiologic condition of the patient is satisfactory. The cumulative survival with this cell type and stage II is approximately 30 percent. If liver metastases are confirmed, then chemotherapy is indicated, e.g., VP-16, adriamycin, and Cytoxan (Chapter 15).

Selawry: I would consider laparoscopy and liver needle biopsy under vision to rule out hepatic metastasis. I would consider resection of the primary tumor if there are no metastatic lesions.

Straus: If liver metastases are not demonstrated, we would proceed to thoracotomy. If liver metastases are present, we would consider irradiating this large primary with conservative ports. We are particularly likely to use radiotherapy in well-differentiated epidermoid carcinomas, since few respond well to chemotherapy. There is no chemotherapy combination that is preferred at this time, and outside of a study situation, therapy associated with severe side effects may be unwarranted.

Case 3

A 42-year-old male presented with a 4-cm *large cell anaplastic carcinoma* of the LLL; mediastinoscopy was positive. Metastatic workup was negative, and the patient was fully ambulatory.

Lee: The patient's stage is T2 N2 M0. If the nodes are low and ipsilateral, surgery may be considered, although the 5-year survival only slightly exceeds the surgical mortality rate. If there is involvement of other nodes, postoperative radiotherapy is indicated. It is helpful if the surgeon marks the location of the nodes. If the subcarinal nodes are positive, it is best to treat the entire mediastinum or at least 7 cm below the carina. The technique is as described for Case 1. We use anterior and opposing posterior ports to encompass the mediastinum with at least 1-cm margin of apparently normal right lung. We would include an 8-cm-wide portal overlapping the left cavity superiorly from the suprasternal notch to at least 8 cm below the carina or to the inferior extent of the mediastinum if so indicated by surgical findings.

Selawry: By definition the patient is inoperable. I would suggest giving maximum tolerated doses of radiotherapy to the tumor, the mediastinum, and both supracalvicular areas. Follow-up with chemotherapy is attractive in principle, and it might include combinations that contain adriamycin. However, there is no evidence in well-controlled trials to suggest superiority of such an approach over radiotherapy alone.

Straus: In this situation we prefer combination chemotherapy, as for Case 1. We have noted a response rate slightly in excess of 50 percent for large cell carcinoma, although complete responses are uncommon. Furthermore, almost all of the responders had a good initial performance status, as in this case. This patient has an evaluable or measurable lesion. When progression occurs we would use either radiotherapy or chemotherapy. Drugs that may provide some therapeutic benefit include adriamycin, procarbazine, and hexamethylmelamine. In cases where a response has occurred, we sometimes alter therapy soon after there is evidence that the tumor is again increasing in size, rather than waiting for a 50 percent increment above the original size of 4 cm (Chapter 2).

Case 4

A 62-year-old male presented with severe chronic obstructive pulmonary disease. Physical examination was negative. He had a 2-cm RUL lesion centrally located on x-ray that was identified as *well-differentiated epidermoid carcinoma* on cytology. On bronchoscopy the lesion was seen to be 3 cm from the right mainsteam bronchus. Bone scan and liver scan were negative.

Lee: The pulmonary physiologic status of the patient should be assessed as described by Dr. Mountain (Chapter 14). If pulmonary function contraindicates surgery, then a perfusion lung scan should be done to assess adequacy of function in non-tumor-bearing tissue. Radiotherapy will induce a functional pneumonectomy and might result in a further deterioration of pulmonary function.

Radiotherapy should be given as anterior and posterior opposing ports to encompass the tumor, keeping the ports as small as possible, with a superior extension to include the ipsilateral supraclavicular region. We would include the mediastinum from the suprasternal notch to at least 5 cm below the carina and 1 cm of contralateral lung. During this radiotherapy an anterior and posterior cervical lead block over the larynx and spinal cord extends down to the level of the suprasternal notch. During the second course a posterior lead block over the spinal cord is used in the posterior port to prevent overdosage of the spinal cord. This block is used for the number of days indicated from the maximum dosage to the spinal cord determined from a sagittal isodose plot of the patient.

Straus: Our approach is similar. We would be reluctant to use chemotherapy even if radiotherapy is contraindicated, since responses are so few. Our choice of drugs would not include those that might cause prolonged anorexia, such as adriamycin. We would certainly avoid drugs associated with pulmonary fibrosis, particularly Bleomycin.

Case 5

A 53-year-old ambulatory male presented with a 4-cm LUL lesion; *small cell carcinoma* was identified by bronchoscopy. Multiple areas in the pelvis and ribs were positive by bone scan, and a small discrete right parietal lesion was seen on brain scan.

Lee: We favor combination chemotherapy (Chapter 15). If osseous metastases are painful or if pathologic fracture is imminent, then palliative radiotherapy is given. Kilovoltage equipment could be used, but I favor megavoltage radiotherapy. Presuming the lesion is in the vertebrae, I would use a posterior port encompassing the involved vertebra and at least one adjacent verte-

bra above and below, administered at a dose of 1500 rads in 5 days. If the cerebral metastasis is symptomatic, then megavoltage radiotherapy is used for its skin-sparing advantage. I prefer 48 hr of preparation with Decadron if possible, 4 mg q.i.d., to be continued during radiotherapy. We use right and left lateral portals to encompass the entire brain, as multiple metastases are likely. An acceptable course would be 2000 rads in 5 days treating both ports daily.

Selawry: Standard treatment includes polychemotherapy with one of the three- or four-drug combinations of established value together with radiotherapy to the equivalent of 5000 rads over 5 weeks to the entire brain. I would propose the following modifications to the above standard approach: radiotherapy to the bulk of the tumor mass in case of pronounced response to chemotherapy, limitation to a two- or three-drug combination such as CCNU, cyclophosphamide, and methotrexate, to be given for approximately 4 months (a time distinctly shorter than the median duration of time to progressive disease in prior trials) or to progressive disease, whichever comes first. I would then change to a mutually non-cross-resistant drug combination (including, for example, adriamycin, vincristine, and imidazole carboxamide) in the hope of further reducing the tumor cell population and prolonging response.

Straus: This is a more typical case of small cell carcinoma with extensive disease at the time of diagnosis. For small cell carcinoma without brain metastases we generally use the drugs Cytoxan and methotrexate. These drugs are well tolerated, and dose adjustments are designed so that few patients develop serious toxicity. These drugs, however, are ineffective for brain metastases, and in this situation a nitrosourea such as CCNU is preferred. Hansen et al.[5] demonstrated good results in small cell carcinoma using the combination of CCNU, Cytoxan, and methotrexate. In our hands, using slightly higher doses than Hansen, the survival time of patients with small cell carcinoma with this three-drug combination was as good as we have seen with the Cytoxan and methotrexate combination. However, the addition of CCNU results in substantially more toxicity. Myelosuppression from the nitrosoureas can be prolonged and cumulative over a number of doses and often comes at unexpected times. Thrombocytopenia is much more of a problem when CCNU is added.

In our experience the combination of high-dose CCNU and radiotherapy results in objective responses in over 75 percent of patients with brain metastasis from lung cancer. Even though this patient does not have CNS symptoms, we would be strongly inclined to treat him initially with brain irradiation and CCNU. We generally favor whole brain irradiation up to 5000 rads in 5 weeks, although there is no evidence that this higher dose results in longer survival. The initial dose of CCNU we use depends on the presence of disease outside the brain. If the only manifestation of the lung tumor is the brain metastasis, aside from perhaps a very small primary lung lesion, then we would use CCNU alone at a full dose of 120 mg/m² orally. CCNU, however, is realtively ineffective as a single drug for disease outside of the brain. Therefore, in the presence of liver or bony metastases, as in this patient, we would start the patient on three-drug chemotherapy. For the first course a dose of CCNU up to 70–80 mg/m² is possible, with an initial dose of Cytoxan of 700 mg/m² i.v. Subsequent doses of methotrexate can be given at a level of 10–15 mg/m² orally twice weekly. Cytoxan is then given at 3-week intervals at 500–700 mg/m², and CCNU is given at 6-week intervals at 50–70 mg/m². After 6 weeks, if the patient has not achieved an objective remission and there are no CNS symptoms, the CCNU may be omitted for a number of courses and the Cytoxan increased to maximum doses. Osseous metastases are treated by radiotherapy as described by Dr. Lee. This patient illustrates the different approaches that one may need to take in treating this widely metastatic, rapidly proliferative disease.

Case 6

A 48-year-old male presented with very early superior venal caval syndrome. A 3-cm lesion in the appropriate area was diagnosed as *small cell carcinoma* by bronchoscopy. Liver scan was positive by biopsy.

Lee: This patient has stage III extensive disease with liver metastases. We would favor multiple-drug chemotherapy and palliative megavoltage radiotherapy to the right hilar mass and mediastinum to relieve the superior vena caval obstruction. We would give 2000 rads in 5 days and review after 3 weeks; if the superior vena caval obstruction has not regressed we would proceed with a second course of 2000 rads in 5 days. For the second course, we would use a posterior thoracic spinal cord block to prevent overdosage of the spinal cord.

Selawry: The basic approach is the same as in Case 5. Most radiotherapists would prefer to give radiotherapy as indicated by Dr. Lee.

Straus: In patients with superior vena caval syndrome secondary to small cell carcinoma who have very mild symptoms we often begin with systemic chemotherapy rather than radiotherapy (Chapter 18). Most of these patients will have symptomatic improvement. If the symptoms become worse we will then use radiotherapy in a split course. For cell types other than small cell carcinoma we use radiotherapy as the initial therapy.[6]

Case 7

A 66-year-old ambulatory male presented with mild dyspnea and a 4-cm LUL lesion diagnosed as *poorly differentiated epidermoid carcinoma* (> 2 cm from carina by bronchoscopy). Mediastinoscopy was negative. Bone scan showed rib destruction over the area of the lesion. All other tests were negative.

Lee and Straus: This patient has epidermoid carcinoma stage T3 and is a candidate for surgery, assuming lung function tests are satisfactory (Chapter 14). In a study by Geha[7] the 5-year survival in similar patients was 32 percent. Other studies have indicated the potential value of adjuvant postoperative radiotherapy. Certainly stage III disease should be considered for adjuvant chemotherapy, although there is no current evidence that demonstrates its value.

Selawry: I would consider eradicative surgery as a primary approach.

Case 8

A 56-year-old female smoker presented with right-side chest pain and moderate shortness of breath. Physical examination revealed dullness to percussion two-thirds of the way up the right side of the chest; there were no other abnormalities. Chest x-ray revealed right-side pleural effusion consistent with the physical examination. Pleural tap revealed effusion that contained numerous adenocarinoma cells. Post-tap chest x-ray suggested a possible peripheral RLL mass. Sputum cytology properly collected was negative; bronchoscopy was negative.

Straus: This patient demonstrates some of the problems associated with determining the etiology of an adenocarcinoma presenting in the chest. In the absence of GI or urinary symptoms the most likely etiology in a female is lung cancer or breast cancer. A good cytologic preparation stained positively for mucicarmine, and further diagnostic workup for renal carcinoma is not considered necessary. Tomography of the right chest post tap was only slightly more helpful in outlining a RLL mass. The patient underwent mammography which demonstrated a 1.5-cm right upper quadrant mass. On careful reexamination this mass was palpable. A biopsy revealed the presence of a primary breast cancer. This case illustrates the importance of a very careful history and physical examination; they cannot be replaced by sophisticated scanning techniques and other laboratory tests.

SUMMARY

Dr. Lee, Dr. Selawry, and I have provided some personal viewpoints regarding the management of specific cases. Often there are circumstances that may militate against a particular diagnostic approach or therapeutic modality. Some patients will refuse surgery. Other patients technically may qualify for surgery, but our feeling may be that the patient is at too high a risk considering the possible benefits of surgery. In some cases the wisest course may be to withhold therapy.

Few patients with unresectable disease and few patients with disease recurring after surgery survive 2 years. The nonsurgical treatment modalities may improve the patient's status, delay tumor growth, or induce remission, but they do not cure. No less important than the treatment we choose is the care and attention we provide for our patients. Support must continue during remissions and when failure occurs. The emerging field of oncology is beginning to supply the much-needed physicians who not only diagnose and treat lung cancer in a more sophisticated way but who are committed to supporting these patients from the beginning of their illness to its end.

REFERENCES

1. Miller AB, Fox W, Tall R: Five-year follow-up of the Medical Research Council. Comparative trial of surgery and radiotherapy for the primary treatment of small-celled or oat-celled carcinoma of the bronchus. Lancet 2:501–505, 1969
2. Abramson N, Cavanaugh PJ: Radiation therapy in carcinoma of the lung: The short-course method. Presented at XIIth International Congress of Radiology, Madrid, Spain, Oct 15–19, 1973
3. Bates M, Hurt R, Levison V, et al: Treatment of oat cell carcinoma of the bronchus by pre-operative radiotherapy and surgery. Lancet 1:1134–1135, 1974
4. Straus MJ: Combination chemotherapy in advanced lung cancer with increased survival. Cancer 38:2232–2242, 1976
5. Hansen HH, Selawry OS, Simon R, et al: Combination chemotherapy of advanced lung cancer: A randomized trial. Cancer 38:2201–2207, 1976
6. Kane R, Cohen MH, Broder LE, et al: Superior vena caval obstruction due to small cell anaplastic lung carcinoma. JAMA 235:1717–1718, 1976
7. Geha AS, Bernatz PE, Woolner LB: Bronchogenic carcinoma involving the thoracic wall. J Thorac Cardiovasc Surg 54:394–402, 1967

Stephen W. Lagakos

20

Prognostic Factors for Survival Time in Inoperable Lung Cancer

The importance of prognostic factors in the evaluation of medical studies is well known to clinical investigators. Failure to account for these factors when comparing treatments can greatly increase the chances of either "seeing" a difference that does not really exist or not detecting a real difference.[1] Prognostic factors are also important in the planning and design aspects of studies in that they can be used to achieve better sample balance between the treatment arms being evaluated.[2,3]

The need to identify and account for prognostic factors is especially important in studies of inoperable lung cancer. First, this category constitutes the vast majority of lung cancer cases and hence involves a great number of patients. Second, since cure rates in inoperable patients are so low, new therapies are constantly being advanced, and substantial numbers of clinical trials are required for thier evaluation.

This chapter will discuss what are thought to be the most important prognostic factors for survival time in patients with inoperable lung cancer. The results have been derived from recently completed lung cancer studies conducted by the Eastern Cooperative Oncology Group (ECOG). The ECOG is a multi-institutional cooperative group

This work was supported by NIH Contract R10 CA-12721.

Special acknowledgment should be given to particular individuals and institutions in the Eastern Cooperative Oncology Group (ECOG) for their efforts in the individual studies from which these results were obtained. These are Paul P. Carbone, M.D. (ECOG Group Chairman); Leo Stolbach, M.D., and Arnold Mittelman, M.D. (Lung Committee Chairmen); and John H. Edmonson, M.D., Charles Perlia, M.D., and Edward Knight, M.D. (Protocol Chairmen). Participating ECOG institutions are (in alphabetical order) Albany Medical College, Albert Einstein College, University of Alberta, American Oncologic Hospital, Boston University, Brookdale Hospital, Brown University, Case Western Reserve University, Chicago Medical School, Georgetown University, Hahnemann Medical College, Jackson Memorial Hospital, Jefferson Medical College, Johns Hopkins University, Lahey Clinic, University of Manitoba, Massachusetts Medical Center, Mayo Clinic, University of Minnesota, Mt. Sinai Medical Center of New York, New York University Medical Center, Northwestern University, University of Ottawa, Centre Hospitalier Universitaire-Paris, Pennsylvania Hospital, University of Pennsylvania, University of Pittsburgh, University of Pretoria, University of Rochester, Roswell Park Memorial Institute, Rush Presbyterian St. Luke's Medical Center, State University of New York at Stony Brook, Tufts University, Virginia Commonwealth University, and Yale University.

I am also grateful to Marvin Zelen and Marc Straus for their beneficial suggestions and to Terry Wagner for her assistance in the preparation of this manuscript.

Table 20-1

Estimated Median Survival (in Weeks) by Initial Performance Status in Patients with Inoperable Lung Cancer

Histologic Type	Ambulatory		Nonambulatory		Reference
	No. of Patients	Median Survival	No. of Patients	Median Survival	
Epidermoid	123	22.4	101	8.9	9
Large cell anaplastic	59	21.4	49	8.2	9
Small cell	118	25.8	96	10.9	8
Adenocarcinoma	86	33.2	80	10.0	8

conducting controlled clinical trials in cancer that primarily involve chemotherapeutic agents. Approximately 60 percent of ECOG lung cancer patients have had no prior treatment on entry into an ECOG study, while the remaining 40 percent have received prior treatment with surgery and/or radiation. Hence, ECOG patients represent a fairly general cross section of inoperable patients.

INDIVIDUAL PROGNOSTIC FACTORS

Performance status. Initial performance status[4,5] is perhaps the single most important and consistently significant prognostic factor for survival in patients with inoperable lung cancer. One of the first detailed accounts of this correlation was given by Zelen.[1] Since then, nearly every

investigation in which performance status has been examined has reconfirmed this relationship.[6-10]

To illustrate, Table 20-1 gives estimated median survival by performance status (ambulatory versus nonambulatory) for each of the four major histologic types. The data are from two recently completed ECOG studies. Note that median survival for initially ambulatory patients is more than twice that of nonambulatory patients in each cell type. These differences are highly significant from both statistical ($p < 0.001$ in each case) and clinical viewpoints.

Extent of disease. Another factor that has consistently demonstrated a significant correlation to survival time is extent of disease.[1,6-10] For example, Table 20-2 gives median survival by

Table 20-2

Estimated Median Survival (in Weeks) by Extent of Disease in Patients with Inoperable Lung Cancer

Histologic Type	Limited		Extensive		Reference
	No. of Patients	Median Survival	No. of Patients	Median Survival	
Epidermoid	33	21.5	115	9.2	7
Large cell anaplastic	24	21.8	83	11.7	9
Small cell	44	29.0	184	17.1	8
Adenocarcinoma	28	43.4	143	17.8	8

Table 20-3

Estimated Median Survival (in Weeks) by Weight Loss in Patients with Inoperable Lung Cancer

Histologic Type	Weight Loss $< 5\%$		Weight Loss $> 5\%$		Reference
	No. of Patients	Median Survival	No. of Patients	Median Survival	
Epidermoid	134	18.8	84	11.2	9
Large cell anaplastic	69	16.2	37	7.0	9
Adenocarcinoma	87	17.3	37	11.1	9

Table 20-4

Estimated Median Survival (in Weeks) by Sex Type in Patients with Inoperable Lung Cancer

Histologic Type	Males		Females		Reference
	No. of Patients	Median Survival	No. of Patients	Median Survival	
Small cell	159	17.6	69	24.5	8
Adenocarcinoma	123	21.3	48	24.5	8

extent of disease for the four histologic types, again based on recent ECOG protocols. Patients with limited disease (that is, confined to a single hemithorax) have a median survival from 70 percent to well over 100 percent longer than that of patients with extensive disease ($p < 0.01$ in each case). Comparable results have been found in other studies.[1,9,10] Moreover, the differences in survival between patients with limited disease and those with extensive disease cannot be explained by differences in performance status, age, sex, etc., between these two groups.

Weight loss. It was demonstrated by the Veterans Administration Lung Group (VALG) that patients experiencing pretreatment weight losses of at least 10 lb have significantly poorer survival than those with weight losses less than 10 lb.[1,10] The ECOG records pre-treatment weight loss in terms of percentage of body weight lost in the 6 months preceding treatment. Using this measure they have demonstrated that patients whose weight losses exceeded 5 percent in the 6 months preceding treatment had significantly worse prognoses than those whose weight losses were less than 5 percent.[9] This is illustrated in Table 20-3. Even though weight loss was measured somewhat differently by the ECOG and VALG, their results are quite consistent. In both cases the apparent importance of weight loss cannot be explained by other patient characteristics.

Sex. For early stages of lung cancer, females tend to have uniformly better prognoses than males.[11] This more favorable prognosis, however, has not manifested itself in every type of inoperable patient. In particular there has not been clear and consistent evidence that females have better prognoses than males in epidermoid carcinoma and large cell carcinoma.[7,9] For small cell carcinoma and adenocarcinoma, however, the general trend has been that females have somewhat more favorable prognoses than males.[6,8,9] Table 20-4 gives median survival by

sex for the small cell carcinoma and adenocarcinoma patients treated in a recent protocol of the ECOG. In each case there is clinically moderate, yet statistically better, survival for females. Note, however, that the magnitude of this difference is not as great as that obtained from performance status or extent of disease.

Other factors. Several other individual factors have demonstrated significant correlation with survival time in particular studies. However, none has appeared as consistently as performance status, extent of disease, weight loss, or sex. For example, in one ECOG protocol[8] small cell carcinoma patients with prior surgical treatment survived significantly longer than those without it, and adenocarcinoma patients with nonmeasurable disease survived significantly longer than those with measurable lesions. Although these results may well reflect real differences, we will not emphasize them in this chapter, simply because they have not yet been corroborated to the extent that performance status, etc., have.

MULTIFACTOR PROGNOSIS

The preceding section was concerned with factors that are individually correlated to survival time. This section will consider multifactor prognosis, that is, the combined effect of several individually important prognostic factors. For example, how does the prognosis for ambulatory patients with extensive disease compare with that for nonambulatory patients with limited disease?

All results in this section were obtained from ECOG protocol 0671, a prospective and centrally randomized clinical trial involving 698 patients with inoperable lung cancer.[7,8] A discussion of the results of this trial, particularly with respect to therapy comparisons, has been presented by Edmonson et al.[7,8] It should be noted that weight loss was not recorded by the ECOG at the time of

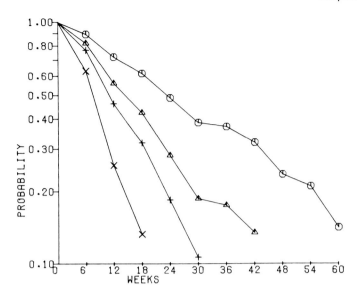

Fig. 20-1.   Estimated survival for patients with inoperable epidermoid carcinoma.

this study, and so its combined effect with other factors is not given. However, the combined effects of initial performance status, extent of disease, and sex type (where applicable) are included. All estimates given arise from modeling patient hazard[12] as a function of prognostic variables. The method used is that of Cox.[13]

Epidermoid carcinoma. In patients with inoperable epidermoid carcinoma, initial performance status and extent of disease have each consistently demonstrated a significant correlation with survival time. Figure 20-1 gives predicted survival curves for the four categories of

patients obtained by combining these two factors. Table 20-5 gives the corresponding median survivals as well as 24- and 36-week survival probabilities. The categories are ordered by decreasing median survival.

Also listed in Table 20-5 is the median ratio index (MRI); i.e., the ratio of each category median to the largest category median. Defined this way, the MRI is a dimensionless quantity taking values between 0 and 1. Similar MRIs indicate categories with similar prognoses, while large (or small) MRIs denote categories with more favorable (or less favorable) prognoses.

As expected, ambulatory patients with limit-

Table 20-5
Predicted Survival for Patients with Inoperable Epidermoid Carcinoma

	Category	Median Survival (weeks)	24-Week Survival Probability	36-Week Survival Probability	MRI*
1	Ambulatory, limited disease	23.2	0.48	0.37	1.00
2	Ambulatory, extensive disease	14.4	0.28	0.17	0.62
3	Nonambulatory, limited disease	10.9	0.18	0.09	0.47
4	Nonambulatory, extensive disease	7.5	0.05	0.01	0.32

*Ratio of category median to largest median.

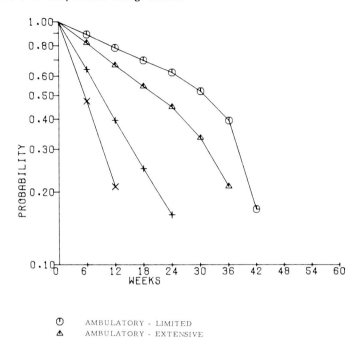

⊙   AMBULATORY - LIMITED
△   AMBULATORY - EXTENSIVE
+   NONAMBULATORY - LIMITED
×   NONAMBULATORY - EXTENSIVE

Fig. 20-2. Estimated survival for patients with inoperable large cell anaplastic carcinoma.

ed disease have the best prognoses (23.2-week median survival, 37 percent 36-week survival probability), while nonambulatory patients with extensive disease have the poorest prognoses (7.5-week median survival, 1 percent 36-week survival). Note also that ambulatory patients with extensive disease have more favorable prognoses than nonambulatory patients with limited disease. In this instance, initial performance status is the more dominant factor in determining prognosis.

Large cell anaplastic carcinoma. As is the case in epidermoid carcinoma, initial perfor-

mance status and extent of disease were consistently demonstrated to have significant correlations with survival time in large cell anaplastic carcinoma. Figure 20-2 gives the predicted survival curves for the four categories of performance and extent, while Table 20-6 gives some corresponding statistics. The *pattern* of results is similar to that for epidermoid carcinoma. Note that performance status is again the dominant factor. In fact, given that a large cell carcinoma patient is nonambulatory, there is little difference in prognosis between the limited and extensive categories (medians of 9.1 and 5.6 weeks).

Table 20-6
Predicted Survival for Patients with Inoperable Large Cell Anaplastic Carcinoma

	Category	Median Survival (weeks)	24-Week Survival Probability	36-Week Survival Probability	MRI*
1	Ambulatory, limited disease	30.9	0.62	0.39	1.00
2	Ambulatory, extensive disease	20.4	0.44	0.21	0.66
3	Nonambulatory, limited disease	9.1	0.16	0.02	0.29
4	Nonambulatory, extensive disease	5.6	0.04	< 0.01	0.18

*Ratio of category median to largest median.

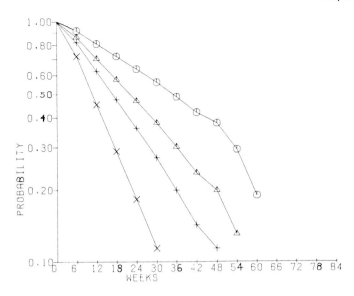

⊙   AMBULATORY - LIMITED
△   AMBULATORY - EXTENSIVE
+   NONAMBULATORY - LIMITED
✕   NONAMBULATORY - EXTENSIVE

Fig. 20-3.   Estimated survival for males with inoperable small cell carcinoma.

Small cell carcinoma. In addition to performance status and extent of disease, sex type has demonstrated a significant correlation with survival time in small cell carcinoma. The 8 (2^3) predicted survival curves for patients with all combinations of these three factors are given in Figs. 20-3 (males) and 20-4 (females). Table 20-7 gives the corresponding median survivals, 24-week and 36-week survival probabilities, and MRIs. Perhaps the most striking aspect of Table 20-7 is the variability in prognosis depending on category. For example, the 36-week survival probability for ambulatory females with limited disease is 10 times that of nonambulatory males with extensive disease (60 percent versus 6 percent). Another observation is that performance status is again the dominant factor, with four of the five most favorable categories representing ambulatory patients. This is also reflected by the similar prognoses of extensive-disease females and limited-disease males within performance status category. That is, the MRIs of these two groups among ambulatory patients are quite similar (0.63 and 0.70), as are their MRIs among nonambulatory patients (0.30 and 0.34).

Adenocarcinoma. Performance status, extent of disease, and sex have consistently dem-onstrated a significant correlation with survival time in patients with inoperable adenocarcinoma. Figures 20-5 and 20-6 give the predicted survival curves for the 8 (2^3) combinations of these factors. Table 20-8 gives the corresponding median, 24-week and 36-week survivals, and MRIs. Note the similarities between Table 20-8 and Table 20-7 for small cell carcinoma. First, there are immense differences in median survival between the eight categories; second, the relative positions of the eight categories are *exactly* the same here as they are for small cell carcinoma. For example, ambulatory females with extensive disease constitute the third most favorable category among adenocarcinoma patients, as well as among small cell carcinoma patients. In fact, the actual MRI values for corresponding categories in the two tables are even quite similar. This suggests that, while the *absolute* prognoses of patients may differ with cell type, the *relative* prognoses of any two categories are roughly the same. For example, if males have a median survival that is 70 percent of that for females among ambulatory patients with limited-extent adenocarcinoma, then for ambulatory patients with limited small cell carcinoma the median survival for males is also about 70 percent of that for females.

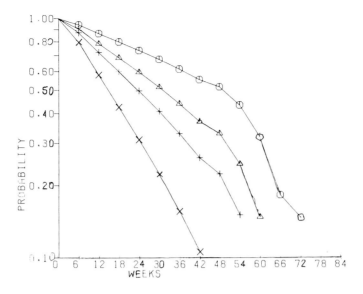

⊙	AMBULATORY - LIMITED
△	AMBULATORY - EXTENSIVE
+	NONAMBULATORY - LIMITED
×	NONAMBULATORY - EXTENSIVE

Fig. 20-4. Estimated survival for females with inoperable small cell carcinoma.

Relative Prognosis. The particular median survivals, as well as the 24- and 36-week survival probabilities, given in this section depend on the treatments used in ECOG protocol 0671. For example, Table 20-5 gives an estimated median survival of about 23 weeks for ambulatory patients with limited-extent inoperable epidermoid carcinoma. Implicit in this estimate, when used to predict survival in a similar group of patients, is that they receive a treatment of equal therapeutic benefit to those used in this study. If a superior treatment were given, one would expect the corresponding median survivals for each category in Table 20-5 to increase. It is likely in such cases, however, that the *relative prognoses* of the categories would remain unchanged. For example, ambulatory patients with limited disease would still tend to survive longer than nonambulatory patients with extensive disease, etc. While actual median values for each category might

Table 20-7
Predicted Survival for Patients with Inoperable Small Cell Carcinoma of the Lung

	Category	Median Survival (weeks)	24-Week Survival Probability	36-Week Survival Probability	MRI*
1	Female, ambulatory, limited	48.7	0.73	0.60	1.00
2	Male, ambulatory, limited	34.1	0.63	0.48	0.70
3	Female, ambulatory, extensive	30.7	0.59	0.43	0.63
4	Female, nonambulatory, limited	23.2	0.49	0.32	0.48
5	Male, ambulatory, extensive	21.9	0.46	0.30	0.45
6	Male, nonambulatory, limited	16.8	0.36	0.19	0.34
7	Female, nonambulatory, extensive	14.5	0.30	0.15	0.30
8	Male, nonambulatory, extensive	10.6	0.18	0.06	0.22

*Ratio of category median to largest median.

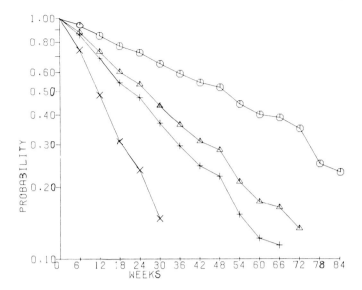

⊕   AMBULATORY - LIMITED
△   AMBULATORY - EXTENSIVE
+   NONAMBULATORY - LIMITED
✕   NONAMBULATORY - EXTENSIVE

Fig. 20-5.   Estimated survival for males with inoperable adenocarcinoma.

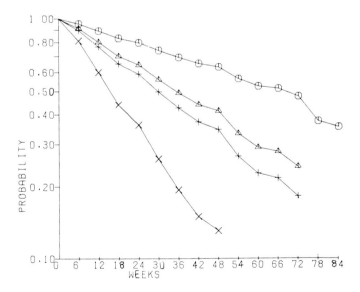

⊕   AMBULATORY - LIMITED
△   AMBULATORY - EXTENSIVE
+   NONAMBULATORY - LIMITED
✕   NONAMBULATORY - EXTENSIVE

Fig. 20-6.   Estimated survival for females with inoperable adenocarcinoma.

Table 20-8
Predicted Survival for Patients with Inoperable Adenocarcinoma of the Lung

	Category	Median Survival (weeks)	24-Week Survival Probability	36-Week Survival Probability	MRI*
1	Female, ambulatory, limited	67.6	0.79	0.69	1.00
2	Male, ambulatory, limited	49.5	0.72	0.59	0.73
3	Female, ambulatory, extensive	34.5	0.64	0.49	0.51
4	Female, nonambulatory, limited	29.2	0.58	0.42	0.43
5	Male, ambulatory, extensive	25.7	0.53	0.36	0.38
6	Male, nonambulatory, limited	21.3	0.47	0.29	0.32
7	Female, nonambulatory, extensive	15.2	0.36	0.19	0.22
8	Male, nonambulatory, extensive	11.5	0.23	0.09	0.17

*Ratio of category median to largest median

differ with different treatments, the MRIs (being *relative* measures) would tend to remain unchanged. Expressed more formally, MRIs are invariant to therapeutic changes that affect category medians in a scalar (e.g., a 20 percent increase) manner. This would suggest that as far as differential prognosis is concerned the MRI is a more applicable quantity to consider than the raw median.

DISCUSSION

The main purposes of this chapter are (1) to identify the most important prognostic factors for survival time in inoperable lung cancer, (2) to discuss their relative importance, and (3) to provide survival estimates for patients having every combination of these factors. This section will briefly discuss how this type of information can be used in the planning, design, and evaluation aspects of medical studies. A much more thorough and detailed discussion of these ideas is given by Zelen.[2,3]

Consider first the comparison of two treatments in patients of a particular cell type. Since the variability in prognosis between the categories in each cell type is so large, it is clear that even small imbalances in the treatment samples with respect to these categories can yield misleading results. For example, suppose epidermoid carcinoma is being investigated and the proportions of patients in categories 1–4 for the first treatment are 40, 40, 10, and 10 percent, while for the second treatment they are 10, 10, 40, and 40 percent (see Table 20-5). Then if the two treat-

ments are actually therapeutically equal, the results will tend to favor the first treatment simply because of the sample imbalance. On the other hand, if the second treatment is actually better than the first, the imbalance may cause the two to *appear* to be equal. In either case an incorrect interpretation of the data can result. The easiest way to avoid this type of error is to make treatment comparisons *within* prognosis categories. For example, how do the treatments compare in ambulatory patients with limited disease? This approach does not require balance between samples and so will lead to unbiased comparisons of the treatments.

Next consider the use of prognostic factors in the design aspects of a randomized clinical trial. Suppose two treatments, A and B, are to be compared with respect to their abilities to prolong survival time. The simplest and most commonly used form of randomization scheme is to assign each incoming patient either A or B with equal chances (without regard to his prognostic category). Such an approach will tend to produce balanced samples "on the average" when sample sizes are large. However, in a particular trial it can often lead to imbalances.[2,3] Better balance can be achieved by randomly assigning equal numbers of patients to the two treatments *within each prognostic category.* Such a scheme is called *stratified randomization,* and it leads to better balance while preserving the randomness of the treatment allocation procedure. While stratified randomization schemes are usually better than simple randomization schemes, they can become impractical when the number of prognostic categories is large relative to the number of patients being randomized.[2] In such circumstances one remedy is to "collapse" the original number of prognostic categories into clusters that have similar prognoses. For example, we see from Table 20-7 that small cell carcinoma patients can be grouped into five prognostic clusters corresponding to categories (1), (2,3), (4,5), (6,7), and (8). In such a way the categories within each

cluster have similar prognoses, and a stratified randomization can be done on the five clustered strata. Since this reduces the total number of strata from 8 to 5, it will enable better sample balance to be achieved in cases where an 8-category stratified randomization might be impractical.

REFERENCES

1. Zelen M: Keynote address on biostatistics. Cancer Chemother Rep (Part 3) 4:31–42, 1973
2. Zelen M: The randomization and stratification of patients to clinical trials. J. Chronic Dis 27:365–375, 1974
3. Zelen M: Importance of prognostic factors in planning therapeutic trials, in Staquet MF (ed): Cancer Therapy: Prognostic Factors and Criteria of Response. New York, Raven, 1975
4. Karnofsky DA, Abelmann WH, Craver LF, et al: The use of nitrogen mustards in the palliative treatment of cancer. Cancer 1:634–656, 1948
5. Zubrod CG, Scheiderman MA, Frei E, et al: Appraisal of methods for the study of chemotherapy of cancer in man: Comparative therapeutic trial of nitrogen mustard and triethylene thiophosphoramide. J Chronic Dis 11:7–33, 1960
6. ECOG Protocol EST 1572: A phase II study of adriamycin in patients with bronchogenic carcinoma (Knight EW, study chairman).
7. Edmonson JH, Lagakos S, Stolbach L, et al: Nitrogen mustard plus CCNU in the treatment of inoperable squamous and large cell carcinoma of

the lung. Cancer Treatment Rep 60:625–629, 1976
8. Edmonson JH, Lagakos S, Selawry OS, et al: Cyclophosphamide and CCNU in the treatment of inoperable small cell and adenocarcinoma of the lung. Cancer Treatment Rep 60:925–932, 1976
9. ECOG Protocol 1573: A phase III comparative study of adriamycin and Cytoxan in patients with inoperable squamous cell, large cell anaplastic, and adenocarcinoma of the lung (Perlia C, study chairman).
10. Amick R, Wolf J, Rohwedder J, et al: An analysis of background variables as prognostic determinants in incurable pulmonary carcinoma, in Proceedings of American Society for Clinical Oncology. Houston, 1974
11. Axtell LM, Cutler SJ, Myers MH: End Results in Cancer, Report No 4. Washington, D.C. DHEW (NIH), 1972, pp 73–272
12. Lagakos SW: Interpretations of survival type data arising from clinical trials. Semin Oncol 1:279–287, 1974
13. Cox DR: Regression models and life tables. J. Royal Stat Society B 26:103–110, 1972

Index

AAT. *See* α-Antitrypsin
Acanthosis nigricans, 90
ACTH (adrenocorticotropic hormone)
  "big." *See* "Big ACTH"
  ectopic production of, 34–36
  K cells and, 50
  production of in lung cancer diagnosis, 263
Adenocarcinoma, 49
  atelectasis in, 187
  bronchiolopapillary forms of, 59–60
  chemotherapy in, 205–206
  Clara cells in, 76
  combination chemotherapy in, 211–212
  development of, 51
  diagnosis of, 58–60
  glandular or acinar structures in, 60
  Golgi complex in, 75
  incidence of, 53–54
  Klebsiella infection and, 59
  mesothelioma and, 81–82
  metastatic sites in, 138–139
  microvilli in, 75
  mortality in, 60
  mucin-producing, 75
  osteoarthropathy in, 90
  papillary vs. glandular tumors in, 60
  peripheral nature of, 85
  pleomorphic zones of, 80
  psammoma bodies in, 60
  radiographic patterns in, 134
  regional lymph nodes and, 60
  roentgenologic findings at presentation of, 86
  site of origin of, 58
  staging system in, 153
  surgery considerations in, 195
  survival following surgery in, 187
  survival in inoperable cases of, 276, 279
  ultrastructure of, 73–76
  well-differentiated, 74
Adenosquamous cell carcinoma, 49
  incidence of, 54
ADH (antidiuretic hormone)
  ectopic production of, 35, 38
  K cells and, 50
  sustained, inappropriate secretion of, 38
Adrenal metastases, 146
Adrenocorticotropic hormone. *See* ACTH
Adriamycin, 202
  in adenocarcinoma, 206
  in epidermoid carcinoma, 203
  in large cell carcinoma, 207
  in small cell carcinoma, 204–205, 265
  toxicity of, 204
Aerosol lavage, 96
AFP (α-fetoprotein), in hepatocellular carcinoma, 39
Air pollution, role of, 7
ALL (acute lymphoblastic leukemia), in immunotherapy studies, 231
American Joint Committee for Cancer Study and End Results Reporting, 132, 151, 161
  definitions of TNM categories by, 158–159

Anaplastic carcinoma. *See* Large cell carcinoma
Anorexia, in various types of cancer, 91
Antidiuretic hormone. *See* ADH
Antigen-antibody responses, 226
Antismoking campaigns, 13
α-Antitrypsin, homozygous deficiency of, 12
ARG (autoradiographic analysis), 20, 26
Argentaffine cells, 50
Arsenic, as carcinogen, 6, 9, 11
Arsenic trioxide, 11
Arterial thrombosis, in bronchogenic carcinoma, 89
Aryl hydrocarbon hydroxylase, 9
    inducibility of in lymphocyte cultures, 12
Asbestos
    in adenocarcinomas and large cell carcinomas, 51
    as carcinogen, 6, 9, 11
    mesotheliomas and, 64
    synergism with cigarette smoking, 11
    tobacco smoke and, 1
Atabrine, in pleural effusions, 246
Atelectasis, in large cell carcinoma, 187
Autoradiographic analysis, 20
    doubling time and, 26
Azygous vein, 117
    in dogs, 252

Basal cell hyperplasia, 51
BCG (Bacille Calmette Guérin)
    in immunotherapy studies, 229–235
    intralesional immunotherapy and, 233
BCNU
    in adenocarcinoma, 206
    in epidermoid carcinoma, 203
    large cell carcinoma and, 207
    in small cell carcinoma, 205
Benz[α]anthracene, 6
Benzo[a]pyrene, 4, 6
    concentration of, 8
    metabolism of, 8
    NO_2 and, 7
    SO_2 and, 7
    synergistic action with N-methyl-N-
        nitrosourea, 5
^{3}H-benzo[a]pyrene, binding of to DNA, 5
Benzo[a]pyrene 4,5-oxide glutathione
    transferase, 9
Benzo[a]pyrene 4,5-oxide hydratase, 9
Benzo[b]fluoranthene, 6
Benzo[j]fluoranthene, 6

Beryllium, as carcinogen, 51
"Big ACTH," as marker, 41
"Big insulin," as marker, 41
Bilobectomy, defined, 193. *See also* Surgery
Biological determinants, in survival, 186–188
Bis(chloromethyl)ether, as carcinogen, 9
Bleeding disorders, in lung cancer, 90
Bleomycin
    in adenocarcinoma, 206
    in epidermoid carcinoma, 203–204
    labeling of, 147
    in large cell carcinoma, 207
    in small cell carcinoma, 204–205
Bone marrow biopsy, 262
Bone marrow studies, metastatic diagnosis
        and, 140
Bone metastases
    detection of, 139–142
    skeletal X-rays and, 141–142
Bone scans, 141
    accuracy of, 262
Brain metastases, 144–145
    in bronchogenic carcinoma, 176
    histology and, 145
    radiotherapy and, 176
Brain scans
    in diagnosis, 145–146
    in lung cancer management, 262, 265
    roentgenographic findings and, 136
Bronchial carcinoids. *See also* Bronchogenic
        carcinoma
    age factor in, 62
    cytoplasmic secretory granules in, 81
    diagnosis of, 62–64
    metastasis in, 63
    staging system in, 153
    ultrastructure of, 80–81
Bronchial mucosa, lining of, 50. *See also* Mucosa
Bronchial studies, 8–9
Bronchioles, respiratory, 50
Bronchioloalveolar carcinoma
    chemotherapy in, 205
    columnar cells and basal nuclei in, 75
    intraalveolar papillary processes in, 59
    proliferation of, 51
Bronchogenic carcinoma
    anorexia and, 91
    arterial thrombosis in, 89
    carcinomatous myopathies in, 91
    cerebral encephalopathy in, 91
    cerebral metastases in, 176
    coagulation disorders in, 89
    cortical cerebellar degeneration in, 91

Bronchogenic carcinoma, *continued*
  dermatomyositis in, 90
  disseminated intravascular coagulation in, 90
  dysphagia in, 88
  endocarditis in, 90
  extrapulmonary nonendocrine manifestations
    of, 89
  extrathoracic findings due to metastasis in, 135
  glycoprotein-tropic hormones and, 36
  hemoptysis in, 176
  hilus enlargement in, 133
  human chorionic gonadotropin in, 41
  hypertrophic pulmonary osteoarthropathy and,
    90
  intrathoracic spread of, 87–88
  local tumor symptoms in, 87
  lymph node involvement in, 188
  medical emergency in, 88
  metastatic lesions to bone and organs in, 136
  metastatic symptoms and signs in, 88–89
  neurologic paraneoplastic syndromes in, 91
  obstructive emphysema in, 135
  operable, 133–135
  paraneoplastic syndromes in, 89–92
  pericardial involvement in, 88
  peripheral neuropathies in, 91
  phrenic nerve involvement in, 88
  production of markers in, 33–41
  prognosis in, 91–92
  radiographic abnormalities associated with, 133
  radiotherapy for, 167
  regional disease symptoms and signs in, 87–88
  scleroderma in, 91
  signs and symptoms in, 85–92
  site in, 85
  superior vena caval obstruction and, 254
  survival in, 167
  susceptibility to, 12
  thrombophlebitis in, 89
  vascular syndrome associated with, 88
Bronchogenic tumors, clear cells in, 80
Bronchopulmonary buds, 49
Bronchoscope
  material collected through, 97
  multilumen, 87

Cadmium, as carcinogen, 51
Calcitonin, ectopic production of, 35–38
Calmette-Guérin bacillus. *See* BCG
Cancer. *See also* Lung cancer
  immunotherapy and, 227–236

  prevention of, 14
  as social disease, 14
Candida, in immunocompetence studies, 225
Carcinoembyronic antigen
  in bronchogenic carcinoma, 39–40
  chemotherapy and, 202
Carcinogenesis. *See* Chemical carcinogenesis;
    Respiratory carcinogenesis
Carcinogens
  environmental. *See* Environmental
    carcinogens
  pathologic changes and, 51
  physical. *See* Physical carcinogens
Carcinoids, 49
Carcinomatous myopathies, in bronchogenic
    carcinoma, 91
Cardiac disorders, lung surgery and, 190
Cavitation, tonograms in detection of, 135
CCNU, 202
  in adenocarcinoma, 206, 211–212
  in epidermoid carcinoma, 203
  in large cell carcinoma, 207
  in small cell carcinoma, 205, 209–211, 265, 267
CEA. *See* Carcinoembryonic antigen
Cell cycle distributions, doubling time and, 28
Cell kinetics, protocols based on, 30
Cell typing
  accuracy of, 101–104
  in lung cancer management, 262
Cellular kinetics, in radiotherapy, 178–179
Cellular macromolecules, carcinogen binding to,
    3–5
Central lesions, histopathology of, 261
Central nervous system
  computerized tomography and, 146
  metastasis in, 144–146
Central nervous system symptoms, brain scans
    and, 265
Cerebral encephalopathy, in bronchogenic
    carcinoma, 91
Cerebrospinal fluid, markers in, 41
Cervix cancer, tumor antigens in, 226
Chemical carcinogenesis, 2–4
Chemical carcinogens
  binding of to cellular macromolecules, 3–5
  direct and indirect, 3–4
  intersection with physical carcinogens, 5–6
  metabolism of, 8–9
Chemotherapy, 199–217. *See also* Combination
    chemotherapy
  CEA level in, 202
  cell-cycle-phase-sensitive single agents in, 215
  choice of drugs in, 200

Chemotherapy, *continued*
  combination with other treatment modalities,
    213–217
  drug combinations in, 206–213
  duration of treatment in, 200–201
  evaluation of response in, 201–203
  "improvement" in, 201
  indications for, 199–200
  intensity of treatment in, 200
  local, 206
  "partial regression" in, 201
  radiotherapy and, 175, 178, 180, 215–217
  single drugs in, 203–206
  surgery and, 213–215
  thrombocytopenia in, 204
Chest pain
  pleural effusions and, 243
  as tumor symptom, 87
Chest roentgenology, 130
Chest wall, percussion of, 96
Chlorambucil, radiotherapy and, 215
Chlorpropamide, SIADH syndrome and, 38
Choriocarcinoma, markers in, 41
Chorionic somatomammotropin, 37
Chromates, as carcinogens, 9
Chronic obstructive pulmonary disease, 12
Chrysene, 6
Cigarettes, types of, 9
Cigarette smoking. *See also* Tobacco smoke
  asbestos and, 11
  lung cancer and, 9
Cigarette tar, carcinogens in, 9
Cigars, lung cancer and, 9
Cirrhosis, liver metastases and, 142
Clara cells (of bronchioles), 50
  adenocarcinoma and, 76
Classical clinical lung cancer, 97–98
Cocarcinogens, in respiratory carcinogenesis, 7
Coke-oven gas, as carcinogen, 9
Collagen-vascular diseases, 90
Colon cancer, tumor antigens in, 226
Columnar cells, 51
Combination chemotherapy, 19, 206–213. *See also* Chemotherapy
  in adenocarcinoma, 211–212
  in epidermoid carcinoma, 208–209, 266
  in large cell carcinoma, 212–213
  other treatment modalities and, 213–217
  in small cell carcinoma, 209–211, 267
Committee for Radiation Therapy Studies, 172
COPD. *See* Chronic obstructive pulmonary disease
Cord compressions, in lung cancer, 145

Cortical cerebellar degeneration, in bronchogenic carcinoma, 91
Corynebacterium parvum, 229–235, 264
Cough
  in lung cancer diagnosis, 95–97, 265
  spontaneous, 95–97
  as tumor symptom, 87
Cushingoid features, 33
Cushing's syndrome, ectopic ACTH and, 34
Cyclophosphamide
  adenocarcinoma and, 205–206, 211
  administration of, 204
  in epidermoid carcinoma, 203
  in large cell carcinoma, 207
  radiotherapy and, 215–217
  SIADH syndrome and, 38
  in small cell carcinoma, 204–205, 213, 265
  as surgical adjunct, 213–214
Cyclophosphamide-methotrexate combination, in radiotherapy, 217
Cytarabine, efficacy of, 207
Cytokinetic growth parameters, 19
Cytopathologic diagnosis, 95–104
  accuracy of cell typing in, 101–104
  methods in, 95–97
Cytoxan, 30, 265, 267. *See also* Cyclophosphamide

Dactinomycin
  efficacy of, 207
  radiotherapy and, 217
Dehydroemetine
  in adenocarcinoma, 206
  in epidermoid carcinoma, 203
  in small cell carcinoma, 205
Delayed hypersensitivity, tumor immunity and, 226
Dermatomyositis, in bronchogenic carcinoma, 90
Diamine oxidase. *See* Histaminase
Dibenz[*a,h*]acridine, 6
Dibenz[*a, j*]acridine, 6
Dibenz[*c*]carbazole, 6
Dibromodulcitol
  in adenocarcinoma, 206
  in epidermoid carcinoma, 203
  in small cell carcinoma, 205
  therapeutic margin for, 204
DIC (disseminated intravascular coagulation), 90
Dichloromethotrexate, 207
Diethylnitrosamine, 6–7
7,12-dimethylbenz[*a*]anthracene, 7

Disseminated intravascular coagulation, 90
Dizziness, in brain metastases, 144
DNA
　^{3}H benzo[a]pyrene binding to, 5, 8
　carcinogen binding to, 3
　in small cell carcinoma, 56
DNCB, in immunotherapy studies, 231–232
Doubling times, 19–27
　benign vs. malignant lesions and, 26
　cell cycle distributions and, 28
　comparison of, 25
　labeling index and, 27–28
　radiosensitivity and, 26–27
　symptoms and prognosis in relation to, 24–26
　therapy response and, 26
Drugs and drug combinations. *See*
　　　Chemotherapy; Combination chemotherapy
DT. *See* Doubling time
DTIC. *See also* Imidazole carboxamide
　efficacy of, 207
DTIC immunotherapy, 231
　as chemotherapeutic agent, 206
Dysphagia
　in bronchial carcinoma, 88
　radiotherapy and, 176
Dyspnea
　pleural effusions and, 243
　radiotherapy and, 176
　as tumor symptom, 87, 265

Early Lung Cancer Cooperative Group, 130
Early occult lung cancer, 97–98
ECOG protocol #0671, 273–274
Ectopic hormones
　histologic cell type and, 35
　as marker substances, 33
　production of, 33–40
Electron microscopy, in lung neoplasm diagnosis,
　71
Embryology, of lung, 49–50
Emetine
　in adenocarcinoma, 206
　in epidermoid carcinoma, 203–204
　in large cell carcinoma, 207
　in small cell carcinoma, 205
Emphysema, obstructive, 135
Empyema, good prognosis and, 233
Endocarditis, nonbacterial thrombotic, 90
Environmental carcinogens, identification of,
　12
Enzymatic markers, 33

Epidermoid carcinoma, 49. *See also* Squamous
　　　cell carcinoma
　blind needle biopsy in, 266
　combination chemotherapy in, 208–209
　diagnosis of, 54–55
　distant metastases in, 138
　identification of, 56
　incidence of, 53–54
　initial diagnosis in, 140
　keratin formation in, 55
　mortality in, 56
　radiotherapy in, 267
　response to single drugs, 203–204
　roentgenologic findings at presentation, 86
　squamous metaplasia in, 55
　survival following surgery in, 187
　survival in inoperable cases of, 274
Epidermoid thickening, in acanthosis nigricans,
　90
Epipodophyllotoxin
　in adenocarcinoma, 206
　in large cell carcinoma, 207
Epipodophyllotoxin-ethylidene-glucoside, in
　　　small cell carcinoma, 204–205
Erythropoietin, ectopic production of, 35, 39
Erythrocythemia, lung cancer and, 39
Esophagitis, in split-course radiography, 169
Esophagus
　compression or invasion of in bronchogenic
　　　carcinoma, 88
　in mediastinoscopy, 117–119
Esophagus cancer, cigarettes and, 9
Estradiol, ectopic production of, 35, 39
Estrogens, in osteoarthropathy, 90

Fetal antigens, tumor type and, 40
Fetoproteins, as markers for bronchogenic
　　　carcinoma, 39–40
α-Fetoproteins, in hepatocellular carcinoma, 39
Fiberbronchoscope, flexible, 107–109
Fiberbronchoscopy, 107–111
　flexible instrument in, 107–109
　in lung cancer diagnosis, 261
　open-tube instrument in, 108
　outlook for, 111
　radiologically occult tumor in, 109–110
　specimens in, 110–111
　techniques in, 108
　X-ray visible tumor and, 109
Fiberoptic bronchoscopy. *See*
　　　Fiberbronchoscopy

Filter cigarettes, reduced risk from, 9–10, 13. *See also* Cigarette smoking
Fluorodeoxyuridine, radiotherapy and, 217
Fluoroscopy, in lung cancer diagnosis, 97
Fluorouracil (5-fluorouracil), 175, 230
    in adenocarcinoma, 206
    in epidermoid carcinoma, 203–204
    in large cell carcinoma, 207
    radiotherapy and, 217
    in small cell carcinoma, 205
Fossa, suprasternal, in mediastoscopy, 116
Fractionation, in radiotherapy, 178–179
Gallium citrate, 147
Gastrin, ectopic production of, 39
GF. *See* Growth fraction
Giant cell carcinoma, 61. *See also* Large cell carcinoma
Glucagon, ectopic production of, 35, 39
Glycoprotein-tropic hormones, 36
Goblet cells, 50–51
Growth fraction, defined, 28
Growth hormone, adenocarcinoma and, 90
Gynecomastia
    human chorionic gonadotropin and, 36
    malnutrition and, 37

Hamartoma, in chest roentgenograms, 135
Hamster, lung cancer in, 4–8
hCG. *See* Human chorionic gonadotropin
Headache, in brain metastases, 144
Head and neck cancer, tumor antigens in, 226
Hemoptysis
    in bronchogenic carcinoma, 176
    as tumor symptom, 87
Hexamethylmelamine
    in adenocarcinoma, 206
    in epidermoid carcinoma, 203–204
    in large cell carcinoma, 207
    in small cell carcinoma, 204–205
High-risk individuals
    identification of, 13
    roentgenographic screening of, 130
Hilus enlargement, in early bronchogenic carcinoma, 130, 133
Histaminase (diamine oxidase), in bronchogenic carcinoma, 40
Histology
    bone lesion and, 141
    in therapy and prognosis, 137–138
Hodgkin's disease, liver biopsy in, 143

Hormone production
    ectopic. *See* Ectopic hormone production by nonendocrine tumors, 33–40
HPO. *See* Hypertrophic pulmonary osteoarthropathy
Human chorionic gonadotropin, ectopic production of, 35–37
Human growth hormone
    adenocarcinoma and, 90
    ectopic production of, 35–37
Human placental lactogen, ectopic production of, 36–37
Human tissues, model systems using, 8
5-Hydroxytryptophan, ectopic production of, 38
Hydroxyurea, efficacy of, 206–207
Hypercalcemia, 33
    in bronchogenic carcinoma, 37
    skeletal involvement and, 141–142
Hyperfractionated radiotherapy, 179–180
Hyperkeratosis, 90
Hypertrophic pulmonary osteoarthropathy, in bronchogenic carcinoma, 90
Hypoglycemic factor, in bronchogenic carcinoma, 39
Hypokalemic alkalosis, 33
Hyponatremia, 33

ICRF-159
    in adenocarcinoma, 206
    in epidermoid carcinoma, 203
    in large call carcinoma, 207
Imidazole carboxamide. *See* DTIC
Immune RNA, 232
Immunocompetence
    Candida in studies of, 225
    immunoreconstitution of, 228
    prognosis and, 224–226
    rebound or overshoot in, 229
    regional, 225
Immunoglobulins, in multiple myeloma, 41
Immunopotentiation, 228
Immunoreconstitution, 228
Immunosuppression, 228
Immunosuppressive serum factor, 225
Immunotherapy, 223–236. *See also* BCG
    active-specific, 227, 235
    as additive or synergistic therapy, 228
    advances in, 223
    BCG in, 229–231
    DNCB in, 231

efficacy of, 223–224, 235
empiric nature of, 229
major approaches to, 227–228
modern era of, 229
monitoring of, 229
radiotherapy and, 175–176, 180
recent progress in, 228
regional, 236
tumor immunobiology and, 229
of tumors other than lung cancer type, 229
Indium chloride, radioactive, 147
Inhalation exposure studies, 6
Inoperable lung cancer
multifactor prognosis in, 273–279
relative prognosis in, 277–278
sex as survival factor in, 273
stratified randomization in, 279–280
survival time in, 271–280
Insulin, ectopic production of, 35, 39
International Union Against Cancer, 123
Interstitial pneumonitis, 51
Interstitial pulmonary fibrosis, lung cancer and, 12
Iodine-fibrinogen, radioactive, 147
Iodized talc, in pleural effusions, 247
ITI Mechanical Precursor, 96

Jaagsietke disease, of sheep, 6
Johns Hopkins University, 130

K-type cells (Kulchitsky cells), 50
in small cell carcinoma, 79
tumors arising from, 51

Labeling index, 20, 27–29
Laparotomy, 144
Large cell carcinoma, 49
atelectasis in, 187
chemotherapy in, 205–207
combination chemotherapy in, 212–213, 266
development of, 51
diagnosis of, 60–62
giant cell subtype of, 61
incidence of, 53–54
metastasis in, 138–140
mortality in, 62
peripheral location of, 85
radiotherapy in, 164
roentgenologic findings at presentation of, 86
surgery indications in, 195
survival following surgery for, 187
survival in inoperative form of, 275
tumor composition in, 61
ultrastructure of, 80
undifferentiated, 153
Laryngeal nerves
in mediastinoscopy, 117
vagi and, 120
Laryngotracheobronchial tree, origin of, 49
Larynx cancer, cigarettes and, 9
Leukemia
immunocompetence and prognosis in, 224
tumor antigens in, 226
Leukopenia, nitrogen mustard and, 246
Levamisole, as surgical adjunct, 214
LI. See Labeling index
Liver biopsy
peritoneoscopy and, 143–144
ultrasound and, 146
Liver chemistries, need for, 262
Liver metastasis, detection of, 142–144
Liver needle biopsy, in epidermoid carcinoma, 266
Liver scans, 142–143
need for, 262
Lobectomy. See also Surgery
defined, 193
enlargement to pneumonectomy, 189
indications for, 194
Lung
embryology of, 49
histology of, 50
lymphatic drainage of, 118–119, 165–166
respiratory portion of, 49–50
Lung buds, 49
Lung cancer. See also Adenocarcinoma;
Carcinoma; Epidermoid carcinoma; Large
cell carcinoma; Small cell carcinoma;
Squamous cell carcinoma
abnormal roentgenologic patterns in, 134
advanced, 135–136
"aggressive therapeutic approach" in, 137
air pollution and, 7
animal models of, 4–8
asbestos and, 11
bleeding disorders in, 90

Lung cancer, *continued*
  brain metastasis in, 144–145
  breast and other cancers accompanying, 263
  bronchographic manifestations of, 129–130
  cell kinetic determinants of, 20–29
  cell types in, 53–54, 164
  cellular atypia in, 85
  and cellular disorganization in mucosa, 51
  central lesion histopathology in, 261–262
  central nervous system symptoms in, 265
  chemical carcinogens in, 2–4
  chemotherapy in, 199–217
  cigarette smoking and, 9–13
  clinical classification of, 152
  cough in, 95–97
  "curative" resections in, 138
  cytokinetic study of, 19
  cytopathologic diagnosis of, 95–104
  deaths from, 1, 9, 56, 58, 60, 62, 163, 190
  diagnosis in. *See* Lung cancer diagnosis
  diseases associated with, 12
  doubling times in, 21–27
  early occult vs. classical clinical, 97–98
  early roentgenographic manifestations of, 129
  epidemiology of, 2
  etiology of, 1–2
  exploratory findings vs. survival in, 193
  growth characteristics of, 19–30
  host determinants in, 11–12
  human vs. other forms of, 9–12
  human bronchial studies and, 8–9
  hypercalcemia and, 33, 37, 141–142
  immunocompetence and prognosis in,
    224–226
  immunotherapy in, 223–236
  incidence of by cell type, 1, 53–54
  individuals at high risk in, 12–13
  inoperable, 271–280
  intervention in, 12–13
  kinetic studies in, 27–29
  major cell types in, 49, 52–53, 153
  mediastinal spread in, 124–125
  mediastinal tumors in, 113
  mediastinoscopy assessment of, 113–126
  metastasis in, 137–147
  neoplastic transformation in, 2
  new cases of, 1
  as number one cancer killer, 163
  occupational, 1
  operable, 133–135
  operability determinants in, 189
  papillary tumors and, 59
  pathogenesis of, 50–52

  pathologic changes caused by, 51
  pleural effusions in, 243–247
  postoperative empyema in, 233
  prevention of, 12–14
  primary tumor symptoms and signs in, 86–87
  progression in, 26
  pulmonary obstruction in, 96
  radiotherapy for, 163–181, 263–264
  relative risk of in smokers, 13
  respiratory carcinogenesis in, 1–14
  roentgenographic manifestations in, 129–136
  screening programs for, 130
  signs and symptoms in, 85–92
  site of origin in, 50–51
  skeletal involvement in, 141–142
  skin response in, 225
  smoking and, 1, 9–13
  as social disease, 14
  staging in, 123–125, 151–161
  superior sulcus tumors in, 196
  surgical therapy for, 185–197
  survival in, 1, 157, 187, 193, 196
  three stages of, 85
  tobacco smoke in, 1, 9–13
  treatment of, 19, 163–181, 199–217, 223–236
  tumor progression in, 2
  tumor regression in, 202
  as worldwide problem, 1
Lung cancer diagnosis
  accuracy in, 98–100
  ACTH production and, 263
  bronchoscopy in, 99, 261
  CNS symptoms in, 263
  cytopathologic results in, 101–104
  establishment of, 124
  fiberoptic bronchoscopy in, 261
  fluoroscopy in, 97
  location of lesion in, 100
  in lung cancer management, 261–262
  mediastinal nodes in, 114
  mediastinoscopy in, 124
  neoplasm size and type in, 100
  number of specimens in, 100
  pleural and pericardial tap in, 97–100
  roentgenography in, 114–115
  scalene node biopsy in, 114
  sputum in, 95–99
  thoracotomy in, 114–115, 188, 192
  TNM staging system in, 124
  tracheobronchial instrumentation in, 97
  transthoracic needle aspiration in, 97–99
Lung cancer management, 261–269
  case review in, 265–269

Lung cancer management, *continued*
  cell type in, 262
  treatment in, 263–265
Lung cancer staging, work sheet for, 160
Lung neoplasms. *See also* Adenocarcinoma;
    Lung cancer; Lung tumors; Mesotheliomas
  electron microscopy in diagnosis of, 71
  ultrastructure of, 71–83
Lung tumors, signs and symptoms of, 86–87. *See
    also* Lung cancer
Lymphangiography, bipedal, 146
Lymphangitic tumor growth, 201
Lymphatic collecting system, in
    mediastinoscopy, 118
Lymphatic drainage, of lung, 118–119
Lymphatic metastases, routes of, 165–166
Lymph node involvement
  in bronchogenic carcinoma, 188
  mortality in, 189
Lymph nodes, in SVC obstruction syndrome,
    251
Lymphocyte blastogenic responses, to tumor
    cells, 225
Lymphocytic function studies, 225
Lymphomas, 153

Malignancies, biologic products produced
    by, 33–40
Malignant lymphoma, immunocompetence and
    prognosis in, 224
Markers
  in cerebrospinal fluid, 41
  production of by bronchogenic carcinoma,
    33–42
  value of in estimation of tumor response, 41
Mayo Lung Project, 130
Mechlorethamine, 202
  in adenocarcinoma, 206
  administration of, 204
  in epidermoid carcinoma, 203
  in large cell carcinoma, 207
  in plural effusions, 245–246
  radiotherapy and, 217
  in small cell carcinoma, 205
  as surgical adjunct, 214
Mediastinal lymph nodes
  cancer spread to, 114, 124–125
  N2 stage in, 156
  surgery for, 194
Mediastinal tumors, origin of, 113

Mediastinoscope, 115
  lighted fiberoptic, 120
  view through, at innominate artery, 122
Mediastinoscopy
  anatomy and, 116–120
  connective tissue and fascia in, 118
  histology in, 124
  history of, 115–116
  in lung cancer assessment, 113–126
  in lung cancer management, 262
  lymphatic lung drainage and, 118–119
  lymph nodes in, 119–120
  mediastinum in, 116–117
  mortality in, 116
  peritracheobronchial group in, 119
  precautions in use of, 123
  pretracheal fascia in, 122
  proposed classification in, 124–125
  superior vena caval obstructive syndrome in,
    122–123
  suprasternal fossa in, 116
  technique in, 120–122
  vs. thoracotomy, 115
  TNM staging system in, 124
  trachea in, 122
Mediastinum
  anatomy of, 116
  anterior, 116
  middle and posterior, 116–117
Medical Research Council of Great Britain,
    166
Melanocyte-stimulating hormone, ectopic
    production of, 35–36
Melanoma, tumor antigens in, 226
Memorial Sloan-Kettering Cancer Center, 130
MER. *See* Methanol extraction residue
Mercaptopurine
  in adenocarcinoma, 206
  efficacy of, 207
  in epidermoid carcinoma, 203
  in large cell carcinoma, 207
  in small cell carcinoma, 205
Mercury chloride, radioactive, 147
Mesenchyme, development of, 49–50
Mesothelial cells, 50
Mesotheliomas, 49
  adenocarcinomas and, 81
  age factor in, 64
  desmosomes in, 81
  diagnosis of, 64–65
  histochemical analyses in, 65
  metastases in, 65
  ultrastructure of, 81–82

Metastasis(-es). *See also* Metastatic sites
  adrenal, 146
  in brain, 144–145
  brain scanning in detection of, 145
  in bronchogenic carcinoma, 88–89
  CNS, 144–146
  doubling times in, 21–24
  in epidermoid carcinoma, 138–140
  in large cell carcinoma, 138–140
  preferred sites of, 138
  in small cell carcinoma, 138–140
  subclinical, 180
Metastatic lung lesions, doubling time of, 20–24
Metastatic sites
  in bone, 139–142
  diagnosis in, 137–147
  new procedures for detection of, 146–147
Methanol extraction residue, 175–176
  in immunotherapy studies, 230
Methchrysenes, 6
Methotrexate, 202
  in adenocarcinoma, 205–206, 211–212
  cell kinetics and, 30
  cross-resistance to, 204
  efficacy of, 204
  in epidermoid carcinoma, 203
  in large cell carcinoma, 207
  leucovorin and, 204
  radiotherapy and, 217
  in small cell carcinoma, 205, 265, 267
Methyl-CCNU
  in adenocarcinoma, 206
  in epidermoid carcinoma, 203
  in large cell carcinoma, 207
Methylbenzo[a]pyrenes, 6
Methylethylnitrosamine, 6
Methylfluoranthene, 6
N-Methyl-N-nitrosourea, 4–5
Mithramycin, efficacy of, 207
Mitomycin C
  in adenocarcinoma, 205–206
  in epidermoid carcinoma, 203
  in small cell carcinoma, 205
Mitosis, in tumor growth, 19
Model systems, human tissues in, 8
MSH. *See* Melanocyte-stimulating hormone
Mucosa
  cellular disorganization in, 51
  origin of tumors in, 51
Mucoepidermoids, 153
Multinodal therapy, 19
Multiple endocrine syndromes, 36
Multiple myeloma, immunoglobulins in, 41
Mustard gas, as carcinogen, 9

Mycobacteria, as carcinogens, 51
Myelitis, radiation, 176
Myocarditis, radiotherapy and, 176–177

N1 stage, spread to lymph nodes in peribronchial
    and ipsilateral hilar regions, 156
N2 stage, spread to mediastinal lymph nodes in,
    156
β-Naphthylamine, 6
National Cancer Institute, 130
National Cancer Institute-Veterans
    Administration Medical Oncology Branch,
    143
Neoplasms
  typing of by bronchoscopic specimens, 103
  typing of by sputum specimens, 102
Neoplastic transformation, 2
Neuroectodermal cells, 79
Neurologic paraneoplastic syndromes, 91
Neurophysins, in bronchogenic carcinoma, 38
Nickel, as carcinogen, 9
Nitrogen dioxide, benzo[z]pyrene and, 7
Nitrogen mustard. *See* Mechlorethamine
Nitrosonornicotine, 6
Nitrosopiperidine, 6
N-Nitrosopyrrolidine, 6
Nitrosourea. *See* BCNU; CCNU; Methyl-CCNU
NSD (nominal standard dose), 179

Oat cell, composition of, 56
Oat cell carcinoma. *See* Small cell carcinoma
Oral cavity cancer, cigarettes and, 9
Osteoarthropathy, in adenocarcinoma, 90
Oxytocin, 38

Palliative radiotherapy, 176. *See also*
    Radiotherapy
PAP. *See* Placental alkaline phosphatase
Papillary adenocarcinoma, 59
Papillary tumors, vs. glandular, 60
Paraneoplastic syndromes, in bronchogenic
    carcinoma, 89–92
Parathyroid hormone, ectopic production of, 35,
    37
Parietal pleura, involvement of, 165
Percent labeled mitosis curves, 28–29
Pericardial involvement, in bronchogenic
    carcinoma, 88

Pericardial tap, diagnostic accuracy and, 99
Pericarditis, radiotherapy and, 176–177
Peripheral lesions, histopathology of, 262
Peritoneoscopy
    laparotomy and, 144
    liver biopsy and, 143–144
Peritracheobronchial group, in mediastinoscopy,
        119–120
Phlebotomy, in superior vena caval obstruction
        syndrome, 257
Phrenic nerve, in bronchogenic carcinoma, 88
Physical carcinogens, interaction of with
        chemical carcinogens, 5–6
Pipe smoking, lung cancer and, 9
Placental alkaline phosphatase
    in bronchogenic carcinoma, 40
    ectopic production of, 36–37
Pleura
    development of, 49
    lining of, 50
Pleural cavity, anatomy of, 116–118
Pleural effusions, 243–247
    in adenocarcinoma and oat cell carcinoma, 187
    atabrine and, 246
    iodized talc in, 247
    nitrogen mustard in, 245–246
    nonneoplastic causes of, 244
    pathophysiology of, 243–245
    radiotherapy in, 247
    sclerosing agents in, 245–247
    surgery in, 247
    tetracycline in, 246–247
    treatment in, 244–245
Pleural malignancies, morphology of, 49–66. See
        also Lung cancer
Pleural mesotheliomas, 64–65. See also
        Mesotheliomas
Pleural space, infiltration of with tumor cells,
        243
Pleural tap, diagnostic accuracy of, 99
Pleuritis, radiotherapy and, 177
PLM curves, 28–29
Pneumocytes
    hyperplastic type II, 76
    types I and II, 50
Pneumoconiotic dusts, in adenocarcinoma, 51
Pneumonectomy. See also Surgery
    defined, 193
    indications for, 194–195
Pneumonitis, radiotherapy and, 177
Polonium 210, in tobacco smoke, 6
Polyamines
    in bronchogenic carcinoma, 40
    as markers, 41

Polychemotherapy, in small cell carcinoma, 267.
        See also Combination chemotherapy
"Popcorn" calcifications, 135
Postoperative empyema, good prognosis and, 233
PPD (purified protein derivative), in
        immunotherapy studies, 232
Prednisone, 201
Prethoracotomy, laparotomy and, 144
Pretracheal fascia, in mediastinoscopy, 122
Primary lung lesions, doubling times for, 24
Primary tumor
    histologic subtype of, 87
    roentgenologic findings at presentation of, 86
    T3 lesions in, 155
Procarbazine
    in adenocarcinoma, 206
    in epidermoid carcinoma, 203–204
    in large cell carcinoma, 207
    radiotherapy and, 217
    in small cell carcinoma, 204–205
Procarcinogens, 3
Prognosis
    immunocompetence and, 224–226
    relation of symptoms to, 92
Progression, measurement of, 26
Progressive system sclerosis, lung cancer and, 12
Prolactin, ectopic production of, 35, 38
Psammoma bodies, in adenocarcinoma, 60
Pseudoacinar spaces, mesothelioma and, 81–82
Pulmonary bullae, 51
Pulmonary fibrosis, 51
Pulmonary malignancies, morphology of, 49–66.
        See also Lung cancer
Pulmonary nodules, in chest roentgenograms, 134
Pulmonary obstruction, in lung cancer diagnosis,
        96
Pulmonary scars, 51
Putrescine, 40

Radiation, as carcinogen, 9
Radiation myelitis, 176
Radiation Therapy Oncology Group, 176
Radiographic abnormalities, classification of, 133
Radiologically occult tumor, fiberbronchoscopy
        in, 109–110
Radionuclides, in bone scanning, 141
Radiopharmaceuticals, in liver scanning, 142, 147
Radiotherapist
    responsibility of, 163
    role of, 163
Radiotherapy, 163–181
    in bronchogenic carcinoma, 167

Radiotherapy, *continued*
  cell type and stage in, 164–165
  cellular kinetics in, 178–179
  chemotherapy and, 174–175, 178, 180, 215–217
  clinical trials in, 180–181
  complications of, 176–178
  continuous vs. split course, 170–171
  cost-effectiveness of, 163
  dose in, 168
  elective, 180
  in epidermoid carcinoma, 266–267
  future developments in, 178–181
  high-let radiation in, 180–181
  hyperfractionated, 179–180
  immunotherapy and, 175–176, 180
  isodose plots in, 172
  management principles in, 164–168
  Mayo Clinic technique in, 171
  minor complications of, 177–178
  myelitis and, 176
  myocarditis and pericarditis in, 176–177
  normal standard dose in, 179
  with other modes of treatment, 172–176
  palliative, 176–177
  in pleural effusions, 247
  pleuritis and, 177
  pneumonitis and, 177
  postoperative, 174
  preoperative, 173–174
  rationale for, 263–265
  selection of patients in, 167
  short-course, 169
  skin reactions in, 177
  in small cell carcinoma, 265
  split-course, 168–170
  superior pulmonary sulcus tumors and, 174
  surgery and, 166, 172–174
  techniques in, 168–172
Radon daughters, as carcinogens, 9, 11
Rat, larynx cancer in, 6
Regional disease symptoms, causes of, 87–88
Renin, ectopic production of, 35, 39
Resectability. *See also* Surgery
  prediction of in mediastinoscopy, 115–116
  technical determinants related to, 192–197
Respiratory carcinogenesis, 1–14
  cocarcinogens in, 7
  human bronchial studies and, 8–9
  inhalation exposure and, 6
  vitamin A deficiency and, 5
  vitamin A prophylaxis in, 7–8
Respiratory bronchioles, 50
β-retinyl acetate, 7. *See also* Vitamin A

Rheumatoid lung disease, 51
RNA, immune 232
Roentgenographic manifestations, 129–136
  abnormal patterns in, 134
  in advanced lung cancer, 135–136
  bronchographic, 129–130
  early, 129
  infiltrates in, 132
  inoperability findings in, 135
  pleural effusions and, 135
  pulmonary nodules in, 134
Roentgenography, in lung cancer diagnosis,
    114–115
Roentgenologic findings, for primary tumors, 86

Sarcoidosis, 12
Scalene node biopsy, in lung cancer diagnosis,
    114
SCE. *See* Squamous cell epitheliomas
Scleroderma
  adenocarcinoma and, 51
  lung cancer and, 12, 91
Selenite, radioactive, 147
Serotonin
  ectopic production of, 35
  in small cell carcinoma, 38
Serratia marcescens, 229
Serum creatine phosphate, in dermatomyositis,
    91
SGOT (serum glutamic-oxaloacetic
    transaminase), in dermatomyositis, 90–91
SGPT (serum glutamic-pyruvic transaminase), in
    dermatomyositis, 91
Short-course radiotherapy, 169. *See also*
    Radiotherapy
Shortness of breath, pleural effusions and, 243
SIADH (sustained, inappropriate secretion of
    antidiuretic hormone) syndrome, 38
Sinus tachycardia, in bronchogenic carcinoma, 88
Skin pigmentation, as ectopic hormone marker,
    33
Skin reactions or response, 177, 225
Small cell carcinoma, 49
  adenocarcinoma and, 57
  anatomic extent of, 153
  CCNU in, 209–211, 267
  chemotherapy in, 204–205
  combination chemotherapy in, 209–211, 267
  cytoplasm granules in, 79
  diagnosis of, 56–58
  desmosomes in, 79

Small cell carcinoma, *continued*
  dissemination of, 186
  elongated cells in, 78
  incidence of, 53–54
  Kulchitsky cells in, 79
  light microscopy in, 76–78
  liver metastases in, 268
  metastasizing in, 58, 138–140, 268
  mortality in, 58, 265
  oat cell in, 56
  operative mortality of, 265
  pathogenesis of, 51
  polychemotherapy in, 267
  primary site of, 57
  radiotherapy in, 164
  roentgenologic findings at presentation of, 86
  smoking and, 51
  subtypes of, 58
  surgery with cyclophosphamide in, 213
  survival following surgery in, 187, 265
  survival in inoperable cases of, 276–277
  tumor cells of, 77
  tumor identification in, 58, 77
  ultrastructure of, 76–80
Smokers
  roentgenographic screening of, 130
  thoracotomy for, 135
Smoking
  lung cancer and, 9–13
  small cell carcinoma and, 51
Spermidine, 40
Spermine, 40
Split-course radiotherapy, 168–170
Sputum
  cytology screening of, 130
  diagnostic accuracy and, 98–99
  early morning, 95–96
  evaluation of, 98
  induced, 96–97
  neoplasm typing by, 102
  postbronchoscopic, 96
Squamous cell carcinoma, 49. *See also*
    Epidermoid carcinoma; Lung cancer
  early roentgenographic detection of, 131
  intercellular bridges in, 72–73
  junction of with small cell carcinoma, 78
  morphogenesis of, 4
  poorly differentiated, 73
  ultrastructure of, 72–73
  well-differentiated, 72
Squamous cell epitheliomas, radiotherapy and,
    164
Squamous cell metaplasia, 51

Stage I disease, radiotherapy for, 166
Stage II disease, radiotherapy for, 166
Stage III disease, radiotherapy for, 166–167
Staging, 151–161
  work sheet for, 160
Split-course radiotherapy, vs. continuous, 170
Stratified randomization, in inoperable lung
    cancer prognosis, 279–280
Streptonigrin, in large cell carcinoma, 207
Subclinical metastases, elective radiotherapy of,
    180
Sulfur dioxide, synergistic action with
    benzo[*a*]pyrene, 7, 11
Superior pulmonary sulcus tumors
  radiotherapy for, 174
  surgery for, 196
Superior vena caval obstruction syndrome,
    249–257
  cancer types related to, 254
  diseases causing, 252–253
  history of, 249
  invasive diagnostic maneuvers in, 255–256
  in lung cancer diagnosis, 263
  mediastinoscopy and, 122–123
  natural history of, 252–255
  neoplastic etiologies in, 253
  obstruction-pressure relationships in, 252
  pathophysiology of, 250–252
  phlebotomy in, 257
  survival in, 256–257
  symptoms and signs in, 250
  treatment in, 256–257
  venography in, 255
Suprasternal notch incision, 121
Surgery
  angina and, 190
  biologic, physiologic, and technical
      determinants in, 185–197
  bundle branch block and, 190
  chemotherapy as adjuvant in, 213–215
  cyclophosphamide and, 213
  five-year survival rate in, 262
  justification for, 188
  mechlorethamine and, 214
  mediastinal node involvement and, 194
  mortality following, 190
  physiologic age in, 190
  physiologic determinants of operability in,
      189–192
  postoperative empyema in, 233
  postsurgical treatment stage in, 189
  pulmonary function study in, 190–191
  pulmonary insufficiency following, 189–190

Surgery, *continued*
   radiotherapy in, 172–174
   reduced ventilatory function in, 189
   in squamous cell carcinoma, 265
   survival following, 187, 190, 193–196, 262
   technical determinants related to resectability
      in, 192–197
   thoracotomy and, 192
   type and extent of, 193–194
   ventilating function in, 190–191
Survival
   biological determinants related to, 186–189
   five-year, following surgery, 262
   in inoperable lung cancer, 271–280
   prognostic factors in, 271–280
"Sutton's law," 137
SVC. *See* Superior vena caval obstruction
      syndrome

T1 lesions, in solitary tumor, 154
T3 lesions, in primary tumor, 155
Talc, iodized, 247
Task Force on Carcinoma of the Lung, 153
T cells, 175
^{99m}Technetium-pertechnetate, 145
Tetracycline, in pleural effusions, 246–247
Therapy response, doubling times and, 26
Thiazide diuretics, in superior vena caval
      obstruction syndrome, 257
Thiotepa, 202
   efficacy of, 207
Thoracentesis, in pleural effusions, 245
Thoracostomy, in pleural effusions, 244
Thoracotomy
   diagnostic and exploratory, 192
   in lung cancer diagnosis, 114
   vs. mediastinoscopy, 115
   mediastinotomy prior to, 188
   mortality from, 114
Thrombocytopenia, chemotherapy and, 204
Thrombocytopenic purpura, 90
Thrombophlebitis, in bronchogenic carcinoma, 89
Thymidine, tritiated, 20
Thymus-dependent lymphocytes, 175
TIC. *See* Trypsin inhibitory capacity
TNM categories
   AJC definitions of, 158–159
   in lung cancer staging, 151–161
   in mediastinoscopy, 124–125
   postsurgical stage in, 189

Tobacco smoke. *See also* Cigarette smoking
   bronchogenic carcinoma and, 12
   carcinogens identified in, 6
   polonium 210 in, 6
   radon daughters and, 11
   in rat larynx cancer, 6
   role of in lung cancer, 1
   uranium and, 11
Tomography
   computerized, 136, 146
   for pulmonary nodules, 134
Tonofilamentous structures, 50
Trachea
   anatomy of, 116
   bifurcation of, 116
Tracheobronchial instrumentation, in lung cancer
      diagnosis, 97
Tracheobronchial tree, division of, 118
Transthoracic needle aspirations
   cell type accuracy and, 104
   in lung cancer diagnosis, 97
Trypsin inhibitory capacity, 12
Tumor(s)
   ACTH production in, 34–36
   anatomic extent of, 151
   histologic cell type and, 87
   hormone production by, 33–40
   primary. *See* Primary tumor
   radiosensitivity of, 26–27
Tumor antigens, tumor immunity and, 226–227
Tumor cells, 87–88
   lymphocytic blastogenic responses to, 225
Tumor growth
   definitions of, 19–20
   mitosis in, 19
   measurement of, 20–29
Tumor immunity, 226–227
Tumor immunobiology, immunotherapy and,
      229
Tumor induction, of chemicals, 3–4
Tumor progression, 2–3
Tumor regression, survival and, 202
Tumor-seeking markers, 33–40
   scanning with, 147
Tumor size, doubling times for, 26

Ulcer diathesis, 144–145
Ultrasound, liver biopsy and, 146
Urine, polyamines in, 40
Urograms, excretory, 136

Vagi, anatomy of, 120
Vagotomy, 90
VALG. *See* Veterans Administration Lung
    Cancer Chemotherapy Study Group
Vascular syndrome, in bronchogenic carcinoma, 88
Vasopressin, 38
Vena cava. *See* Superior vena caval obstruction
    syndrome
Venography, in SVC syndrome, 255
Veterans Adminstration Lung Cancer
    Chemotherapy Study Group, 52–53, 173
Veterans Administration Surgical Adjuvant
    Group, 53
Vinblastine
  in epidermoid carcinoma, 203–204
  in large cell carcinoma, 207
  radiotherapy and, 217
  in small cell carcinoma, 205
Vincristine
  SIADH syndrome and, 38
  in small cell carcinoma, 204–205, 265

Vinyl chloride
  liver cancer and, 11
  lung cancer and, 11
Vitamin A, prophylactic effect of, 7–8
Vitamin A deficiency, respiratory carcinogenesis
    and, 5
Vomiting, in brain metastasis, 144

Weight loss, survival time and, 273
Working Party for Therapy of Lung Cancer
    (WP-L), 52–53, 76–77, 145, 169–170,
    225
World Health Organization classification, 33, 52,
    76

X-ray–visible tumor, in fiberbronchoscopy, 109